THE HUMORAL HERBAL

THE HUMORAL HERBAL
A practical guide to the Western
Energetic system of health,
lifestyle and herbs

Stephen Taylor

AEON

First published in 2021 by
Aeon Books
PO Box 76401
London W5 9RG

British Library Cataloguing in Publication Data

A C.I.P. for this book is available from the British Library

ISBN-13: 978-1-91280-710-9

Typeset by Medlar Publishing Solutions Pvt Ltd, India
Printed in Great Britain

www.aeonbooks.co.uk

CONTENTS

CREDITS

Cover design: Anna Jarvis Design & Illustration: acjjarvis.carbonmade.com

Pictures:
Picture 1. Wellcome Library, London. Wellcome Images. images@wellcome.ac.uk
http://wellcomeimages.org

Picture 2. Wellcome Library, London. Wellcome Images . Portrait of Nicholas Culpeper Culpeper's complete herbal and English Physician Published: 1813. images@
wellcome.ac.uk http://wellcomeimages.org

Picture 7. The Metropolitan Museum of Art, New York. Rogers fund. 1955.

Picture 10. The Metropolitan Museum of Art, New York. The Cesnola Collection,
Purchased by subscription, 1874–76.

Picture 21. Archaeological museum, Iraklion.

Picture 25. Wellcome Library, London. Wellcome Images. images@wellcome.ac.uk
http://wellcomeimages.org

Herbal images:
Bay: Alison Taylor Photography.
Lavender: heidelbergerin. Pixabay

All other attributable herbal images:
Brain Robinson: The Petersfield Physic Garden, Petersfield, Hampshire, U.K.
Brian Fellows: Brook Meadow Conservation group, Emsworth, Hampshire U.K.
Stephen Taylor.

ACKNOWLEDGEMENTS

If we are fortunate, we may be blessed by meeting teachers who truly find a way of drawing out of us our latent potential; Christopher Hedley was one such teacher, who throughout his life showed a generosity of spirit to all of his students and patients. His support and encouragement from the first meeting to the last meeting I had with him was a wonderful gift, and I wholeheartedly thank him and his wife, Non Shaw, for all their love and support. I was fortunate to meet Dylan Warren-Davis at an early point in my herbal development, and I thank him for sharing his insights and passions and sparking in me an ongoing excitement about the works of Nicholas Culpeper. I have been helped immensely through the opportunity to learn Plant Spirit Medicine from Eliot Cowan, and to be trained by him in pulse diagnosis, and I am grateful for his encouragement to explore ancestral traditions of healing. I am indebted to all of those involved in herbal research, and in particular to Graeme Tobyn, his writings and insights into Culpeper have been invaluable in the writing of this book.

Along the way I have had encouragement and support from so many friends and colleagues; I would particularly like to thank Anne Lynn and Anna Richardson for helping me as a fledgling teacher, to Anne Jones and Guy Waddell for helping me with workshops, and to all those who have joined me on the "Exploring herbs" journeys we have undertaken in Chichester. In particular to Vivi, Paul, Susan, Vic, Julia and Ghislaine for sharing their insights and herbal experiences that have helped to deepen my understanding of the herbs that we studied together.

I have been fortunate enough to have had some very supportive colleagues who share my passion for herbs, I would particularly like to thank those who have supported my work at the Medicine Garden over the years and have encouraged me to keep going, I would especially like to thank Elaine Able and Rebecca Theed, two wise women with a huge amount of herbal knowledge. I am truly grateful to the wonderful herbalist Emma Baynes for her proof reading, and for her many helpful suggestions, and to Wendy Budd of the wonderful Budd's Herbal Apothecary for her many years of friendship and for the generous sharing of her herbal knowledge and stories. The early chapters of the book also benefitted greatly from the suggestions and insights given to me by my son Sid Taylor-Jones.

None of what I share in this book would have been possible without the many patients who have trusted the herbs, and have trusted me to guide them in their use, and I am eternally grateful for the opportunity they have all given me.

I bless the Xhosa and Swati Sangomas of Southern Africa for sharing their traditions of dream healing with me, and for welcoming me into the heart of ancient ceremony, ritual, and initiation. I would particularly like to thank the elders Tat' uSukwini, Ma' Ngwevu, Tata Bongani, and my teacher Gogo Nobalile for all their help and encouragement.

This book was a long time in germination, and without it being resuscitated by Oliver Rathbone and Melinda McDougall at Aeon Books, it is unlikely it would have ever grown into a completed work, so huge thanks to them for having faith in my abilities, and having the patience to give me enough time and free reign to run with it, and to finally allow it to blossom and fruit.

Without the companionship and love of my life partner Zoe, I would never have found and developed my calling as a healer. It is through her that I have made strong connections with herbs, healing and massage, and it is because of her consistent support that I have been able to complete this book. So alongside her, I must probably also thank platform 2 on Horsham railway station for bringing us together all those years ago!

Finally I must acknowledge all the many ancestors who stand behind me and speak through me, and for the wisdom they have passed down the ages which made this book possible. May they remain in our hearts, speak to us in our dreams, protect us from suffering, and guide us all to a place of wisdom.

INTRODUCTION

The inspiration for this book originated during a visit to the ancient healing temple known as the Asklepion on the Greek island of Kos. At that time, I already had a vague understanding of what the humours were, and that the medical tradition of which they were a part had first been formalised and written about by early Greek physicians and philosophers. I also knew that Nicholas Culpeper, the most widely known English herbalist had used humoral physiology as the basis for his medical practice.

I had been inspired to delve deeper into the writings of Nicholas Culpeper after going to a lecture at a herbal student support group in London some years before. The lecturer, Dylan Warren-Davis, an already experienced herbalist and astrologer, had opened my eyes to the possibility of using the astrological characteristics of the planets as a symbolic language. He had demonstrated how they are able to seamlessly tie together all the disparate aspects of diseases, herbs, healing, and patients. He explained how Nicholas Culpeper had given each plant a planetary ruler and an elemental quality so that we could understand how the herb would influence and change the humours in the body. I remember travelling home afterwards with my mind buzzing, full of all the possibilities that this new way of looking at herbs could provide. However, since then I had not had a real opportunity to spend time exploring this approach further.

It was some years later while holidaying with my family on the Greek island of Kos that I finally had the opportunity to really get under the skin of humoral philosophy. I had taken with me a copy of Nicholas Culpeper's 'The Compleat Herbal and English Physician Enlarged' hoping that I might be able to take advantage of some free time to get a better understanding of his approach to healing. It so

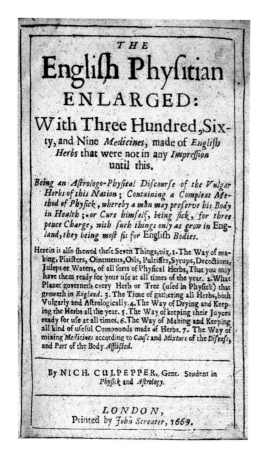

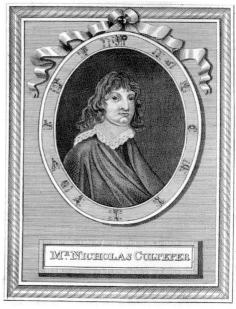

Frontispiece 'The Compleat Herbal'.   Nicholas Culpeper.

happened that while swimming in the sea I had cut my ankle, which had unfortunately become infected, meaning that I was unable to enjoy the beach or the pool, but would be confined to a sun lounger where my leg could be elevated to stop it throbbing. This meant that I now had many hours to do little else but read and study Culpeper's book. The initial excitement that I had felt all those years before was confirmed, the more that I studied the humoral system. It struck me that this truly was a system of medicine that was clear and practical, as complete and as comprehensive as any of the ancient traditional medical systems that had recently become so popular, such as traditional Chinese medicine and Indian Ayurvedic medicine. It seemed an amazing coincidence that my exploration of this ancient system was happening while actually staying on the island where the most famous of the humoral physicians, Hippocrates, had both studied and practiced. I was now exploring this ancient system for myself amongst the hills and bays in one of the places in which it evolved and had been perfected.

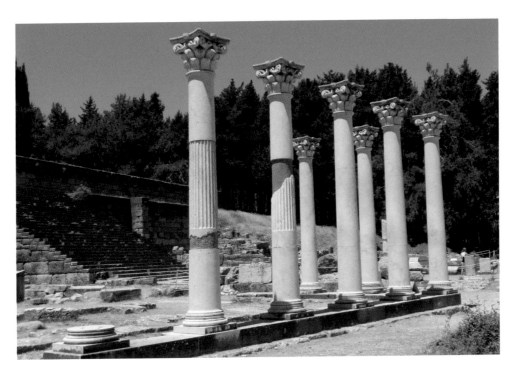

Kos Asklepius.

There are already a multitude of books on herbal medicine available, many are very well researched and written, many of them are very inspiring. There are also those that a wise teacher of mine once referred to as "that herbal book that keeps being written", a repetition of all that was written in an earlier book, just by a new author. There are even books on Culpeper and medieval medicine, many of them academic and erudite, but what it seems that we are lacking is a truly contemporary and practical exposition of the Western tradition of energetic herbal healing.

So this is not just another book repeating the same herbal information in an updated or more marketable format, nor is it an academic text book written for a small number of herbal academics, historians, and professionals. This book is an exploration of Western herbal healing as an art, as a practice, and as a science. It is aimed at everyone with an interest in herbs and healing, from the novice to the professional therapist. It is based on my attempts during my development as a herbalist to make sense of my practice, and comes from my desire to identify the strategies that will best help those who come for help from herbs and natural medicine.

Even though the traditional ancient art of healing as originally practiced throughout Europe has all but disappeared, its world vision and its perception of life are still resonating in our language and culture. When we use phrases such as "let's look at this with a cool head", "I feel in low spirits", or "how easily he loses his temper!" we are using concepts that come from the humoral world view. It begins with the basic premise that all things in nature are underpinned by an order that we can see, feel, touch, and interpret, as we too are part of that natural order. Therefore, the world is not something that can only be explored by experts, scientists and specialists.

When we start drawing on these inherited prescientific concepts to interpret our experiences as herbalists and healers, straight away we find that a template for interpreting these descriptions is already embedded in our language and culture. The Western energetic 'Humoral' model is as precise, subtle, and enlightening of the healing processes taking place as any that I have come across from distant cultures. The advantage is that when we use our own cultural standpoint as a starting point, we don't have to grapple with a foreign language or culture to get going.

Perhaps the greatest challenge for us to overcome when attempting to re-energise this cultural legacy is that it was taught, transmitted, and practiced within a largely non-literate society. We have learnt to conceptualise, record, and explore our world from the standpoint of literate, lineal thinkers and have become dependent on the written word to store and communicate our knowledge. The ancient mystic systems were part of an oral tradition, they were not passed down as a written dogma, but communicated by a teacher to their apprentices in small lineage-based schools. They were an oral and experiential tradition, passed on through myth, story, anecdote, and by watching its application. Remembering the uses of plants was achieved by absorbing stories and myths about them, often poetic in nature, and by connecting them with symbols, which themselves provided a multitude of connections to other aspects of the cosmos. The very essence of these ancient energetic systems is that they are not fixed, they evolve with each healing encounter, with each person who practices them, and with each person who teaches them.

Unlike a written book of rules and laws, oral traditions change each time they are passed on, with the speaker adding a little of their own experience, wisdom and inspiration to the narrative each time they recount it. In this way, traditional systems adapt to the varying needs of new situations and to the differences experienced by the inhabitants of the many places where the tradition is practiced, evolving with the community of which they are a part.

This dynamic evolving nature of traditional knowledge is balanced by it having a foundation of core stories, symbols, myths, and themes that remain constant. These core concepts guide us to look at the world in a particular way, providing an informative, intuitive, and adaptable description. In this way, we become aware of what it is we need to look for and the meaning of what it is we are looking at, enabling us to interpret signs and patterns in the world around us, and to respond to them most effectively.

In the ancient traditional system of education, one learns about things directly, rather than by memorising descriptions of their characteristics. I once heard a Tibetan trained herbalist speak about the first lesson his herbal tutor gave him when he was only four years old; the teacher emptied a sack of plants on the floor and asked the new student to identify a particular plant from the heap. The student couldn't ask a direct question such as "is this the plant, or is it that one?" he had to deduce which one it was by asking questions such as "Are its leaves round or pointed, does it have hairy stems, has it many petals or few petals, has it a strong smell or a subtle smell?" Eventually in this way he found the correct plant by a process of deduction and sensory exploration, and therefore through that process really understood the plants' essential characteristics to enable future identification. When we learn in this way through seeing, tasting, smelling, touching, and using plants, we become competent in knowing them for ourselves and can still identify the plant and its close relatives even if they are in a different location or season, and are looking very different to how we last encountered them.

What I have written is therefore trying in a similar way to suggest a path to get to know things about herbs and healing for ourselves. Hopefully I can encourage an approach that gives us a way of deducing the solutions we need using our own knowledge, wisdom, and intuition when working as healers. I am, therefore, inviting you to explore what you are doing by using a vision that has been seen to be useful to generations of our forebears and former teachers. I ask you not to take this book as the truth, unchangeable and fixed, to be adhered to dogmatically. Rather I suggest it as a pointer as to where we might find the truth that is relevant and appropriate for us at any particular time and situation.

In the ancient traditions of learning, education was seen as a personal journey towards enlightenment. This was never limited to a process of merely memorising information and learning set responses to situations. Education aimed to develop our ability to see each situation as new and unique, to enable us to draw out of ourselves an equally new and unique response. The aim was to become a philosopher; that is a lover (philos) of Sophia, the goddess of Wisdom. The central aspect of this kind of education is focusing on coming from the heart with love, not just from the head with reason alone. During this process we are called to use our feelings, intuition, and divine self to connect with wisdom, rather than just thinking about it. By responding from our heart, the seat of the divine soul, we are enabled to create a spiritually inspired and unique solution for each patient.

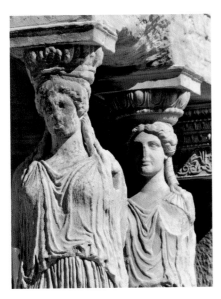

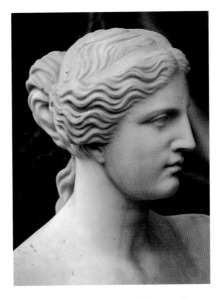

Greek Goddesses, The Acropolis, Athens.   unidentified Greek Goddess sculpture.

The Humoral Herbal has three main themes and sections; the mythical (Mythos), the rational (Logos), and the practice (Ars). In such a way, we acknowledge the role of spirit, mind, and body in healing and also bring them together in one whole exposition.

'Mythos' refers to the word or story associated with the unreal or "otherworld", the world outside of reason. It is the place of poetic inspiration, of imagination and dreaming. It is by connecting to this mystical tradition that we can unlock the symbolic wisdom of ancient storytelling, and renew our belief in the underlying connectedness of all things. In this section, we will uncover the wisdom of European folk and fairy stories, unlocking their symbolism and the teachings that can still inspire and guide us today, we can then weave mysticism, knowledge, and practice together in our healing work.

The rational or 'Logos' section aims to give a practical based working knowledge of the traditional Galenic humoral theory of ancient Greece and post-medieval Europe. "Logos" represents the underlying universal divine reason, an eternal and unchanging truth present from the time of creation, available to every individual who seeks it. In this section, we will explore the rational, structured theories of the European humoral tradition, as practised since the time of Hippocrates and described within the medical tradition of Galen. This is my own adaptation of this system and is the reworking that I have found most helpful for practicing as a twenty first century Western European herbalist. It is not an attempt to present an entirely accurate historical model, but rather a vision for today's practitioners inspired by our ancestors and the way that they practiced this ancient art.

The 'Ars' section covers the art, the skill, and the practice of medicine. It includes therapeutic approaches, identifying temperaments and imbalances of humours. It includes instruction on tongue and pulse diagnosis and explores how to use herbs, diet, and lifestyle to correct imbalances. In these sections I have provided citations to all the quoted texts to assist those who wish to research further into the source material. The book is complemented by the materia medica compendium of herbs, placing the herbs in their traditional and historical context and elucidating how they fit into the humoral model we have explored in the book. In this section I have not provided exhaustive citations as I do not want to interrupt the flow of the narrative of the herbs. I frequently quote from Culpeper's Complete Herbal (1652),[1] and the references in this section are all taken from this source, the quotations coming from the entry in Culpeper for the particular herb that is being discussed. This is also the case with passages taken from Maude Grieve's "A Modern Herbal" (1932).[2] I hope that readers will appreciate the balance that I have tried to strike in this section between an academic presentation and an accessible read, and apologise to those who would have wished for a more rigorous academic presentation. The bibliography provides full details of the publications I have used. Details of all the texts referred to throughout the book will be found in the bibliography. The herbal section does not provide a description of every possible medicinal plant available, but a core group of some of my favourite herbs, as I hope that each reader will find their own group of best known and loved herbs to use. There is a formulary following this section, which offers practical advice about herbal therapy listed by ailment; this is often the most useful tool when we are first learning about the practice of herbal medicine. It gives us a practical starting point so we can learn through our own experimentation and exploration.

Each section stands alone and can be read alone. However, by embracing the complete picture presented I hope that it will act as a catalyst to enable you to make your own connections and enhance your own inspiration as a healer.

My aim is to produce a beneficial contribution to the art and practice of healing with herbs, a contribution that comes out of having had the opportunity to spend many years working with plants and patients and discovering their powerful healing potential. I hope that I can successfully communicate all the knowledge and experience I have gained in a straight-forward way that most readers will find easy to absorb and understand. I have attempted to give a practical guide to using herbs, whilst also giving a narrative that will help us to see why the things we do may be effective, so that we can respond equally well when we encounter a similar pattern of imbalance or similar health issue in a subsequent patient. I have also wanted to open up the possibility of us experiencing our work with herbs as something greater than merely the attempt to free ourselves of troubling symptoms alone. By inspiring the regular use of herbs, I hope for us to all deepen our relationship with nature and through that develop a new respect, love, and care for mother Earth.

CHAPTER ONE

The roots of Western healing practice

There is no single or pure Western tradition of healing from which we might claim inheritance. Traditions change, adapt, and evolve along with the cultures and societies that make use of them. Impermanence and change are the essential nature of the Cosmos, so not having an orthodox rule book to adhere to is an advantage. It not only aligns what we do with cosmic reality, but it also ensures freedom from any single set of beliefs, which inevitably would evolve into a new dogma, a new set of blinkers, reducing our openness to the dynamic aspects of a living vital tradition and practice. However, we will still benefit greatly by finding a clear starting point to our explorations of Western healing practice, and it is also essential to have a common language with which to communicate our discoveries and inspirations. We need to clearly define and identify what we mean when we use words such as element, humour, and spirit, as in this way we can be a part of the revival of a vibrant tradition, developing it through learning it, practicing it, applying it, and talking about it.

Exploration of the rich tapestry of ancient European indigenous beliefs and practices can provide us with this starting point. Through revisiting these old ways, we can find a doorway through which we may rediscover and then regenerate a culture of Western traditional healing, and then through immersing ourselves within it, continue its evolution. The clues as to how these ancient practices functioned can be traced through historical, mythological, and linguistic evidence. Nicholas Culpeper was writing just before conventional medical practice embraced chemical medicine as its new direction, and this book takes its starting point where Nicholas Culpeper finished. We are taking the ideas and practices of the mid to late 17th century as a foundation for an ongoing evolution of our Western herbal practice today, picking up the trail where it was last seen in its completeness.

The philosophy of the body and the medical physiology used in the time of Culpeper evolved out of the medical practices developed by the ancient Greeks and Romans, originally formulated by the Greek philosopher Empodecles and then systemised by the Roman physician Galen.

It is said that the earliest systemisation of medicine was developed by the Greek Asclepeaides, or healer priests, who practiced in the temple complexes of ancient Greece. These complexes can still be explored at a number of locations including Ephesus, Epidurus, and Kos. The Asclepian tradition of healing spanned at least 1000 years, from about 500 BC to 500 AD. Asclepion healing sites were widely dispersed throughout Europe, with 368 individual sites known to have been active within this period.

Hippocrates is said to be the father of Western medicine, and the most influential Asclepeaide. Born on the island of Kos in 460 BC he practiced and studied medicine at its Asclepion, the healing temple that was situated on the island. He also studied in Ionia, the region in which Western philosophy is said to have evolved, as well as travelling to study in Egypt and Asia.

It is said that he taught far and wide, and from this broad background of learning and his years of clinical experience, he developed a concept of illness that was removed from the realm of superstition and instead was based on the concept of a physical imbalance arising from natural causes.

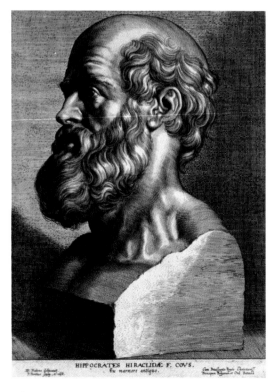

Hippocrates; 460–370 BC.

He proposed that disease was caused by the imbalance of the basic qualities and elements of the universe, earth, air, fire and water, which manifest in the body as the humours, and are all interconnected through the medium of ether.

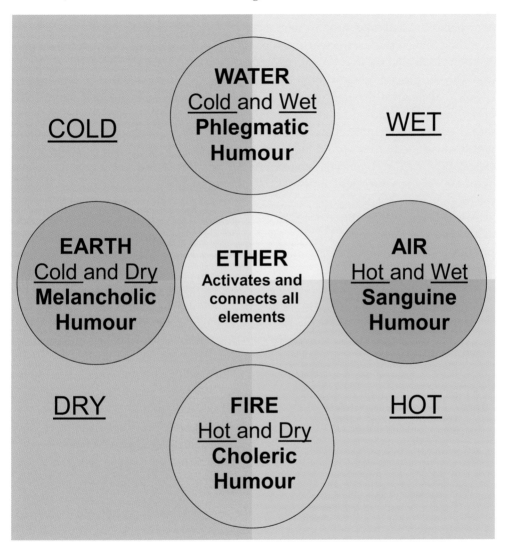

Elements and humours.

Greek medicine at the time of Hippocrates was both practiced by local and itinerant physicians, as well as at organised centres of medical excellence. The treatment involved the application of a range of therapies applied over a period of time aimed at restoring the natural good health and balance of the patient's humours and vital spirit. Physical wellbeing, as well as emotional and spiritual restoration was promoted. The patients who had the good fortune to attend one of the temple centres would be treated through diet, internal medicines, exercise, bathing, and surgery where necessary. To help to strengthen and restore the patients psyche; theatre, debate, music, and singing were all recommended. The period of preparation would include fasting and cleansing practices, the drinking of pure water and abstinence from intoxicants with the temples often being situated on or near ancient healing springs or wells. Patients were charged according to their means, the wealthiest paying more to subsidise the poor who if necessary were treated for free. Women about to give birth, the dying, and those suffering from chronic disease brought about through intoxication were all refused admittance.

Spiritual renewal through daily ritual and prayer was considered a central part of the treatment, leading to a final healing climax of dream incubation in the most sacred part of the temple complex, the Abaton or sleep chamber. When the patient was deemed ready they would be given access to the sacred dream chamber in the expectation of a direct intervention from Asclepius himself, the god of healing, or one of his emissaries, who might appear as one of his daughters, Hygeia or Panacea, or in the form of a serpent or dog.

Aristotle referred to Hippocrates as the leader of the Asclepiads—the name given to the temple physicians. The theories of Hippocrates and other contemporary physicians were recorded in a compilation of about seventy documents known as The Hippocratic Corpus, which was written between the 5th and 4th centuries BC.

The ideas of the Hippocratic School were further developed and formalised by the Roman physician Galen in the 2nd century AC. Although today it is often claimed that the main contribution of the Hippocratic school to Western medicine was to free medical practice from superstition, it is incorrect to believe that spiritual beliefs and practices were not still considered a central part of the healing process, and for healing itself to be a divine gift and skill. For example, in a plea to the healing god Asclepius, Galen says:

> "Have mercy, blessed healer, you who created this remedy, whether you inhabit the hilly ridges of Tricca, O Demi-God, or in Rhodes or in Cos or in Epidaurus by the sea. Have mercy and send your ever kindly daughter, Panacea, to the Emperor, who will offer you sacrifices of good omen for ridding him once and for all from his pain" (Edelstein & Edelstein, 1945).[1]

Up until the late medieval period, many of the ancient texts that contained these medical theories were lost to Europe, partly because the ancient Greek language in which they were written had been forgotten, and also because the texts only remained in a physical form in Arabic translations held in the libraries of the Arabic scholars. It was at this time that the Islamic world was at its cultural peak, and therefore came to supply such ancient ideas and information to Europe via Spain, Sicily and the crusader kingdoms in the Levant. This included Latin translations of the Greek classics and of Arabic texts in astronomy, mathematics, science, and medicine. The translation of Arabic philosophical texts into Latin led to the transformation of almost all philosophical disciplines in the medieval Latin world. The philosophy of Hermeticism also became a significant philosophical system within theology, academic thought, and within medicine at this time, with the eighteen treatises that made up the "Corpus hermeticum" being translated in Florence in 1463. The corpus also gave an underpinning to the practice of alchemy and astrology, and was central to the practice of physicians, such as Nicholas Culpeper.

The philosophy of the Hermetic tradition contained in the corpus was ascribed to Hermes Trismegistus and was originally compiled between the first and third century BC. In both Egyptian and Greek traditions, Hermes and Thoth were considered to be the symbolic keepers of the wisdom traditions of magic, medicine, and communication, and the writings were believed to have come directly from the god Thoth. Hermeticism held that there was one true theology given by a single transcendent God. Creation was manifested in a universal reality in which all things including people, animals, plants, and all living things participate. It proposes a hierarchy of realms all of which emanate from divine light and include angels, celestial bodies, and humans. It also holds that the principle of the macrocosm is reflected in the microcosm, and that all that occurs above is reflected in all that occurs below.

In this Picture Thoth appears three times, from left to right: assimilated with the moon god Khonsu-Harpokrates, in baboon form, and as an ibis-headed crowned figure. The last wears an elaborate mythological kilt like those seen on representations of Roman Period pharaohs at Dendara. Three small panels on the kilt illustrate, from top: a griffin-type form that presumably represents the god Nemesis, an eagle, and a seated baboon.

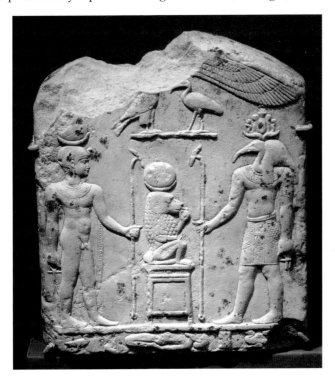

Thoth, Egyptian God. 1st–2nd Century, Egypt.

It is interesting to note the presence of a staff, similar to Hermes and Asklepius, and also the connection to the moon as the bringer of wisdom into the mental realm.

The traditions practiced by the Greeks in temple medicine are also known to have developed out of much earlier traditions, in particular moon goddess worshipping cults that came out of northern Africa and settled on the Greek islands and Malta. These traditions were intimately connected with incubation practices that placed healing dreams, oracular divinatory utterances, and inner journeys to the divine, through silence and contemplation at the centre of healing practice. In Malta at the sacred underground complex of chambers, known as the hypogeum and the labyrinthos potnia dating from as early as 3,800 BC, several figurines known as the sleeping goddess were found, which may possibly have been associated with dreaming and healing traditions similar to those being subsequently practiced in the Greek healing temples.

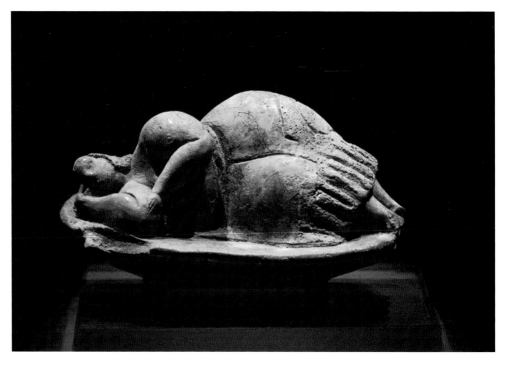

The sleeping goddess of Malta.

When we explore ancestral wisdom traditions, we find that there are often recurring patterns, concepts, and symbols. In our culture where literacy is elevated to being the only medium of information sharing, the potential of symbols to enlighten is rarely fully realised. The great power of symbols is that they can convey a multitude of meanings, insights, and stories, providing a stimulus to our imagination to explore and expand our own unique understanding, they open ideas up rather than limiting and shutting them down. The planets are used as symbols in Culpeper's humoral philosophy, and the way he uses them had developed within hermetic philosophy.

When we look at any ancient mystical, spiritual, or philosophical tradition certain similar symbols seem to constantly arise, coming up again and again, as if these patterns will always present themselves wherever, and whenever a search for wisdom is undertaken. Not only do we see them repeated in human cultures across time, geography, and culture, but we see them recurring in nature, in our dreams, and in the cycles of existence. Amongst these symbols are serpents, spirals, circles, crescents, stars, continual lines and knots, sacred animals—such as dogs, birds and horses—and natural patterns containing leaves, trees, flowers, and fruits. So it is no surprise then, to find them appearing when we explore humoral medicine, ancient philosophy, and Hermeticism.

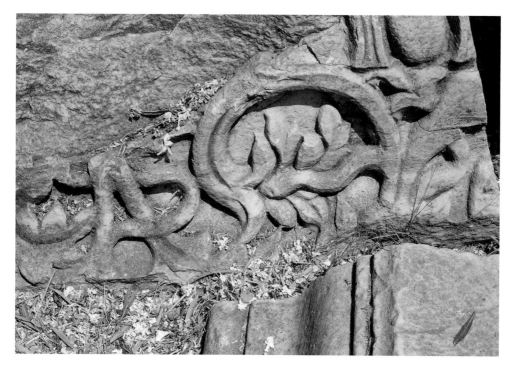

Serpent image and tree of life design, island of Kos.

The spiral is one of the most ancient recurring symbols, not only is it found in ancient Europe but throughout the world. The spiral represents the energy of the life force, the spiritual power of the goddess, and the ever repeating pattern of expansion and contraction. It symbolises the cycles of regeneration and death, summer and winter, the waxing and waning of the moon, and expansive masculine energy being balanced by receptive feminine energy. When we follow a spiral from the centre point, we are guided on an expansive journey from our individual starting point out into the surrounding cosmos, and when we start from the outside of the spiral we experience the contraction and consolidation that occurs on our return to the heart, bringing wisdom and greater vision back to the centre.

When we go on a journey of learning, we ourselves become like a spiral, both bringing the learning experience inside to our centre from the outside, and then by spiralling it out again from the inside to the outside as a changed, new response. We ourselves then become like the serpent, performing a continual spiral dance of absorbing and digesting, then birthing and creating. If we succeed in our endeavour of gaining this wise viewpoint, our openness allows us to respond with clarity and authenticity, enabling us to make the best use of our intuitive abilities while being anchored to the solid ground of experience and knowledge. In Hermetic philosophy the spiral is used to show the passage of divine inspiration from the heavenly realms of divine light to the mundane level of Earth where the elements and people are manifested.

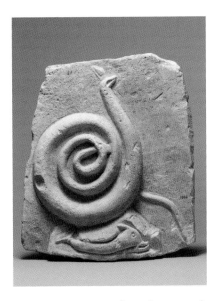

Ancient carving of snake, spiral, and dolphin. 3rd–4th Century Cyprus.

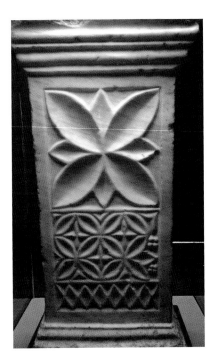

Roman plinth: Cordoba, Spain—symbols of nature, circles, directions and plants.

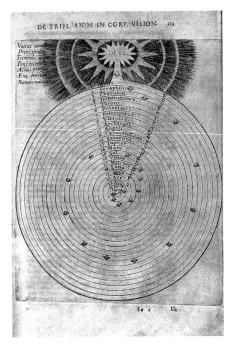

Robert Fludd's three worlds spiral diagram.

Numbers also have symbolic meanings and the number three commonly occurs. We see it in the ancient culture of the European triple white goddess, the three muses, the three stages of life, the three worlds view point, and as a teaching symbol in the myths and stories that lie behind the wisdom tales that we have inherited.

If we look at the symbols left carved on stones by our ancient ancestors we see the number three represented in many ways, perhaps the most striking of these is the triple spiral known as the triskelion, a central symbol of the ancient druidic peoples.

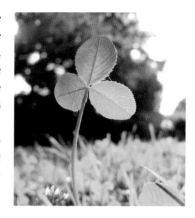

Three leaf clover.

The continuous line of the triskelion travels through each spiral, starting and finishing at the central point of all three, illustrating the continuity between the celestial, spiritual, and physical realms.

As well as symbolising the three realms of existence, the number three also symbolises the way we gain true knowledge of the skills we wish to use in the world, first we are taught by others, then we are taught by our own experience, and finally we are taught by seeing how our learning impacts on the world and people around us. Humans have always been born into existing communities and cultures that teach them what is already known, and then each individual must become familiar with the subject matter for themselves, whether that be medicines, artefacts, or practices. We complete the process of gaining wisdom by observing the impact these things have on others and the world around us, and finally through seeing these effects we can adapt and change what we do, improving and honing our skills. Finally, we will become teachers and elders ourselves and therefore

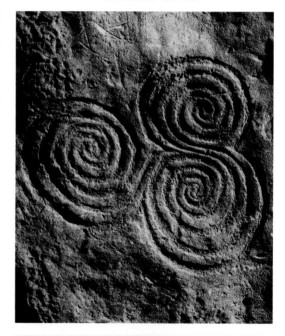

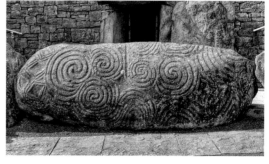

Triskelion carvings at New Grange, Ireland.

also renew and feed the wisdom of our culture, continuing the cycle.

The mythological clues connecting us to "old Europe" and the ancient mystical systems still live on through myths and folk stories, which are retained within our repertoire of modern fairy tales. It seems that although many of these stories were given a Christian slant during the later centuries of the second millennium, the structure and symbols within these mystery tales are still as they always have been. Research has also shown that early linguistic evidence contained in these stories predates the evolution of many of the European languages and therefore is a direct link back the late Neolithic Indo-European cultures.

The cultures of old Europe shared a reverence for a divine figure known as the triple goddess, this reverence continues to send its echoes through the succeeding cultures in various guises, including the three graces of ancient

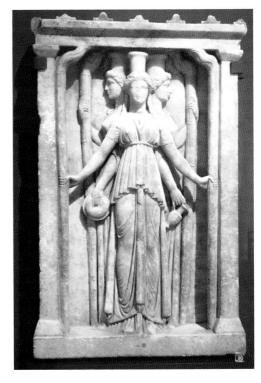

Hecate, triple-headed Greek goddess.

Greek myth, Hecate the triple goddess, and the sacred trinity of Christian theology.

In our exploration of the traditional practice of Western medicine we will find that many of these symbols will become apparent. They will be present when exploring the myths and stories passed down to us through time, and they are particularly significant in the symbolic use of the planetary rulerships and astrology of Culpeper's medicine. We also make use of the number three in this book through working with the three ancient concepts of logos, mythos, and ars—reason, intuition, and practice.

CHAPTER TWO

Asclepius and hygeia, the healing deities and their temples

> "Greetings, Lord Paeeon [Asklepios], who rulest Tricca and hast settled sweet Cos and Epidauros, and also may Coronis who gave thee birth and Apollo be greeted, and she whom thou touchest with thy right hand Hygieia, and those to whom belong these honored altars, Panace and Epio and Ieso be greeted … curers of cruel diseases, and whatsoever gods and goddesses live at thy hearth,"
> —Herondas, *Mimiambi*, IV, 1–5 (P. 227).[1]

Asclepius was not one of the twelve main gods of the Greek pantheon, but a "hero-god", a mortal being, who through heroic acts of healing became immortalised and then worshipped as a demi or lesser god. His name means "he who heals through gentleness" and his status as a hero god was gained by going beyond life, travelling to the land of death, and then returning with otherworld wisdom gained from forging a connection with the goddesses of death and the underworld, Hecate and Persephone. By experiencing human birth, life, and death and by also journeying beyond the realms of life, he became imbued with divine knowledge, whilst remaining more accessible to people than the immortal gods themselves.

There are a number of variants to the story of Asclepius, but what they all have in common is that he was fathered by Apollo and had the nymph Coronis as his mother. Although Coronis was betrothed to the god Apollo, she was also attracted to Ischys, a mere mortal who she made love to when Apollo was absent. In a fit of rage Apollo had Coronis killed by Artemis for her infidelity and it wasn't until the body of Coronis was already on the funeral pyre that Apollo felt any remorse for his actions. However his wife's spirit had already descended to Tartarus, the land of the dead, making it impossible to restore her to life. When he remembered that she was pregnant with his child

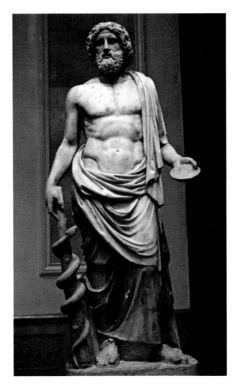

Asclepius.

he instructed Hermes to cut the babe from her womb, and put the child under the care of Chiron the centaur. It was said that Chiron was the one who then taught Asclepius the healing power of plants.

The Epidaurian version of this myth says that Asclepius was nursed by goats on mount Titthon, a place of sacred healing herbs, that he became skilled in the art of surgery and the use of medicines through being trained by both Apollo and Chiron. Whilst in Crete, it was believed that when visiting a tomb Asclepius killed a serpent and then gained his unique herbal knowledge from witnessing another serpent bringing herbs in its mouth to restore it to life. It is also said that Athene gave him two phials of the Gorgon's blood, enabling him to raise the dead by using the blood that had been drawn from the veins of the Gorgon's left side and to kill instantly with the blood taken from her right side.

Zeus, the king of the gods, was enraged when he discovered that Asclepius was using this power to bring the dead back to life, as that was a privilege reserved only for Zeus himself. As punishment he killed Asclepius with a thunder bolt, but following an appeal from Apollo relented and finally placed Asclepius amongst the stars as the constellation of a serpent carrying god. Thus Asclepius became known as the "twice born" god of healing.

Asclepius had fathered five children with the goddess Epione; there were two sons, Machaon and Podilarus, who had both inherited the surgical skills of their father.

According to the Iliad they came to lead an army from Thessaly to fight with the Greeks at Troy and during the campaign they used their medical skills to heal the wounded Greek warriors Philoctetes, Meneleus, and Telephus.

The fact that Asclepius and Epione had five children is a reflection of the central presence of the ancient goddess in the continuing mythology of healing, as five is the sacred number of Venus. As well as their two sons, their five children included three daughters; Aigle, meaning "radiance", Panacea, meaning "cure all", and Hygeia meaning "health". Their mother's name Epione, derives from the ancient Greek word "epios", meaning "to soothe". It was Hygeia who finally came to embody her mother's essential soothing quality. In Greek temple medicine Hygeia was considered an emissary of Asclepian medicine, a provider of health and healing in her own right and was a constant and important attendant in the healing rituals.

Hygeia represents health, nature, and the female creative powers that are rooted in women's natural power to bear children and to create life. Hygieia is perceived as being connected to nature, and like Gaia is lauded as the mother of all things, embodying fertility and the feminine creative principle. She also represents health as being a state of natural cosmic balance, a characteristic said to be represented by Gaia, mother nature herself.

Traditionally, Asclepius is depicted holding a caduceus entwined with a serpent. Like the staff of Hermes this caduceus is made of willow, a plant sacred to the goddess, or alternatively made from the tree of chaste berry, a totem plant of Asclepius himself.

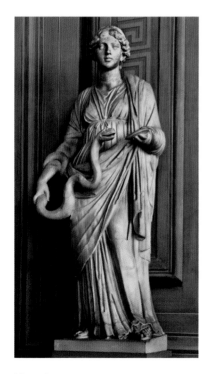

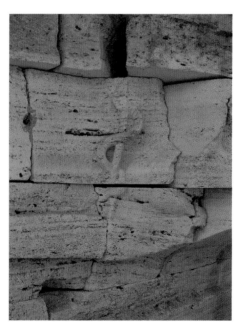

Carving of the staff of Asclepius on Tiber island in Rome where there was a temple dedicated to Asclepius.

Hygeia.

However, unlike the caduceus of Hermes, the stake of Asclepius only has a single serpent and the stake often resembled the trunk or branch of a sacred tree.

Hygeia is usually also depicted bearing a serpent who she feeds from a bowl. The serpent represents divinatory prowess, divine authority, and in Greek culture it was associated with Apollo, who was the god of both divination and healing. Prior to Apollo usurping the goddess as the patroness of healing and divination, serpents had been traditionally considered a powerful symbol of her power. The combination of the stake and serpent was an ancient symbol of the male and female energies of the cosmos being held in opposite but equal balance. The cyclic shedding of the serpent's skin also symbolised death and rebirth and harks back to the serpent as an emblem of the ancient European triple goddess.

Although for the Greeks the world order is presented as naturally favouring a patriarchal hierarchy, they could not expunge the powerful former beliefs surrounding the mother goddess of the many cultures they colonised. There is evidence in the writings of ancient Greek philosophers, such as Aristotle, Aristides, Proclus, and in the Hippocratic corpus, showing that they believed there was a necessity for a balance of female and male creative principles in order for healing to occur. The Greek myths also project and reinforce the perception that women are connected to nature and men to culture; and that both need to be honoured, with Hygeia and Asclepius providing the representation of these two principles.

Asclepius was taught the art and skill of medicine by Chiron the centaur. Chiron is part human, part horse and therefore represents the fusing of the feminine natural world with the masculine world of technical skill and human culture. Chiron is skilled in the art of medicine and because he is half-nature, half-culture, he represents the straddling of both principles and is therefore able to teach Asclepius the art of healing. Because of this training, Asclepius became an extremely skilled surgeon. Although he mastered medical skills, Asclepius could not heal the sick without the essential presence of the female creative principle, which is embodied by Hygeia. Healing requires a return to one's natural state of health, and as nature is embodied by the feminine principle the male healing arts needed always to be balanced by the feminine in order to cure the temple suppliants. Thus the medical skills of Asclepius bring one back to health, a natural state which is both created and symbolised by Hygeia.

One of the functions of the Greek myths is to provide a cultural justification of the Helenic colonisation of the eastern Mediterranean. Underlying the Asclepian myth is the justification of the Helenic suppression of an earlier medical cult presided over by moon priestesses at shrines with oracles.

The Helenistic patriarchal oppression of these earlier matriarchal societies is referenced in the Asclepius myth by the killing of Coronis, pointing towards the ascendance of the new Greek male healing god Asclepius, over the former mother goddess and her priestesses. This is also alluded to in the different versions of the myth. In one, he kills the serpent, representing the dominance of the new patriarchal culture over the pre-existing matriarchal ones. In the other, it is Athene who gives him

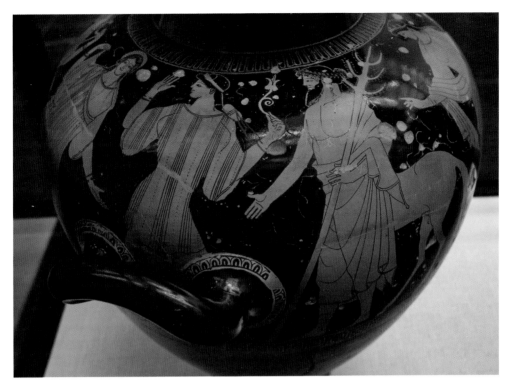

Chiron the centaur.

his miraculous healing powers over life and death, showing that the origination of these powers is from the former moon goddess.

Athene had been patroness of the earlier healing cults and was believed to have been the daughter of a sacred lake. She had originally been introduced to Cretan mythology by immigrant Libyan goddess worshipping tribes. The ancient oracular shrines found throughout the Greek world had also often formerly been dedicated to serpent heroes and female serpent worshipping oracles and crow or raven divinities. The most well-known of these shrines is in Delphi, an oracular site believed to date from at least 1400 BC. There is evidence showing that it was given over to Apollo in the 8th century BC, overturning its earlier dedication to Gaia.

The Egyptian hieroglyph of the goddess of life and healing was a serpent, and in her earlier pre-dynastic form she was called Wadjet, the mother of creation. She appears in the form of a Cobra twined around a papyrus stem, to be later reflected in the Greek symbol of the serpent entwined around the tree branch or stake. Wadjet was also known as the "Serpent Queen of Heaven", and later on was associated with the goddess Isis, and like at Delphi, it was at her temples that divinations were sought from sacred snake priestesses with oracular powers.

There have been a large number of figurines, some dating back 30,000 years, found at many different sites across Europe that depict the goddess as a snake. She is

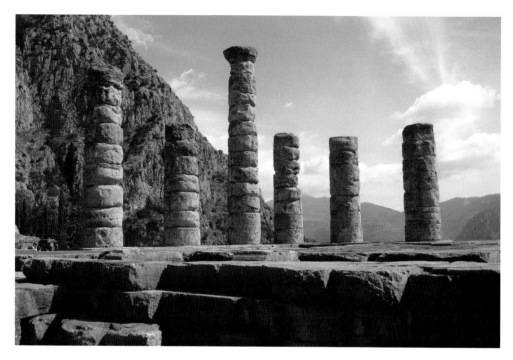

Delphic temple of Apollo.

sometimes directly represented as a serpent, she sometimes has serpent motifs etched into her, or in some cases part of her body has transmuted into a serpent. Often she is depicted in a sitting position with her legs entwined resembling the coils of a snake. The motifs of the serpent are frequently found on pottery and engraved on bone fragments as wavy lines, zig-zags, spirals, and the ourobos, an image of a snake eating its own tail. These images have recurred as a symbol of everlasting life throughout ancient European history. In Crete, snake goddess figurines dating from 1700 BC show her holding snakes or being entwined by them, and are said to resemble Egyptian depictions of Wadjet, the goddess of life.

Coronis, the name of Asclepius's mother, is linked to the crow. Crows were also a sacred bird of the ancient moon goddess cults, considered to be messengers from the otherworld or the land of the dead. They were birds of divination associated with many of the ancient oracular sites and temples. In a similar way to the serpent motif, we find the representation of the bird goddess recurring throughout the ancient artefacts of old Europe, she appears with chevron markings and often in forms that contain bird characteristics, she comes in various combinations of bird, woman, and goddess.

The Greek colonists of the eastern Mediterranean replaced and edited existing myths to justify their place as rulers over new lands with divine provenance. By inserting their own pantheon of gods into these new myths, they could present a cultural and spiritual justification for Hellenistic colonisation. In this way, the Greek rulers

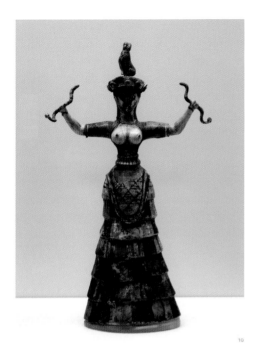
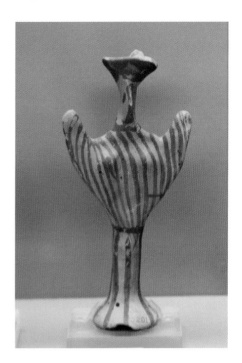

Minoan snake goddess figurine from Crete.   Mycenean bird goddess.

proclaimed themselves to be divinely inspired, and therefore the legitimate holders of authority over the newly colonised tribes.

In the Greek pantheon the patriarchal hierarchy had removed the goddess from her central position. However, the symbols of the earlier moon goddess cult continued to exist, making appearances as the serpent, the crow, and in the form of Hygeia. Even within Greek theology, there was an ongoing reverence for sacred springs and dreaming caves, these being the sacred abode of the goddess. These aspects of the former traditions remained central to Greek healing practices, and although often appearing in a diminished form, continued in the myths and practices surrounding healing.

Ancient healing traditions: the Asclepiades

Hippocrates was a member of a healing tradition known as the Asclepiades. The Asclepiades were graduates of a medical apprenticeship that was likely to have been passed down through an inherited connection to healing clans or schools. Through their apprenticeships they would have learnt medical skills as well as gaining knowledge of medicinal plants and their use. As well as being local medical experts often under the patronage of wealthy families or individuals, they would have practiced as travelling itinerant healers. The Asclepiades are also thought to have practised their art in healing centres or Asclepions throughout the ancient Greek world in conjunction with temple priests or Therapuetes. The former focusing on the physical aspects of medicine and the later on the spiritual, mental, and emotional needs of the patients.

The temple rituals, which engaged the divine realms in the process of healing, were under the authority of the temple priests and priestesses. Entry into the priesthood is likely to have been restricted to certain families who were known for their high spirituality and who jealously guarded their sacred traditions and rites. Within the temple there was a hierarchy of priests and priestesses, the senior priests holding the highest position were elected for a limited period of time and chosen from members of the lower ranks. The most senior of their subordinates were the neocorus or assistant priests, along with another class of assistant priests known as the pyrophoros, or fire bearers. These fire bearers also had assistants called the zacoros, and beneath them were the naophylakes or temple guardians. There were also the heiromanes whose role it was to remember the sacred words, and the aoidoi who were the singers or cantors.

It is likely that the early Asclepion practices of medicine had evolved from the Babylonian healing traditions of the original northern African migrants to the Greek islands. It is therefore also likely that contemporary African tribal cultures that have maintained a clear link to their ancient ancestral practices may well still be utilising similar healing traditions to those practiced in ancient Greek temple medicine. In these African healing traditions, we find a similar division between herbalists who treat illness with a range of therapies based around the use of plants, and the spiritual healers who use rituals, ceremony, and more magical forms of healing. This is likely to correspond to the division between the Asclepiades and Therapeutes in ancient times. Nowadays the priestly healing tradition in Africa is often disparagingly known as the witch doctors, however, they are still greatly revered by traditional people for their skills in divination, prognosis, ritual healing and dream interpretation. Traditional African spiritual healers also still preside over the communal healing ceremonies, in which they call on the healing ancestors to come in dreams and visions, and to bless the supplicants with their healing gifts. They also learn their craft through apprenticeship, and they undergo stages of initiation which are seen to enable them to more easily access the ancestral worlds of the dead where they receive messages, guidance, and often direct healing for their patients. We know that the training of the priesthood of the Asclepions involved a similar system of apprenticeship and is likely to have also included similar initiation rituals, in which they would have experienced a ritual death and rebirth, making them "twice born" like their god Asclepius. Such initiation would make them more able to access the divine realms and open the entrance to the otherworld of the gods for the benefit of their patients. In cultures that still retain ancient healing traditions, it is common for the training, initiations, and practices of spiritual healers to be guarded by complete secrecy. As well as showing respect to the healing deities, such secrecy protects against imitators. However, it also means that there are unlikely to be any records of these esoteric traditions left when the cultures disappear. This would account for us having found so little information about the training, rituals, and practices of the temple Therapuetes and Asclepiads

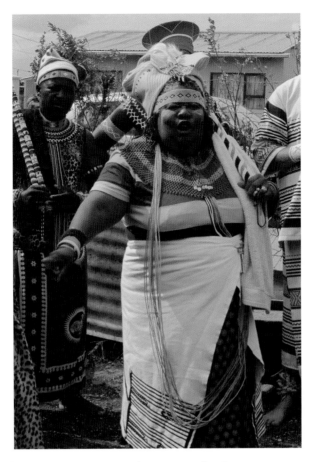

Contemporary African Sangoma, presiding over a healing ceremony.

from 2000 years ago. However, by gathering information from a range of written, archaeological, and mythological sources there is a lot we can confidently say about what took place in the ancient healing temples.

The Asclepion temple healing centres were situated in places that had the benefit of good climate, fresh air, healing springs, and were placed in areas where divine energy was believed to be strong. Many of them were built on the sites of former oracular and divinatory shrines, which had been placed on natural fault lines where springs, thermal waters, and vapours arose, with natural cracks, caves, and crevices through which one might more easily connect with the underworld.

The temples were also famous for being the abode of sacred serpents, which were used by the Asclepiades and Therapuetes in their healing rituals. Each time an Asclepian complex was opened, serpents from the main Asclepian centres, such as Epidaurus, would be bought, bringing the sacred power of the god and goddess with them.

The sacred Asclepian serpents were chosen from a breed of native non-venomous snakes known as *Elaphe longissima*. They can grow to up to 2 metres in length and have

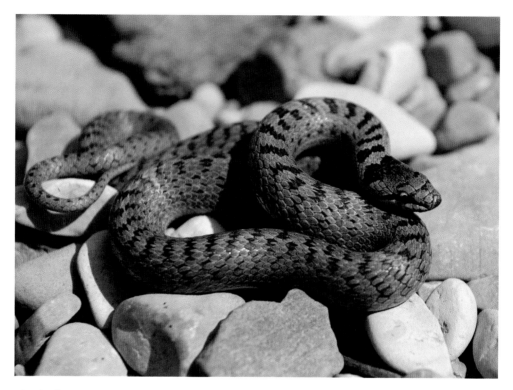

Elaphe longissima.

a diameter of 3.1cm. The actual snakes at Epidaurus, the main centre for Asclepian worship, are thought to have had a larger diameter possibly due to a process of selective breeding. This serpent eats small mammals and rodents and is often to be found living in trees and hanging from branches awaiting the passage of its prey. The serpent was both a mystical embodiment of the healing gods, and an actual living healing tool used in the healing rituals themselves.

The Asclepions were large complexes, containing thermal baths, exercise areas, treatment areas, theatres, sleeping quarters, and as a central focus had temples, shrines, and altars. The most important and potent healing structure in the temple complex was the incubation chamber. It was a place of dreaming and divination, and was known as the "abaton" a word connected to the lair or resting place of animals.

Those visiting the Asclepion would hope to be prepared for admittance into the abaton, and there be guided on a mystical journey to the otherworld, in search of divine healing through dream healing (enkoimesis). Through taking this journey to the otherworld, they too could directly experience the healing power of the under-world goddesses and divine beings. Through visiting the underworld, they could leave behind all that ailed them and while allowing it to remain in the world of the dead, return as a new resurrected and healed person, becoming twice born like the god Asclepius himself.

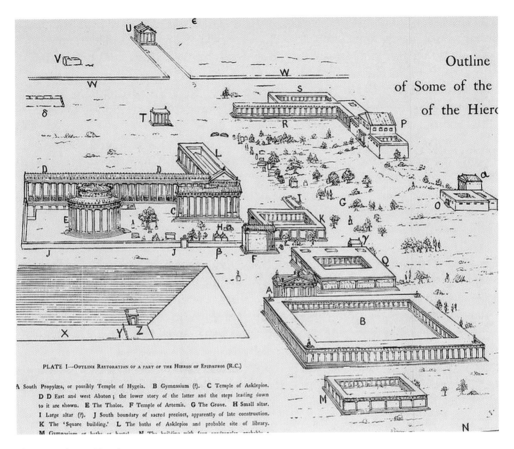

PLATE I—Outline Restoration of a part of the Hieron of Epidauros (R.C.)

A South Propylæa, or possibly Temple of Hygeia. B Gymnasium (?). C Temple of Asklepios.
  D D East and west Abaton; the lower story of the latter and the steps leading down
  to it are shown. E The Tholos. F Temple of Artemis. G The Grove. H Small altar.
  I Large altar (?). J South boundary of sacred precinct, apparently of late construction.
  K The 'Square building.' L The baths of Asklepios and probable site of library.
  M Gymnasium or baths or hostel. N The building with four spandrels, probably a

The temple at Epidaurus.

The famous Asclepion on the island of Kos where Hippocrates was a practitioner has been excavated and can give us a good impression of how it must have been to be a visitor to one of these healing sites.

In the fresh light of dawn, the initiates coming for healing at the island of Kos would have sailed into its harbour. In front of them, a magical vista of green hills and mountains silhouetted against a clear blue Mediterranean sky arose out of the crystal clear waters of the ocean. The hopes and prayers nurtured for years in their hearts for healing and enlightenment would seem to have been answered when they caught site of the sacred island rising out of the cool mist. Although the sacred Healing temple of Asclepius was some distance from the harbour and the town that surrounds it, its marble paved streets were charged with an aura of celebration and hopefulness. Even those who were bought on stretchers would likely find the energy to stretch and rise up to catch their first glimpse of this wondrous place. Many of the pilgrims had travelled great distances, crossing land, mountains and seas to get to this special place. The tales of healing that travelled the lands of Europe and Asia acted like a magnet to bring the infirm, the desperate, and the seekers of enlightenment to the island.

On leaving the harbour, the route to the temple would take the supplicants through the large bustling city that had been built as a model of Greek civil life; grand marble buildings lined the main street, adorned with columns, porticoes, and fine statues of the pantheon of the twelve Greek gods.

Once they had left behind the bustle and the noise of the market with its multitude of traders, the procession of pilgrims would make its way through groves of olives and cedars, reverberating to the songs of the birds, themselves sacred messengers from the otherworldly realms. The sound of honey bees searching out the wild mountain flowers would envelop them, and the occasional short burst of the sharp rattle of a cicada warming up for the day would cut through the bees' quiet hum. The procession would then enter the mountain groves, which exuded the enlivening aroma of pine resin. The warmth of the rising sun would begin to release the heady perfume of wild sage and basil, freshening their nostrils and awakening their minds.

Well before arriving at the temple, the sounds of the holy complex could be heard. The singing and drumming of tambourines would come in waves towards them, preparing the pilgrims for the first sight of the magnificent complex and the great entrance portico.

Passing through the grand portico into the holy shrine, its power had already impressed the procession with the importance of the experience that awaited each and every one of them. As the pilgrims take their first steps into the sacred compound, they are required to utter a vow to maintain a clean body, remain free of intoxicants and to cultivate a mind that only entertains thoughts of purity and reverence for the god of healing, Asclepius himself.

> ... and the loud cry both of those who are present and of those who are arriving, shouting this very well-known refrain, "Great is Asclepius"
>
> —Aristedes, Oratio.[2]

The priests and priestesses of the temple await the arrival of the pilgrims, passing amongst them using a sprig of sacred bay laurel to sprinkle all the newcomers with the holy water from the sacred spring. The air inside the great cloistered plaza is thick with incense. The chanting and the singing of the priests is joined by the pilgrims as the new arrivals are each accepted into the holy shrine. At the back of the courtyard is the holy spring itself. It is here that each patient is anointed and cleansed with the holy water from the sacred spring for the first time. Passing the stone basin in which the water is collected, a ritual cup of the cool water is poured onto each bowed head.

The water has come from a spout that protrudes from the feet of a statuette of Pan, the god of nature, alluding to the importance of nature as the maintainer of health. The small statue releases a crystal clear stream of spring water, which glistens and sparkles in the morning sunshine.

> "... this [spring] was discovered by and belongs to the great miracle worker [Asclepius], he who does everything for the healthy wellbeing of humankind and for many it takes the place of drugs. For many who have bathed in it recovered

their eyesight, while many by drinking were cured of chest ailments and regained vital breathing. For in some cases it cured their feet, while for others it cured some other part of the body. One patient who had been mute drank it and straight away recovered his voice, just as those who drink sacred waters turn into prophets. For some patients the process of drawing off the water was itself therapeutic. What is more, it not only provides a remedy and salvation for the sick, but even to those who are enjoying good health, it renders the use of any other water inappropriate"
—Oratio.[3]

Alongside the arch that shelters this sacred spring, the whole back wall is punctuated with many other arches so that it resembles a long cloister. Out of each archway statues of hero gods, goddesses, nymphs, and divine beings look down, and devotees stand transfixed at their feet.

Once each person has been accepted into the holy complex and has been cleansed of all outside influences, it is time for each of them to offer to the shrine of Asclepius a votive object. Each of these objects depicts the body part to be healed or the gift requested. They are made of silver plates engraved or shaped like a limb or body part. Not all of the little silver plates are so literal, as some of them are symbolic, patterned with images associated with fertility, health, or success.

Having made offerings, there is time to offer personal prayers to the gods whose shrines and statues line the back wall. Some spend time in front of the beautiful Hygeia, some in front of Panacea, two of the daughters of Asclepius. The statues are beautifully painted so that their life-like compassionate faces exude the promise of comfort and a long awaited respite from the pain and distress that has driven so many to make this journey.

Each person has their own reason for coming to this holy place, where the gods themselves walk amongst the people. This is their opportunity to honour, praise, and bless the divinities, to request their support in the healing endeavour. This is done in various ways, in rituals involving calling out to the god one's personal entreaties, and in ceremonies involving moments of quiet personal rapture, while incense is burnt, and prayers are sung to the various healing gods and goddess.

This is the first ritual in a sacred journey of preparation. There follows a process of preparing the body through the physical treatments of massage, herbal baths, and hydrotherapy. This is helped by the use of diet, medicines, and exercise.

As each day passes the pilgrims become more used to the temple routine. A rhythm develops of rising at dawn, bathing, praying, and meditating on the rising sun. Once this first communal ritual is complete the treatments begin. Some people must take herbal drinks before food, and others after eating. The diet is light, containing fresh fruits, green salads of celery, fennel, and chicory with olives, pine nuts, and freshly gathered herbs. Beans are eaten fresh or cooked with grains such as barley and oats. Yoghurt and cheese from sheep and goats milk accompanies fresh fish and wild meat. Depending on the individual constitution of each person a particular diet is prescribed. Diet is the first foundation of providing the maintenance of "good humour" throughout the body, and stopping a loss of correct temperament starts with the foods that we eat.

Gluttony is frowned upon, and those who have made themselves unwell through over-indulgence are expected to have changed their ways, or are not allowed admittance to the Asclepion at all.

The morning is also the time for the healing baths and gentle exercise. Time is spent following the personal healing rituals, which the "therpeutes" have prescribed for each person according to their needs. After the midday meal, a quiet hush descends over the whole temple complex as people rest, sheltering in quiet rooms away from the searing heat of the afternoon.

As the day cools, people once again can be seen strolling in the piazzas, engaging in debate, and listening to the teachers of philosophy. In the cool of the evening it is time for theatre and music, and at the Auspicious times of the month when the full moon illuminates the whole shrine the important rituals and ceremonies will take place, preparing pilgrims for the powerful dream rituals.

Emotions are cleansed by catharsis provided through the dramatic performances in the theatre and through the music that resonates around the mountainsides on the cooler evening breezes. Minds are strengthened, clarified, and calmed through meditation, chanting, philosophy, and debate.

If the preparation is done correctly, if the cleansing diet and regular bathing prescribed by the priests is followed, if patients have consistently taken the herbal steams,

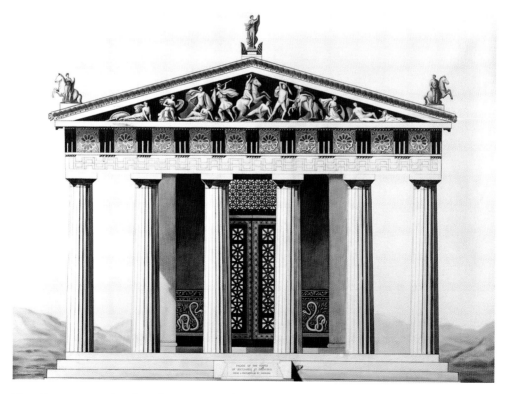

The Abaton, temple of Asclepius at Epidaurus.

and have dutifully purged their bodies with the daily herbal concoctions, then the possibility exists to be allowed entrance to the Abaton itself. This is the holy space of incubation, where in a dream the God himself may lick one's soul clean. His serpent tongue may also clear their eyes so that one may attain divine vision, and therefore find the answer to the prayers of healing.

However, there was a long period of preparation before a pilgrim would be given the chance of entering the sacred space of dream incubation, where the priests and priestesses were possessed of the divine nature of gods. For in the Abaton healers were no longer mortal but were transformed into divine beings attending to mortals with the assistance of the divine creatures of healing; the serpent and the dog. It will only be when the temple Therapeutes considered a patient ready that they are introduced to the Abaton. This may take a month of preparation or longer. All they can do is to continue to follow the treatments prescribed, and pray to the healing God while awaiting the omen that will indicate readiness for this final sacred ritual.

Once given admission to the sacred dream incubation room, the dream rituals would begin. Prayers, drumming, and chanting fill the incense suffused atmosphere. The acoustics and echoes of the chamber change and twist the rhythms and melodies so it begins to sound like the gods themselves are adding their voices to the ritual. The chants produce harmonics that are amplified as they bounce around the chamber from stone wall to stone wall. It sounds like heavenly voices have joined in, transporting the whole company to another realm. The low light from flickering oil lamps adds to the ethereal feel of this most sacred place, a place where magic and transformation of the soul may truly be possible.

Periods of fasting and prayer have heightened senses, allowing patients to be open to the trance inducing effects of these ancient songs and chants. Finally, they hope to slip into sleep with the hypnotic chanting lulling their minds into a world of magical dreaming. Already they are on the great journey to the otherworld of the divine beings and the great ancestral spirits.

The priests and priestesses dress in Egyptian sandals, white robes, and their hair is tied with white bands. The world of healing and dreaming is a place of clear vision, clarity, and purity and the white adornments mark them out as the mediums of this otherworld. They continue their singing as they bring the sacred ancestral energy into the Abaton. To help the pilgrims make the final preparations for the sacred dreams, they are given a brew of holy dreaming herbs, a recipe received through dreams of the gods themselves. It has a slightly bitter and sharp taste, which is only partially mollified by the sweetness of the honey and wine that has been added to it. The priests and priestesses have now become manifestations of the gods and goddesses themselves, passing amongst the sleepers carrying sacred serpents and attended by the other animal companion of Asclepius, the divine dog. They are the sacred mediums and manifestations of Asclepius, or of his daughters Hygieia and Panacea. It is possible that the dream experiences that arise are aided by the physical sensation of being licked by these serpents and dogs during the time of sleeping. But when one experiences such a thing in our dreams, we know that the two worlds have merged, the gods have become physical and we have become divine.

Asclepius is the god of healing and the source of healing wisdom, a wisdom that may be imparted in the healing dreams that occur in the Abaton. The Asclepiades and Therupeutes were adept at dream analysis and for a supplicant the greatest wish was to be blessed by a healing dream in which Asclepius himself comes to them in his serpent form. The dream cure could provide spontaneous healing, or the healing remedies, offerings, or practices would be found within a prophetic dream. Many illnesses were cured and votive offerings attesting to the power of the gods were presented to the temple. Every shrine would glisten with silver medallions showing the healing miracles that had occurred. It was common to have dreams about specific herbs that should be used as well as dreams within which healing would occur, due to the touch of the god or the effect of being licked by the serpent itself.

In this way, the healing experience reached its pinnacle with patients either receiving the completion of their healing journey through such a dream, or being directed as to how to continue the healing process.

Although the temples fell into disuse in the middle of the first millennium, the tradition continued to influence and reappear in religious and healing symbolism in the subsequent centuries. The depiction in Christian iconography of angels dressed in white robes is a good example of the continuing cultural memory of the Therapuetes and their divine healing rituals.

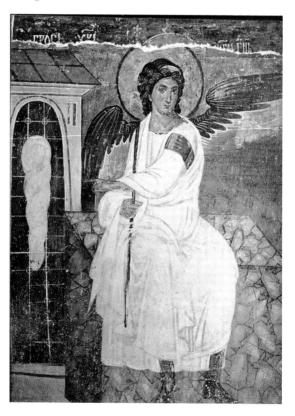

13th century white angel mosaic, Serbia.

MYTHOS

CHAPTER THREE

Mythos, creation, ancestors, and healing

"In the beginning … Gaia, the Earth, came into being, her broad bosom the
ever-firm foundation of all"

—(Hesiod, 117).[1]

Hesiod is considered the earliest of the Greek poets, writing in about 750 BC, he was
the first to recount the myths of the classical Greek culture of the Olympian gods. It is
said that before the Greek culture there existed a culture known as the Pelasgians, and
the following is their story of creation:

In the beginning, Eurynome, the goddess of all things, arose naked out of chaos.
Finding nothing substantial to rest her feet upon, she divided the sea from the sky and
danced alone across the ocean waves. She danced towards the south, and the wind
that was set in motion behind her became the north wind, this was the first of her
creations. She grasped this wind and rubbing it between her hands created the great
serpent, Ophion.

Eurynome then danced wildly to warm herself, she danced and danced until she
was in a state of ecstasy. As Ophion watched her wild dance he felt lust and passion
arise in him. Finally, he could hold back no longer and entwining his coils around her,
he coupled with her. From the mixing of their two energies she became ready to birth
the second of her creations. She assumed the form of a white dove and flew over the
stormy waters of the ocean bringing peace and harmony. Then, in this calm place she
lay the great universal egg. She then called the serpent Ophion, commanding him to
coil around the egg seven times and germinate it with his warmth until it hatched.
The universal egg split into two and out tumbled all the things that exist, with all of
them becoming her children; she had birthed the sun and the moon, the planets, the

stars, and the earth itself, with all its rivers, oceans, forests, plants, and all the living creatures that roamed, flew, and swam on its surface.

Eurynome thus became the original Earth mother, and by creating all the future mothers on Earth, now watches over us all like a grandmother. We feel her body with every step that we walk, she gives us life with every breath that we take, and she nourishes us with every meal that we eat. She is the earth from which all life is continually generated. She appears in the form of the wise old hag that has witnessed so many lives, so many generations of her children being born, growing, and finally dying. She is the great repository of history, the story of all beings, the songs of all creation, and she knows the cycles and changes of this world before they come. She has always shown us how to survive and continue even in the darkest of times.

In one of her manifestations, she is the winter goddess of death and takes on the appearance of the old ugly hag, dwelling in deep crags and caves. She carries with her our death, but also promises our regeneration. She is seen flying above us as the sacred dove, carrying the great golden egg of rebirth. We must visit her sacred lairs to hear messages from the underworld, these lairs are the places of death and dreaming, and like the abaton in the temples of healing, they are the lair of magical creatures and offer gateways of transition between the worlds. It is by going within them that we may return healed and renewed. Her cycle of renewal is symbolised by the sacred serpent of the Asclepiads, representing the goddess's energy of rebirth, hibernating each winter, and reawakening each spring with a new skin and new life force.

Eurynome's daughter, the moon, manifests in the fertile waters that flow around her body. She is seen in the new life of spring, she brings us rain and fertility, and presents us with the gift of rivers, springs, rainbows, and oceans. Like the new moon she embodies the maiden, like the full moon she embodies the mother, and like the waning moon she embodies the crone. She is the dream that keeps evolving, the doorway to the wisdom of intuition and visions. She fills us with poetry and song, flowing through us stirring up romance, compassion, and kindness. She used to manifest as the bird goddess of fertility and creation of new life. In later times, she appeared as a fate, fairy, or sometimes as a swan or bird, often being associated with the waters of a magical lake. When fulfilling her role as the primeval nurturing mother, she often appears in stories and myths as a magical dear, or as in the story of Goldilocks, appears as a bear giving shelter and food.

Eurynome's male child, the sun, has become the father that shines down on us by day, the source of warmth that brings life and fills our hearts with joy and passion. His light wakes us in the morning, filling us with the enthusiasm to be creative and to fulfil our potential, giving us the energy to provide a strong and safe home for our families, clan, and tribe. He is generous and warm, welcoming us every morning with his bright return; when young he is the adventurer, exploring and expanding our world vision and setting us out on our journey of finding truth and wisdom.

Our grandfather is the sky, continually observing all that goes on in the world below, his infinite vision making him wise and far-sighted. He inspires us by opening up new horizons, bringing fresh ideas, shinning light on new paths and opportunities.

He symbolises the elders, teachers, our human ancestors, and the enlightened mind. Along with our grandmother the earth, he holds us in an eternal embrace, their arms enfolding us above and beneath, earth and sky forever encircling us.

This is the family of our greater ancestors, grandfather Sky and grandmother Earth giving us a home in which the dreams of the Moon mother are realised, and the creations of our Sun father are manifested.

These four elemental ancestors appear and reappear in the fairytales and myths that have been passed down to us today, even when the original stories have been absorbed, digested, changed, and regurgitated by countless cultures across time many of the original themes remain intact.

We can still hear the voice of the triple goddess of old Europe calling to us today through our European folktales, beliefs, and traditional rituals and songs. These ancient tales and ways of being in the world connect us to the beliefs held by those who lived before the Indo European colonists came from the Eurasian steppes with their domesticated horses carrying armies of oppression. They hark back to a time before Christianity demonised nature worship and paganistic beliefs. We still find the ancient goddesses in our fairy tales, in our cultural symbols and folk tradition, and we find memories of her in the healing springs and wells and the sacred lore that surrounds them.

Wherever you go in the world, you will find stories of how medicine arose, and I will now tell a story from a village in a small mountain valley in south west Wales, which still carries within it the echoes of the wisdom and enlightenment myths of old Europe.

The magical lake of Llyn y Fan Fach

The story begins in the spring, with the people of the small village of Myddfai rejoicing as winter draws back her snowy cloak from the tops of the Black Mountains. When the winter's darkness lifts, the villagers' hearts are filled with hope and joy, as they celebrate the returning warmth of spring and look forward to the summer that it heralds. This is also the time when the livestock are returned to the mountain pastures once again, being set free to roam and graze on the fresh herbs and flowers that grace those beautiful slopes.

So, it was that on the first day of spring that a young farmer called Gwyn eagerly began to travel with his sheep and cattle to the pastures that lie around the magical lake of Llyn y Fan Fach. The magical nature of the lake lies in the fact that it has always been known to be the abode of powerful lake fairies. Like all young spirits, Gwyn was ready to start on the adventure of the journey, for although the young farmer had made this journey many times with his own father, today he was alone. His father was now an old man and the seven-mile trek along the tracks and lanes of the valleys from their village of Myddfai to the foot of the mountains was now too far for his father's aching bones to carry him. It was time for Gwyn himself to grow tall and strong, to rise up from the earth like a strong young sapling and to take on the challenges of

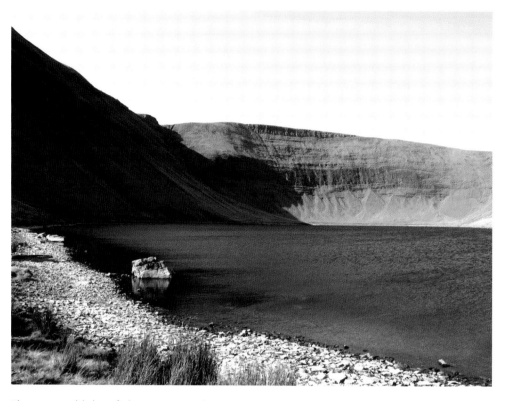

The magical lake of Llyn y Fan Fach.

adulthood, facing the tasks that will surely come to test us all, and through testing us, unfold our inner wisdom as we embark on our journey through life.

Gwyn had a spring in his step, he was singing to himself as he breathed the fresh morning air, as he once again felt the joy of heading up into the hills. Each year for as long as he could remember he had travelled this way bringing the animals up in the spring, then taking them down later in the summer to shear their wool and to check and count the lambs. Then before the onset of autumn he would return with the flocks to let them feed on the last of the summer grasses, with him finally bringing them down again before the rough weather of winter sets in.

He knew the tale of the magical lake beings, and he had spent many summer days playing on the lake shore as a boy, but neither sight nor sound of the fairies had ever come his way.

The well trodden track travels up beside the mountain stream that flows down from the lake. Llyn y Fan Fach sits in a small bowl carved out of the mountains by glaciers countless years before, so that the peaks around it hold it in a tight embrace. The slopes rise steeply up behind its waters like a protective parent holding the lake in its lap, challenging all comers to regard this place with respect. On the walk up to the lake, the waters only come into sight as you finally mount the small knoll that has held back the clear fresh mountain waters since the beginning of time.

Although on that early day of spring the sun shone brightly, it had little strength to warm the heart. However, Gwyn felt carefree and his heart was gladdened at the thought of seeing that magical place once more. He sat on a rock on the shore of the lake to take a rest from the long trek up and took in the sight of the glistening lake. He let the sounds of the sighing winds blowing freshly down from the mountain tops roll over him, mingling with the rhythm of his own breath, and he sunk into a gentle reverie of the happy times past he had spent in this place. As he broke this trance by looking up and gazing along the shore line he caught his first glimpse of something strange at the far end of the lake. He lifted his hand to shade his eyes from the sun as he peered at what seemed to be a small figure sitting on a large rock at the edge of the water.

Intrigued, he decided to make his way around the lake edge to where the strange figure sat. There were two choices; he could take the longer route around travelling through lower but marshier ground to the north of the lake, or he could follow the direct route that skirted the bottom of the steep slope that bordered the other side. He chose the latter shorter route, but after a few minutes began to regret his choice as he found that the narrow mountain path along the side of the steep hills demanded more attention than he thought would have been necessary. He had to keep looking down to check that his foothold was secure and that he wouldn't slip and go tumbling into the lake. This meant that he wasn't able to keep the figure in sight, which was made worse every time he had to negotiate one of the small ravines that cut into the cliff face, as then the figure was completely lost from view while he was wrapped in one of the deep folds cut into the mountainside.

As he approached it became clear that the figure was in fact a young woman. She sat sunning herself, allowing her long hair to be gently caressed by the breeze that was blowing across the lake. At first Gwyn rushed along the path, desperate not to lose sight of her lest she disappear. As she seemed to be in no mood to leave her seat, he worried less, but kept his pace brisk nonetheless. Finally, as he rounded the last fold in the hillside, he slowed down. He felt a bit self-conscious wiping the sweat from his brow and panting slightly from the exertion. Then he tried to gather his composure as he made directly across the flat ground at the water's edge toward her. He was now worried that he may frighten her and that she would run off, so he tried to put on a slightly unconcerned frivolous but jolly air. His intention was to make it seem that he was just on a gentle stroll around the lake and that this was a chance meeting with her, in such a situation he reasoned that it would be entirely appropriate to offer a good day to her, in fact it would be rude not to acknowledge her in the circumstances.

His approach was a little haphazard, as he negotiated the last of the reeds at the water's edge and slipped a few times on the rocks along the shore. At last he was next to her, blushing slightly, having been aware of the close regard she had been giving his recent progress, a regard barely hidden under her long lashes. Now that he could see her clearly he became transfixed by her stunning beauty, he took in her long dark flowing hair, the beautiful green shimmering material that adorned her lithe body, and the perfectly worked slippers on her feet and he admired the way the satin ribbon that held them on was so daintily tied at her ankle.

He had seen all this in a short moment, which had already seemed to last an age. Flustered, he was unable to think of what to say. There were only a few young maidens in the valleys and he knew them all so well that conversation with them had never been a problem. However, to be presented with such a stunning beauty and to have no introduction made for him, left him completely speechless.

"I must give her something" he thought "present her with a gift, that's what I must do!" he quickly felt in his bag and fishing around in it brought out the only thing that he had with him. The look of slight amusement on the maiden's face at these strange antics soon turned to one of utter disdain when he handed her all that he had; a rather hard dry crust of barley bread grabbed from the scullery when he had left the farm before dawn that morning.

His hopes of pleasing her were very soon dashed, as she flung the crust at his feet saying "Sir, thy bread is much too dry, I'm not that easy to catch!" Then, stretching herself down off her perch on the rock, she slipped a foot into the water, and without a single shiver trembling her body, she began to walk away from him, deeper and deeper into the still ice cold mountain lake. Soon all he could see was the top of her head, a small black point protruding out of the water, it was as if she were an otter or a bird about to dive, and then she was gone. The ripples closed around the point where the top of her head had finally disappeared, and to his surprise she did not resurface there or anywhere else. He sat there, his unflinching gaze fixed like a hawk upon that very spot, until this body began to ache and the chill of the mountain breeze began to penetrate into his very core.

He returned to the village in a kind of daze, no longer sure if he had imagined the extraordinary encounter or whether the beautiful maiden had actually been there. He reasoned that she had seemed too solid, too real, and too vivid to have been a dream, but he didn't dare tell anyone knowing that they would only laugh at him, calling him a fool who believed in his own wild fancies.

The following morning he set out early, not wanting to alert anyone to his strange desire to spend the whole morning unproductively walking to a mountain lake instead of getting on with the many unfinished jobs on the farm.

He arrived at the edge of the lake with a sense of excitement and hope, wishing that beyond all possibility the magical being would be there once again. The sweat that trickled down his back moistening his shirt was caused not just by the exertion of the walk, but also his growing anticipation and anxiety.

He strained his eyes as soon as the lake came into sight, trying to make out whether the small figure he thought that he could see sitting by the far end of the lake was actually a person and not a large rock or a clump of marsh reeds. With growing excitement, he began to walk around the edge of the lake as he had done on the previous day and soon he had no doubt that it was the young beauty herself. Encouraged by seeing her there again he felt confident that she wouldn't disappear before he could reach her, so today he took a more measured pace in his approach.

Still with some trepidation, he once again approached the beautiful fairy maiden, unable to stop asking himself if this really could be happening and hoping that it wasn't just a trick of his imagination. But as he came close he could have no doubt that this breathing living being, smiling coyly at him was quite as real as himself.

He knelt down in front of her trying to be as respectful and as polite as he could, then reaching into his bag, he produced a soft, sweet smelling ball of dough. She took it with a glint in her eye, but no sooner had she taken it did she turn to him saying with laughing disdain;

"Thy bread is too moist young sir … you'll have to try a lot harder than that!"

With those words she once again slipped off the rock and gracefully walked into the lake and finally disappeared beneath its surface, leaving Gwyn both dumbstruck and terribly disappointed. However, he didn't allow his dark mood to stay for long as he was quickly back on his way down to the village with a plan. He went straight to the baker pleading with him to bake the sweetest, freshest loaf of bread that he had ever produced for the following morning, and he promised to pay him handsomely.

It was with this special loaf that he left the farm at dawn for the third time, making his way up to the lake in the thin morning light. It was with a feeling of growing confidence that he followed the now familiar lakeside path to the place where once again he could see the small figure sitting. As soon as he arrived in front of her he produced the loaf with a flourish, and it was with growing excitement that he witnessed a smile cross her face as she took the gift in her hands. However, she uttered not a single word, but slipping the loaf under her arm she daintily skipped back into the lake, casting approving glances back at him before disappearing once again under its silvery, still waters.

He waited for a moment, confused by the unexpected turn of events. Suddenly, his confusion turned to fear as a towering water spout rose up out of the lake in front of him, twisting and spraying a mist of cold rain down upon him. It then crashed back down into the lake as quickly as it had appeared, and revealed standing within its centre a sumptuously dressed fairy king, his clothes emanating rainbow colours, shimmering like iridescent fish scales, and his golden crown sending out a bright golden light like the sun rising on a spring morning. He stood tall for a fairy, seeming to tower above Gwyn as in a booming voice he declared; "So you are the young mortal who has set his heart on my daughter, you're not the first, and I'll bet that you'll not be the last! Many have tried to win her hand and all have failed, so I'll give you an equal chance to pass the test I give each of her suitors. If you succeed I'll give you a fine wedding and a dowry of magical creatures that will ensure that your farm will always prosper … However, before I set her free to marry there will be one condition you must agree to accept; You must undertake to never strike your wife, and if you do so, even if done in error, she will disappear after the third blow is struck." Gwyn could never imagine that such a thing would happen, he was sure that he would always treat her with kindness and love, and that they would never come to blows, so he readily agreed to the deal. The King accepted his agreement, and then turned to the lake saying; "So young mortal, here is your task …"

At that point, out of the lake the fairy princess reappeared, but to Gwyn's surprise she was closely followed by a second fairy, the two of them seating themselves side by side on the usual rock by the lake. The king turned to Gwyn saying "The challenge is for you to tell me which one it is of my two daughters that has stolen your heart."

At first Gwyn thought he would easily be able to tell them apart, but soon his initial confidence waned as he realised that the two maidens were undoubtedly identical twins. In fact so alike were they that each mirrored the other exactly, even down to the placing of the freckles on their cheeks, the colour of their eyes and the way that their hair seductively fell down over their shoulders. The more that Gwyn studied them the less sure he became about which one was the beauty that he had fallen for, he looked from one to the other searching for a clue, but there was nothing at all that set them apart. The Fairy King began to chuckle, "You see, many have tried and all have failed, your time for guessing is up, so say which one it is!"

At that point as Gwyn looked back at the fairies in desperation, one of them slightly moved her foot. His gaze fell on the movement and to his joy he realised that he recognised the exact way that the satin ribbon on her fairy shoe was tied, just like on the first day he had seen her, and in triumph he shouted "that is her, she is the one!"

The King could not deny that Gwyn was correct, and in an instant they all seemed to be back in the village organising a great wedding celebration. The allotted day came quickly and people from the whole valley came, as word had spread quickly about the fairy princess come to marry a lowly shepherd. The extraordinary celebration was made all the more memorable due to the fairy food and wine that never ran out, the fairy music that never stopped and the ability of the people to dance and sing and party night and day without ever becoming exhausted. After three days and nights of celebration, quiet finally returned to the small village of Myddfai and everyone could finally rest.

With the benefit of fairy sheep that were always fat and healthy, fairy oxen who could plough night and day, and horses that could travel for days without tiring, the farm began to prosper. Gwyn and his fairy wife lived in great happiness and out of their joy and love three sons were born.

It was some time later that they were invited to the christening of their neighbour's child, the fairy was ready to mount her horse when she realised that she had left her riding gloves in the farmhouse, and she asked Gwynn to fetch them for her. As she waited she became transfixed by the beauty of the fairy horse beside her, it seemed to hover above the ground and exude a magical glow. When Gwynn came out he saw her standing there like a statue, it was as if she had been turned to stone. In panic he grabbed her arm shaking her to get her attention, it was then that she turned to him saying; "You have struck me for the first time. I know it's not your fault, and that as a mortal you are unaware of how much more sensitive we fairies are, often crossing between the worlds, having visions and insights that mortals can rarely understand …"

Gwyn was determined that such a thing would never happen again and he was mindful of his every action lest he should once again make the same mistake. Some months later they were invited to the wedding of a neighbour. The celebration went well and the wedding barn was packed with joyful friends and family when a terrible screeching and wailing cut through the happy sounds. Everyone turned to look at the source of the awful noise, and there sobbing and wailing in the corner was the fairy, Gwyn quickly rushed up to her and grabbing her pulled her to her feet. She then turned to him with tears in her eyes, saying: "You have struck me a second time, you can't see what I can see, and so you don't understand; I can see that this sweet couple's future path is full of tragedy and sadness, and that is why I could not help but to cry."

Even more determined to be vigilant Gwyn and the fairy returned to the cottage. It was almost a year later that an old, well respected neighbour died and along with the rest of the village they attended her funeral. The wake began with everyone releasing their grief and recounting the many good actions of the old wise woman who had died. Their tearful valedictories were suddenly interrupted by a sound of laughing and cackling, which soon grew into howls of laughter and finally shrieks of joy. All in the room turned at that moment to see the fairy rolling on the ground holding onto her sides as if they would burst from the laughter wracking her body. Gwyn quickly jumped on her putting his hand across her mouth to quieten the embarrassing display. It was at that point the fairy turned to him saying; "I can see that the old woman is now in paradise, free of pain and sadness, and so full of joy, and I cannot not contain my happiness for her, seeing her dance so happily in the after world. But now you have struck me for the third time and I must return to the lake as was agreed." And with tears in her eyes she said "Our marriage is now over, goodbye my love."

With those words she sang out to all of the magical beasts, calling them to return with her to the lake, and then she began the long walk back up to the mountains. Gwyn pleaded every step of the way with her to stay, but it was if she had become deaf, caught in a trance, and unable to do anything but take step after step back to the watery kingdom of the lake fairies. The magical horses, sheep, and oxen followed, with the biggest ox leaving the field still tied to its plough. It is said that even today you can see the scar cut into the mountainside by the plough as it was pulled back down to the watery pastures beneath the lake.

Gwyn stayed at the lakeside for three full days and nights, desperate and bereft at the loss of his lovely fairy princess. But cry as he did, praying continually at the lakeside for her return, he never once saw her again.

It was many years later that his sons became the ones to take the sheep and cattle up to the pastures around the magical lake, leaving their now old father at the farmhouse. When they arrived alone for the first time at the lake they could not hold back their tears for their lost mother. As their tears fell into the lake, out of the ripples a mist appeared. The magical mist then twisted, turned, and swirled around, finally forming itself into the figure of their mother. Then she sat with them, patiently teaching them the songs and stories of the healing plants that grew in the mountains. That was her gift to them, and from then onwards they and their descendants became the famous herbalists of Myddfai. So renowned did they become that the Princes of Wales eventually put them under their protection as a way of honouring their great healing knowledge and skills. They passed their recipes down generation to generation until the last of them died out in the middle of the eighteenth century. Some of these recipes were written down and can still be read today.

And so this is the story of the beginnings of our medicine. It is said that because of this magical union between the fairies and us mortals, we also have fairy blood in our veins. They are now part of our ancestry, and we too now have the ability to hear the songs of medicine sung by nature. If we can become still enough, we may be able to hear these songs in the rustling of the leaves in the tops of trees, in the bubbling sounds of the mountain streams, in the songs of birds, or even sometimes in our dreams. It is these songs that can guide us to find the medicines that we need, and it is from them that the ancient healing knowledge of how to work with healing plants comes.

This story is like so many other ancient teaching stories, containing the continuing themes of adventure, challenge, courage, love, hidden messages, magical worlds accessed through divination, and the magic of water and its spirits. These wisdom tales invite us to experience our time on this earth as an unfolding and expanding story, as a myth full of surprise and adventure, of confusion and of enlightenment, of gifts and of loss, to be celebrated and enjoyed while it lasts, as our story like all stories will come to an end one day. We can either experience our lives as a linear journey through time, acquiring experiences as we go along the road, increasingly battered by the challenges and shocks that come our way, or we can embrace our place in this mythic vision of the unfolding cosmos, and see that we too are part of the magical story of life.

I have visited the lake of Llyn y Fan Fach twice. On my first visit I was held up by a queue of traffic on the single track road leading to the mountain, it transpired that we were caught behind a herd of sheep. When we got to the open fields at the foot of the mountains I began the walk up, eventually crossing paths with the shepherd who was herding the sheep. He was riding a red off-road motorbike, which cut back and forth across the path as he harried and searched for the stragglers of the herd. At one point he stopped on the track and we spoke:

"Hello there" he said, "I'm sorry that I kept you waiting on the road behind the herd."

"That's no problem at all" I said, "Have you come far?"

"Oh yes, I had to get up at dawn, as our farm is seven miles down the valley in a small village that you probably won't have heard of, it's called Myddfai … you see we first bring the sheep up in the spring, take them down later for a shear, then up again for the last of the grass before the winter sets in … My family has farmed in the valley for generations so we're always up and down this way."

I had just learnt the story of the lake, and I smiled to myself, enjoying the experience of myth and reality intermingling, one dissolving into the other, always able to surprise and excite us. Here was another message from the cosmos, a confirmation from the land, from the ancestors, and a signpost that we are on track with destiny.

On my second trip ten years later, I was visiting the lake with a group of herbalists. On the way back down, as we drove along the narrow lanes, the minibus we were in hit a large boulder on a sharp bend, which blew out the rear tyre. We all got out of the bus to assess the situation, and at that point a couple of farmers on quad bikes came past, stopping on the bend to see what was happening. It was only then, when I looked down the road that I saw the same shepherd on his red off road motorbike coming into view. He had changed very little in the intervening years, apart from having a slightly more rugged and wind-blown complexion, and here on the same road we had once again crossed paths as he made his way to round up the cattle and sheep from the mountain pastures around the magical lake of Llyn y Fan Fach. It seems that as has always been the way, magical moments, like rainbows, are always just around the corner.

LOGOS

CHAPTER FOUR

The humoral cosmos

The central concepts of Galenic medicine were formalised in the 4th century BC by the Greek philosopher Empedocles, who posited that nature consisted of four basic elements; earth, air, fire, and water. They denote the various interacting patterns of the cosmos, showing how all its aspects interrelate with one another. The four elements provide a means of measuring the balance or imbalances that can arise in the natural world and how one may redress them.

The human race only experienced the world through our five senses when the concepts underpinning Galenic medicine arose. The language used in Galenic medicine describes the world as we see it, using simple and straight forward concepts. This Galenic definition of an element as something that can be directly sensed through our organs of perception was still largely held right up until the time when microscopy and the development of modern chemistry occurred. It wasn't until the late 19th century that Dimtry Mendeleev defined a new kind of "chemical element" based on the atomic number of a substance, and these new "elements" were placed in the periodic table we still use today.

However, this new way of viewing the material world as being made up of a very large number of basic elements doesn't make the traditional Galenic four element description irrelevant. The new model of unseen atomic elements doesn't relate to our daily experience of this world, and can't help us to identify for ourselves when an imbalance arises, or from where it comes, and gives us no clue as to how to adapt to re-align them. When the universe is reduced to a description of its smallest parts in this way, only the chaotic swirl of this sub-matter is observed, and the patterns that arise out of this chaos which produce the world we experience are not given much attention. The atomic description of elements can tell us all kinds of things about the physical universe that we couldn't know without it and has enabled huge techno-logical advances. However, it should not be seen as a replacement for the traditional description of the four elements, which serves quite a different purpose.

We can view the Galenic system of ideas as a model that evolved to give us a way of describing the world as we experience it. It does this by referring to natural cycles and states that we can easily observe. By using the four elemental description of the world it is still possible to recognise how disharmony arises in a person, and by referring to this viewpoint we are able to take account of every aspect of an individual. Taking such a viewpoint can give clear guidance in how to recognise any disharmony in the natural state of a person and how to bring back their balance and health.

The humoral cosmos is not envisioned as merely containing two sets of binary opposites of elements, such as hot versus cold and moistness versus dryness, but as a realm where there is a dynamic and continually changing combination of elements. It is from this dynamic mixing of elemental energies that life then arises. From the combination of fire in the divine light with the waters of the cosmos, living things arise and grow. This energy of life itself, is called the aqua vitae or vital spirit. It is the third energy that is created through the coming together of the two opposites; light and dark, male and female, hot and cold. The story of Eurynome and Ophion, symbol-ises this creative force, from their sacred coupling the world that we live in is created from the world egg. The vital spirit, the life force which arises in the body, is similarly formed by the combination of opposing forces. It is in the heart that the innate heat and the radical moisture are brought together by the action of the divine spirit, travel-ling through the ether as "pneuma" or the breath of life.

It is when two opposite elements come together that they manifest as the third entity of vital spirit, once again reminding us of the power of the symbol of the sacred three. This harks back to the sacred triple goddess, the triskele symbol, the three worlds of Hermetic philosophy, and the triad of birth, life, and death.

When Ether is included we have five elemental aspects, with the number five being an ancient symbol of the goddess in the form of Venus, as her planet follows a five-directional transit through the sky, marking this as her sacred number. It is from her that all fertility and life is birthed.

The four main elements are evident in all the aspects of the cosmos. They have an association with the seasons, the times of day, the stages of life, the organs of the body, the functions and systems of the body, and the activity of all things in relation to one another. In the body the elements manifest as the Humours, and by placing all of these aspects into a circular pattern we can more easily represent their many interactions and connections.

In the diagram, the four main coloured sections represent the four primary quali-ties of hot, cold, dry, and wet.

The circles represent the four elements and their corresponding humours, with the circle for ether in the centre. This shows how each element and its humour is a combi-nation of two of the four primary qualities.

As we move around the circle we can see how each element and humour transform into the next one as the primary qualities change with each seasonal shift.

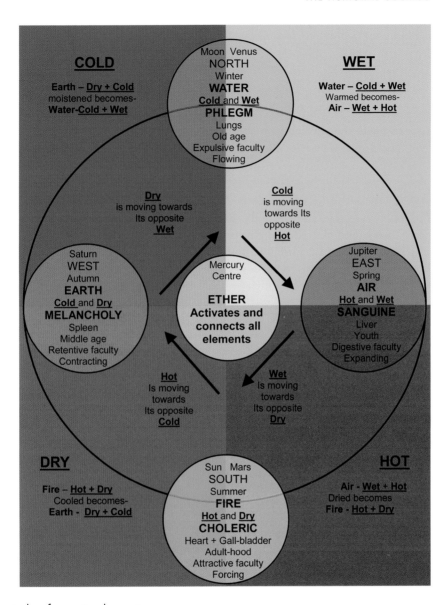

The circle of cosmic elements.

A good place to start exploring our circle is at the east position, the direction of the rising sun seasonally associated with the spring, marking the beginning of the year's cycle of growth. The wet and cold winter, the season of the phlegmatic humour is transformed through the arrival of warmth to the wet and warm season of spring and the sanguine humour. In the ancient calendars, this is when the return of light is celebrated with the ceremony of Imbolc. It is the time when returning warmth brings back growth, movement, and expansion outwards and upwards. The returning warmth of the sun is transforming the cold dampness of winter into a time of warm moist fertility and growth. It is therefore connected to birth, youthfulness, and move-ment. At this point heat returns to the wet earth, vaporising the water to produce the hot and moist air element. The air element is carried in, and therefore associated with the blood, which is made in the liver through the process of digestion. The air element becomes the sanguine humour, and Jupiter is the planetary ruler associated with all of its aspects.

As we move into the summer the increasing heat dries out the wetness carried in the air element, and transforms it into the hot and dry fire element and the choleric humour. It is the time when everything is coming into its fullness, and is at its full strength and vitality. It is therefore connected to adulthood, activity and manifesta-tion. Its energy focuses and distils out the essence of things, accounting for the attrac-tive or apprehensive faculty of the body, a faculty that brings ideas into the mind, and distils nourishment out of food. The choleric humour has its seat in the gall bladder, is seen as the red part of blood, and is ruled by the two hot planets of Mars and the sun. The summer solstice is traditionally celebrated with fires at midsummer, honouring the heat and warmth of the sun. The sun is hot like Mars, but rather than ruling the choleric humour, it rules the vital spirit, which resides in the heart.

It is followed by autumn, which is associated with the earth element. It is the time when the heat of the summer is replaced by the return of coldness, giving us a cold and dry season of contraction, and the falling away and returning of energy to the earth. It is connected to middle age, when energy lessens, and we cool and slow down. At this point, we benefit from the return of the energy to the centre, like the bringing in of the harvest of all that has been achieved and manifested through the activity of our lives. It is associated with the retentive faculty of the body, holding onto nourishment, memories, and to giving substance to tissues. It is the time of contraction and return to the earth, with the earth element in the body becoming the melancholic humour, found in the sediment of blood with its seat being the spleen. It naturally fits well into the western position, the place of the setting sun and the diminishing heat associated with it. The ancient festival of Samhain celebrated at this time of the year acknowl-edges the dying back of things as a necessary part of the cycle of regeneration. The earth element, the melancholic humour, and the spleen are all ruled by the cold, dry planet Saturn.

The winter is placed in the north, and is associated with the water element. It is when the moisture replaces dryness so that we experience the invasion of dampness and condensation. It is the time of old age and dying, when we let go of strong con-cerns and attachments, allowing us to experience the wisdom of flow and release. It is the time when moisture abounds in nature, with puddles, floods, and rivers in full flow. It is the time when the body is prone to becoming colder, damper, softer, and more swollen. It is when we see the beginnings of fertility in the process of ger-mination, like the strengthening return of the sun after the celebration of the winter solstice. Life will return and regeneration will follow this process of death and disso-lution. It is associated with the expulsive faculty, which removes waste and makes the passages slippery. It is seen in the wet portion of blood called the plasma, its seat is in the lungs, and it is ruled by the moon. Venus co-rules the water element and is indicative of the fertility that moisture brings, which is similar to the sun returning after the winter solstice reminding us of the potential for the regeneration that is to come.

The elements are all inimical to each other, which means that they cannot remain the same when they are in contact with each other. This will ensure a continual cycle of change and evolution as they transform from one to the other. However, there needs to be a medium in which they all exist, a medium that takes on the characteristics of whatever element it contains without changing or influencing it. We place this medium in the centre as it provides connection and communication of all things and allows the flow of divine spirit to infuse all parts of the cosmos. This element, therefore, has no qualities of its own, it is neither hot nor cold, and neither wet nor dry. It may be thought of as space or as emptiness, as an element without restriction, which allows both contraction and expansion. We call it ether, it has no specific organ as its seat but is apparent in the body as the animation that comes through the nerves, and the communication of the senses to the brain. It is ruled by the planet Mercury, and is the medium through which the divine spirit activates our soul.

When we look at this humoral circle we can see the inter-relationships of all aspects of the cosmos. We can see them as a continuous cycle, and like the ancient symbols of circles and spirals left by our ancestors, they show the elements continually feeding their own transformation in a never ending cycle of expansion and contraction, energised and enabled by divine energy through the ether.

CHAPTER FIVE

The seven naturals and six non-naturals

In Galenic philosophy, the living body exists and functions through the harmonious interaction of seven natural things. The seven naturals are seen as internal aspects and influences within the body. There are also six non-natural or external factors that directly influence the internal humoral balance.

The seven naturals

1. The Elements
   In humoral cosmology there are four natural elements that combine to form the material world; earth, air, fire, water. There is a fifth entity called ether, which has no physical form of its own, but exists as the medium of connection and communication between the elements. It is within ether that divine spirit travels from the realm of light bringing "anima" or the life force down to the world of matter.
2. The Four Temperaments
   As each element manifests in the body it will have a particular influence on the organ, system, or person. These elemental manifestations are seen as "temperamental" characteristics, as they influence the actual temperature of the person or organ. For instance the influence of the fire element is to heat and dry the temperament, while the water element has a cooling moistening influence. Consequently, earth cools and dries, while air warms and moistens.
3. The Four Humours
   As the elements are the basis for all matter, when they manifest in the body they appear as physically identifiable substances that through their combination form

flesh, bones, organs, and fluids. Each humour corresponds to an element, and it has a place in the body where it naturally resides and collects, with each humour bestowing a "virtue" that enables the various physical functions of the body to function.

The Vital Spirit	Resides in the heart—Ruled by the Sun Comprised of the Innate heat and the radical moisture The manifestation of the divine force in the body			7
The Animal Spirit	Resides in the head—Ruled by Mercury, comprised of Ether Internal intellective virtues– apprehension, judgement, memory			
The Procreative & conservative Spirits		The procreative Spirit The womb and testes	The Natural Spirit The Liver	6
The four Administering virtues	The apprehensive virtue	The expulsive virtue	The Digestive virtue	The retentive virtue	5
The parts	Fore brain, right eye, heart, gall bladder, nose	Head, Left eye, stomach, bowels, reproductive organs, kidneys, bladder, Joints, skin	Mid brain, tongue, Lungs, liver, sides and ribs, sinews	Rear brain, Ears, Spleen, bones	4
Humours	Choleric	Phlegmatic	Sanguine	Melancholic	3
Temperaments	Hot and Dry	Cold and Wet	Hot and Wet	Cold and Dry	2
Elements	Fire	Water	Air	Earth	1

The seven naturals.

4. The Similar Parts

    These are the organs and structures of the body, and each one is assigned a planetary ruler and a corresponding humour and temperament. These help to indicate its character and what is required to keep it in humoral balance.

5. The Administering Virtues

    Each of the humours activates a particular set of functions in the body, these functions are called the administering virtues. They consist of the apprehensive virtue associated with fire, which draws things out and brings them into the body; the digestive virtue associated with blood and air, which breaks things down into their constituent humours for distribution around the body; the retentive virtue associated with earth, which holds onto things and makes them solid; and the expulsive virtue associated with water, which clears waste and makes things slippery so that they can move around the body easily.

6. The Faculties or Spirits of the Body

    The spirits are the manifestation of divine life force, which motivates the activity of each organ and system, guiding it to perform its function. They provide the ability to procreate, to digest and absorb, and to think and feel. The spirits are strong when there is a healthy balance of humours throughout the body.

7. The Vital Spirit

    The vital spirit is the spark of divine light that resides in the heart as the soul. It radiates life force throughout the body and is carried in the arteries to all the organs and structures. In this way, it activates them as well as motivating our desires and aspirations.

The six non-naturals

There are also considered to be six non-natural influences. These are factors that do not arise directly from the nature of the body, but are seen as external factors. They must also be attended to when trying to maintain health or overcome an excess of an individual humour.

1. Air
2. Diet
3. Exercise and rest
4. Sleep and wakefulness
5. Retention and evacuation of waste matter
6. Perturbations of the mind and emotions

We will next address the impact of the six non-naturals.

CHAPTER SIX

The six non-naturals

There are also considered to be six non-natural influences, these are factors that do not arise directly from the nature of the body, but are seen as external factors. They must also be attended to when trying to maintain health or overcome an excess of an individual humour.

1. Air

The air that we breathe has a profound effect on the internal balance of the humours. It is in the air that the pneuma that sustains life in the body is carried. Once it has been inhaled by the lungs, it passes to the heart where it helps make the innate heat. This heat is distributed as a part of the vital spirit to all the individual organs, activating them and enabling them to carry out their essential functions. Hot air disperses pneuma, relaxes the body, and loosens the joints. It also weakens digestion and promotes thirst, so when the air is excessively hot it will weaken the body and dry it out. The lungs are cold and moist in temperament, so they can become excessively moist or phlegmatic when the air is damp and humid and can become irritated when the air is too hot and dry.

The temperament of the air itself will influence the level and balance of the different humours in the body. Its effects are passed into the blood through the breath, so the ambient temperature and humidity of the air must therefore become an important consideration when assessing the influences on any particular individual's temperament. The usual temperament of the air is moist and cool like the temperament of the lungs, and one of its beneficial effects is to cool the heart. Clearly if a person has a weak heart or a cold circulation then they must be particularly careful when being exposed to cold air. However, cold and moist air will strengthen digestion by driving and aggregating heat inside the body. Cold air will also close the pores of the skin, and reduce insensible transpiration, including sweating and movement of heat outwards. Although this can encourage a better appetite (we often feel hungrier in the winter), it can also lead to stasis and constipation through strengthening the retentive virtue. However, as the cold air reduces sweating it will increase elimination of wastes through activating urination.

Excessively cold air is particularly challenging for the head and the brain, which itself has a cold and moist temperament. The cold will increase the "distillation of rheum" in the head, causing an increase in catarrh and potentially exacerbating head pain from a cold cause. A hot moist wind that has the same temperament as the air humour will increase the risk of putrefaction, leading to infections, boils, and abscesses. A very moist air will soften and moisten the tissues, opening the pores, and clearing the skin. It can also slow and dampen the body, bringing on lethargy, making the body slow and heavy, and dulling the brain and senses. A cold and dry air will harden the body and increase the retentive virtue, reducing cleansing and expulsion of wastes and potentially causing blockages in the passages.

The movement and flow of the air is also an important factor. Still, stagnant air is likely to encourage putrefaction in the body, in a similar way to the effects of stagnation in any part of the body. Strong winds can also stir up the internal wind, especially in the head. This can bring on agitation, confusion, and loss of focus.

Any sudden change in the air is considered a difficult challenge, as nature itself abhors sudden variations in environment and is trying to always create gradual change.

Each temperament will benefit from the air that has the opposite quality, as it will balance it; so hot and dry types will benefit from cool moist air, while cold and moist types will benefit from warm dry air and an absence of drafts.

Purity of air is as important as purity of food and water. It is best whenever possible to avoid polluted and degraded air, and to avoid closed spaces where there is no free flow of air.

2. Diet

From the earliest times, diet has been linked with health. Hippocrates said "Let food be thy medicine and medicine be thy food". Hippocrates also recognised that over eating will cause as much sickness as excessive fasting.

It was considered that when the body was in a good balance it would naturally be attracted to the correct foods to maintain health. Clearly that depends on healthy foods both being available and the person being familiar enough with them to recognise the effect that they have upon them.

It was always considered beneficial to eat appropriately with the seasons, not just in the choice of seasonally appropriate foods, but also as to the quantity. Culpeper suggested that one should have more meat in the winter than the summer, as the spirits and the ability to digest are more contained and concentrated in the winter and more dispersed in the summer. It would also be wise to generally eat a diet of foods that would be more heating and drying in the winter, and more cooling and moistening in the summer to balance out the effects of the season. This fits in with our usual preference for lighter salads with cooling vegetables such as lettuce, cucumber and soft fruits in the summer, and to have well cooked warming soups and stews in the winter with warming vegetables, such as leeks and squash, flavoured with warming herbs and spices. Warming foods are generally considered more beneficial for health than cold or cooling foods, as warming foods increase metabolism and leave little residue to be cleared while cold foods tend to diminish metabolism and are more likely to leave residues of crude undigested humours.

Eating appropriately for ones constitution is important, hot constitutions as in choleric and sanguine types generally have stronger digestion than the colder constitutions of the melancholics and the phlegmatics. In the sections on the specific temperaments more guidance is given for foods that help and hinder each constitution. It is also important to match the diet to the person's age; children need plenty of food as they are growing. It is best to give them easily digestible foods and some cooling foods, such as lettuce, barley, and summer fruits to balance the excess heat of youth. Older children need less food, but more moistening foods to temper the dryness of their heat, as they enter the more choleric phase of life. Older people should be given less in a meal as their digestive heat is weaker, and it should be of warmer and moister foods, which are easier to digest and will preserve more of what remains of their radical moisture. The moistening diet appropriate for the elderly and those in convalescence emphasises soft foods, such as yoghurt and milk, cooked barley, rice and root vegetables, with chicken, fish, soft cheeses, asparagus, spinach, and turnips. Wine in moderation is gently warming and therefore is appropriate for adults and older people, with the cooling temperament of beer and cider being more appropriate for younger people.

There are certain foods that are traditionally considered to be easily digestible and nutritious for most people, most of the time. These include bread in moderation, cooked grains such as barley, oats, and rice, chicken, mutton, and berries. These foods were considered wholesome because they avoided the excess of any form, being neither too hard nor soft, too cloying or too insubstantial, too heavy or too light and created few heavy or dense excrements. Bread was considered wholesome as long as it wasn't eaten warm or stale, and only in moderation, otherwise its glutinous quality can clog the digestive tract and cause obstructions.

Meat is generally hot and moist, with the meat from younger animals having more moisture and is softer to digest. Fried and baked meats are harder to digest and should be eaten only in small quantities, chicken is more digestible than duck or goose. Pork from a young animal is thought to be better than cured meat, which is drying and conducive to melancholy. Lamb is considered more digestible than mutton, but beef is considered excessively cooling, difficult to digest, and liable to produce thick melancholy humours.

Fish is considered generally cold and moist and needs to only be eaten in moderation, ideally with the addition of warming herbs, such as fennel, dill, and pepper.

Shellfish are considerably more nourishing than fish, and have a warmer temperament. Phlegmatic constitutions are not well suited to fish, but cholerics may eat them without any concern.

Vegetables vary greatly in their temperaments, with some being very heating such as onions, watercress and cabbage, while others such as lettuce, chicory, cucumbers, and carrots are considered to be cooling. Cooked vegetables are always warmer and moister than fresh vegetables, salads tend to be cooling, and large amounts of raw food can easily overwhelm the digestive heat and leave cold crude humours, which may upset the bowels. Beans, unlike chickpeas, are generally cooling and drying. However, when they are sprouted they become gently warming and moistening, with the enzymes released from them helpful for the metabolism, and the moistness that they contain making them softening, rather than and drying and hardening.

Fruits also vary greatly in their heat and digestibility. Raw apples and pears are both generally cooling, whilst when they are cooked they are warming, moistening, and aid digestion.

Nuts should be eaten as fresh as possible and old dry nuts should be avoided as they are too drying and heating.

Qualities of foods and nutrients

	Heating	*Cooling*	*Moistening*	*Drying*
Meat and fish	Lamb, liver, chicken, goose, duck, goat, shellfish	Beef, rabbit, fish	Fish: plaice, bass, salmon, trout	Dried meats, cured meats, beef, mutton
Dairy products	Sheep's milk, cream cheese, cream, ghee, eggs (esp. yolk)	Cow's milk, goat's milk, butter, dried cheese, cottage cheese	Cottage cheese, soft cheese, butter	Dried cheese
Vegetables and beans	Asparagus, beets, radish, garlic, onions, greens, leeks, cabbage family, peppers, tomatoes, squash, aubergine, chick peas, turnip, artichokes, parsnips	Lentils, carrot, lettuce, celery, courgettes, potatoes, sweet potato, soybeans, peas, cucumber, spinach, mushrooms	Spinach, asparagus, turnip, cucumber, lettuce	Lentils, carrot, cabbage, parsnip, garlic, onions leeks, tomatoes, artichokes
Fruits	Peach, plum, lime, rhubarb, raisins, dates, figs, dried fruit, cooked fruits, mango, pineapple	Cherries, strawberries, raspberries, lemon, orange, damsons, prunes	Cooked apples and pears, figs, damsons, prunes, summer fruits	Citrus fruits, blackberries, bilberries

(Continued)

	Heating	Cooling	Moistening	Drying
Seeds, nuts, grains	Almonds, pistachio, apricot kernels, walnuts, pine nuts, hazelnuts, oats, wheat, rice, buckwheat	Barley	Most nuts when fresh, oats, barley, buckwheat	
Drinks	Black tea, cinnamon, mints, fennel tea, ginger, chamomile, warming herbs.	Green tea, water, lemon juice, rose water, orange blossom water		Lemon juice
Oils	Sesame oil, olive oil	Dripping, rendered oils, coconut oil		
Others	Fresh bread, fresh pasta, honey, sweet things, salty things	Vinegar, bitter foods, pickled foods, refined sugar	Moist bread	

3. Exercise and rest

Gentle exercise will stir up the spirits and activate the innate heat. This improves the digestion and the concoction of the humours, and by opening the pores increases the elimination of waste through the skin and also through the lungs due to increased respiration. From Hippocrates and Galen onwards, it was considered that moderation in the diet and moderation in exercise is the best way to preserve health. It has always been recognised that by being active a person can develop a strong and resilient physique, which will serve to keep the muscles, sinews, organs and bones in good health.

Exercise increases heat, so excessive exercise will have a damaging effect on the body, and will potentially exhaust the radical moisture. Excessive rest increases dampness and the phlegmatic humour, which will slow the activity of the spirits and faculties of the body, potentially causing bloating, congestion and will eventually lead to excess weight gain. The amount of exercise should be consistent with what is most beneficial for the individual and their temperament.

Sanguines benefit from a steady regular regime of exercise to balance their potential for doing all or nothing. They particularly enjoy being involved in group activities, but any form of sustained but steady exercise is good for them.

Cholerics are capable of high intensity exercise but should always keep sessions brief, and take regular rest periods between them. They should not spend long periods sedentary or inactive as their heat will not be released, bringing on agitation and states of internal dryness. Exercise that is naturally cathartic, such as drumming, is very beneficial. They enjoy competitive sports such as tennis, but usually prefer to be team leaders when involved in group activities.

Melancholics benefit from long walks, and being encouraged to do joyful activities, such as dancing and singing, which will stop them becoming too solitary. They enjoy activities that require focus and concentration such as fencing, bowling, billiards and snooker.

Phlegmatics need to ensure that they regularly get their innate heat moving to avoid stagnation. Doing exercise in the morning particularly helps their constitution as it gets them going straight away and clears any stagnation that may have built up overnight. They tend to have good stamina once they are moving so brisk walking, cycling, and swimming are good choices for them.

Children benefit from regular moderate exercise as this helps to balance their ebullient sanguine energy. Young adults are suited to more vigorous activity, but need to be warned against over doing it as they can be prone to doing things to excess as they have an excess of heat, which can make them too focused on achieving goals. Moderate exercise is suitable for older adults, and it is especially important for the elderly to do regular daily exercise as they are most prone to phlegmatic congestion.

Exercise is best taken before food, but gentle exercise after food is always considered helpful.

4. Sleep and wakefulness

In Culpeper's time it was considered that sleep occurred due to the rising up of a sweet vapour, which would condense in the head calming and sedating the mind and senses. If digestion in the stomach isn't complete, then the undigested humours will also produce vapours that will rise up and disrupt the sleep process. So having completed the first digestion of foods in the stomach before bed is very important. Overheated or agitated organs similarly produce disruptive vapours. Sleeping on a stomach that had not received food for some time was considered to be diminishing and weakening, as there would not adequate humours being produced from the concoctions in the liver to adequately sustain the organs.

Sleep benefits the body in a number of ways; it stops the dispersion of innate heat, allowing it to be concentrated in the liver to complete the concoctions of the humours. It allows a period of repose for the senses and the brain, which refreshes and restores. The sweet vapour of sleep has a moistening effect on the brain and nerves, which is particularly helpful as we age, dry, and cool.

Excessive sleep will cause an excessive build up of this otherwise beneficial moisture, as will sleeping too long in the day. It will also reduce elimination, potentially causing a build up of foul and damaging excrements in the system. A short sleep in the day can be restorative, as long as it is not so long that we awaken dulled by the build up of this moisture. A gentle walk after food and before sleeping will help to disperse any residual disruptive humours and their vapours allowing for good sleep to occur, such a walk used to often be referred to as a "constitutional".

Insomnia consumes and dissipates the spirits, drying both the body and the brain. This will lead to an excessively cold, dull brain, and the diminution of innate heat will make a person more prone to diseases coming from a cold cause.

5. Retention and evacuation

The excrements of the body need to be cleared regularly enough so that prolonged retention doesn't occur. The excrements include faeces, urine, sweat, transpiration through the skin, menstrual blood, and semen. Retention may either be caused by excessive retention, associated with the melancholic humour, or weakness of the expulsive virtue. If the innate heat is low, the concoctions in the liver are slowed causing the nutrients held by the retentive virtue in the spleen to remain unprocessed with a backlog ensuing. The blockage of evacuation can also be caused either by excessive heat drying and constricting the channels or by the blocking effects of cold glutinous phlegmatic obstructions. Fermentation follows when these excrements build up, producing irritating vapours leading to colic, distension, and wind. Such excessive retention can lead to loss of bowel tone and activity, bowel spasms, and inflammation from the irritation. The vapours may also rise up and cause headaches, vertigo, and giddiness. If there is inadequate transpiration through the skin, heat will build up in the blood causing fevers and will overload the lungs, leading to pneumonias and pleurisies.

6. Perturbations of the mind and emotions

There is no separation of the mind from the body, it will equally manifest humoral imbalance as any other organ. The brain is susceptible to changes in humour, and the heart, which is the seat of the emotions, is also dependent on a balance of the heat of excitement and stimulation, and the cooling flow of emotions. Excessive emotions will stir up the wind in the brain, causing chaos and confusion, and they will also scorch the heart and the other organs. Cooling cephalic herbs are helpful to calm the mind, and soothing protective cordial herbs are necessary to allay the damaging effects of excessive emotions on the heart.

The maintenance of a calm state throughout the body and mind is most beneficial to health. Reducing stress and releasing extreme emotions through cathartic activities are very helpful. Activities that promote joyfulness, such as empathetic interactions with others, singing, dancing, sharing good conversation, and practicing kindness are as important as any other measure we may take to maintain health.

The non-natural causes of heat, cold, moisture, and dryness

	Causes of heat	Causes of cold	Causes of moisture	Causes of dryness
External causes	External heat—summer, hot baths, overly hot rooms.	External cold—winter, immersion in cold water, cold foods and drinks.	Baths, esp. after meals. Cooling things—causing humours to be retained and dampness to accumulate. Mildly warm applications that liquefy and promote secretions.	External cold, which congeals humours, blocks channels, obstructing the flow of moisture. Excessive heat that that disperses moisture.
Activity and rest	Moderate exercise and movement, friction, massage, warming foods.	Excess exercise depleting heat, excess repose blocking flow of heat.	Resting and sleeping.	Excessive exercise drying out the fluids. Insomnia, insufficient sleep.
Food	Nourishment generally.	Insufficient food.	Moistening foods, food in excess.	Drying foods, insufficient food.
Emotions	Anger, worry, moderate joy, balance of sleep and wakefulness.	Extreme containment of emotions, which strangle the innate heat.	Moderate joy and happiness.	Frequent emotional disturbance and stress.
Internal causes	Putrefaction from the fermentation of excess damp or blockage.	Excessive heat that disperses innate heat leaving a state of cold depletion.	Retention of matter ordinarily evacuated from the body.	
Depletions and evacuations	Depletion of radical moisture to balance heat.	Depletion of vital spirit and innate heat.	Excess evacuation of a dry humour.	Violent evacuations, diarrhoea, excessive sexual activity.

CHAPTER SEVEN

The humoral body

Now that we have been introduced to the seven naturals, which comprise the Galenic humoral body, we can look at them in more detail. At this point it is helpful to have an overview of all of the aspects of the body; however, in later chapters we will explore the temperaments and each of the humours more thoroughly.

1. The elements

Element	Temperament	Quality	Action
Air	Hot and moist	Expanding	Dispersing
Fire	Hot and dry	Activating	Directing
Earth	Cold and dry	Contracting	Retaining
Water	Cold and moist	Flowing	Expelling
Ether	Non-physical	Without substance	Integrates and connects

The four basic elements can initially be put into two opposite pairs; Fire and Air are hot, while Water and Earth are cold. Empedocles said that each of the four basic elements are not just made up of these primary qualities of hot or cold, but also have one of the other primary qualities of moistness or dryness. This means that the hot and cold elements are further differentiated into four separate entities by combining them with moistness and dryness. This produces four distinct possibilities; heat combined with dryness gives us the Fire element, heat combined with moistness gives us the Air element, coldness combined with moistness gives us the Water element, coldness combined with dryness gives us the Earth element. Primary qualities such as hot, cold, wet and dry define the nature of the element, and qualities such as hardness, softness, stability, fluidity, are all called secondary qualities because they are characteristics which flow from that primary essential nature.

Strictly speaking there are only four physical elements, but we cannot consider them without addressing the role of the one non physical element—ether. This is the element that exists in all the other elements but has no substance of its own. It is also the substance that gives us space. Ether acts like a cosmic glue or fluid that connects all things, flowing within and between them, allowing interaction and communication. It is the medium through which divine energy or pneuma travels, through which the inspiration of divine spirit is seen to guide and form all that exists in the cosmos. The physical elements with their separate and contrary qualities also require something non-substantial, such as ether that can flow between them to overcome their separate and opposite natures, enabling them to combine and interact with each other, so that a third dynamic entity can arise giving life and manifestation in the physical world.

Air
Primary qualities—warm and moist.
Secondary qualities—light and thin, mobile, expansive, allowing things to float upwards and outwards.

As moisture warms and evaporates it becomes part of the air element, making air warm and moist.
Associations—spring, youth.

Fire
Primary qualities—warm and dry.
Secondary qualities—bright, illuminating, rarefying, giving absolute lightness.

It allows the natural ripening and transformation of substances, allowing compounds to change into substances with different qualities, such as moisture becoming air through evaporation. It penetrates through air, water, and into earth activating and energising them.
Associations—summer, adulthood.

Earth
Primary qualities—cold and dry.
Secondary qualities—dense, heavy, and hard.

It is immobile, gives stability, form, firmness, and continuity. It is at the centre of all the other elements.

Associations—autumn, middle age.

Water
Primary qualities—cold and moist.
Secondary qualities—soft, adaptable, changes shape to accommodate other objects.

It connects and compounds, it stops the desiccating effect of dryness from making things crumble and fall apart. It is less dense than earth, but heavier than fire and air. So it surrounds the earth, wrapping around it as the oceans.

Associations—winter, old age.

Ether
Primary qualities—emptiness, space, non-physical.
Secondary qualities—connecting, interacting, enlivening, carrying divine spirit.

It exists in all the physical elements and doesn't have any substance of its own. It is the quicksilver through which divine energy flows throughout the cosmos. It enables opposites to connect and to interrelate to one another and for all the disparate parts of the body to be connected and guided.

Associations—spirit, communication, transformation, inspiration.

2. The four temperaments

Element	Temperament	Quality	Life stage	Character
Air	Sanguine	Hot and moist	Youth	Exuberant
Fire	Choleric	Hot and dry	Adulthood	Striving
Earth	Melancholic	Cold and dry	Middle age	Considering
Water	Phlegmatic	Cold and moist	Old age	Accepting

Each individual will have their own mix of elements that is unique to them. This will make them hotter or colder, and wetter or drier. This individual elemental manifestation in the body will influence it in a variety of ways, and will determine the natural "temperament" or constitution of each individual. Each organ of the body also has an expected correct dominant temperament, which governs it and needs to be correctly maintained for optimal health and function.

In each of us one element will be in greater abundance, dominating the others, giving us air people, fire people, earth people and water people. This personal temperament is set for life, although it will vary as we age. In each stage of life there is an element that becomes more dominant at that time; air in youth, fire in adulthood, earth in middle age and water in old age. It is also common that as we age our under-lying or dominant temperament tends to become more prominent. The temperament is named by the humour that it is associated with.

We can define the personality of each temperament by considering its positive and negative attributes and assign to each of them a set of associations:

Temperament/Humour	Positive Attributes	Negative Attributes
Air Sanguine	Embracing, jovial, valiant, friendly, liberal, artistic.	Obsessive, arrogant, addictive, eccentric, sentimental, dispersed.
Fire Choleric	Striving, passionate, generous, direct, active, decisive, driven, fast, focused.	Angry, sharp, intolerant, critical, narrow-minded, aggressive.
Earth Melancholic	Considerate, solitary, studious, careful, conservative, grounded, loyal, trustworthy, supportive.	Fearful, closed minded, stubborn, pessimistic, prejudiced.
Water Phlegmatic	Tolerant, dreamy, relaxed, poetic, empathetic, enchanting, emotional, accommodating.	Distant, sentimental, lazy, sad, grieving, unmotivated.

We also find that some people have a combined temperament, a dominant one and a secondary one. Some temperaments cannot mix and combine; earth and water don't mix as the wetness of water would make the dry earth wet too. Fire and air don't mix as the combined heat in both would dry out the moistness in air.

This gives an extra eight combined temperaments, a total of twelve all together.

1. *Air – Sanguine*
2. Air and water – Sanguine phlegmatic
3. Air and earth – Sanguine melancholic
4. *Fire – Choleric*
5. Fire and water – Choleric phlegmatic
6. Fire and earth – Choleric melancholic
7. *Earth – Melancholic*
8. Earth and air – Melancholic sanguine
9. Earth and fire – Melancholic choleric
10. *Water – Phlegmatic*
11. Water and air – Phlegmatic sanguine
12. Water and fire – Phlegmatic choleric

We will explore more fully the physical, emotional, and mental implications of the temperaments in a separate chapter.

3. The four humours

Sanguine	Air	Resides in the liver
Choleric	Fire	Resides in the gall bladder
Melancholic	Earth	Resides in the spleen
Phlegmatic	Water	Resides in the lungs

"Humour" is the name given to each of the elements as they manifest in the body, they are formed out of the chyle from the stomach, which is the food broken down into its four constituent elements. They are produced in the liver and are carried in the blood. The air element becomes the blood itself, which is the medium within which all the other elements are carried; the fire element becomes the choleric humour and is carried in the red portion of the blood; the water element becomes the phlegmatic humour and is carried in the plasma of the blood; and the earth element becomes the melancholic humour and is considered to be the sediment of the blood, that which remains after the other humours have been made from the digested foods.

Ether is not strictly one of the physical humours, but as it is both contained in all the humours and also provides the underlying medium through which the constituent parts of the cosmos and the body remain in dynamic flow and connection, we need to include it in our list of humours.

Humour	Season	Life stage	Quality	Spirit	Virtue	Organ	Planet
Air – Sanguine: hot and moist	Spring	Youth	Expansive	Natural spirit	Digestive virtue	Liver	Jupiter
Fire – Choleric: hot and dry	Summer	Adulthood	Active		Apprehensive virtue	Heart and gall bladder	Mars
Earth – Melancholic: cold and dry	Autumn	Middle age	Contracting		Retentive virtue	Spleen	Saturn
Water – Phlegmatic: cold and moist	Winter	Old age	Flowing	Procreative spirit	Expulsive virtue	Lungs	Moon and Venus
Space – Ether	Exists in all times and places		Connects and combines	Animal spirit	Intellective and sensitive virtues		Mercury

Humoral imbalances

When the natural balance of the humours is lost, it is due to one or more of the humours becoming excessive. This initially just effects the function of that humour itself and the organs that are connected to it and then leads onto it overwhelming the other humours and interfering with their function. These two states are called dyscrasias, and when the humour is just in excess of itself it is referred to as a qualitive dyscrasia, and when this goes onto overwhelm other humours it is referred to as a quantitive dyscrasia.

Whether the offending humour has affected just a particular organ or system as in a qualitative dyscrasia, or the whole body as in the state of a quantative dyscrasia, the offending humour will have to be ripened and cleared from the body. The ripening is achieved through a process of heating or making mobile the excess humour in an appropriate way. It is then purged through defecation, diuresis, sweating, or vomiting.

As well as reducing the function of an organ, or interfering with the natural processes that sustain the body, the effects of humoral imbalance may diminish the vital spirit of the body and impede the activity of the other life giving spirits of the body.

An imbalance in the humours may occur because there is one humour that dominates, known as the temperament or complexion of the person, because of illness that has increased a humoral imbalance, or because of one of the external causes indicated by the six non naturals that we considered earlier.

4. The similar parts (Anatomy)

Head, eyes, ears, nose, mouth, throat, breast, heart, lungs, stomach, bowels, liver, gall bladder, spleen, reproductive organs, kidneys, bladder, joints, skin, muscles, sinews, limbs, hands, and feet.

Each part or organ has a planetary connection and is said to be under its rulership. It also has a natural temperament, which indicates what elemental balance it has. It may lose its balance either due to one of the humours becoming excessive in the body and overwhelming it, or because of one of the six non-natural things (air, diet, exercise and rest, sleep and wakefulness, retention and evacuation, perturbations of the mind and emotions) have had a negative influence and has upset its natural temperament.

The head

The brain is phlegmatic in temperament, and therefore cold and moist. It is also the seat of the animal spirit, which has a cold and dry nature, making the animal spirit, or what we would now call the nervous system, susceptible to any excess of the cold and moist phlegmatic temperament of the brain. Excess coldness and dampness will cause obstructions in the flow of the animal spirit, leading to lethargy, palsy, paralysis, and epilepsy. When there is coldness or dampness affecting the brain perceptions and sensations are not quickly apprehended and turned into ideas; ideas are not clearly discerned and judged, and memories are not awakened and retrieved. The thoughts and messages in the brain are passed around by a nervous wind, this is where the name for the "ventricles" of the brain comes from, literally "containers of wind". When this nervous wind gets overwhelmed by excess cold and damp, mist and fogginess literally overcome the brain, dulling our wits. The function of the brain can also be put out of balance by an excess of mental wind, this will lead to "frenzy"—over-thinking, obsessions, illusions, and hallucinations. Frenzy of this kind is often caused by an excess of the air humour, overstimulation, or severe emotional agitation.

The brain is divided into three main distinct areas; the forebrain, midbrain, and hindbrain.

1. The front of the brain is where the apprehension of ideas takes place, where the emotions from the heart trigger thoughts. This part of the brain has an association with heat, and if the innate heat getting to it is diminished or weak we have difficulty getting hold of ideas, becoming dull-witted and confused. Head pain can be caused by either excess cold or excess heat in the brain. An excess of heat will also produce a fast agitated mind jumping from one thought to another without being able to concentrate or to hold onto thoughts. When someone is stressed and anxious we often tell them to "chill out", and we consider that the brain is working best when it is cool, calm, and collected. Herbs, such as roses, hops, cowslip flowers, and violets, may all be used to cool, move, and allay excess heat in the brain. When there is an excess of coldness in the brain ideas are not easily apprehended, and we become slowed down, unable to think quickly. Coldness can also be a cause of head pain, with rosemary, sage, vervain, feverfew, and lavender all being beneficial in warming and stimulating the brain when its temperament is too cold.
2. The midbrain is the place of judgement, where the ideas apprehended in the forebrain are digested and divided into the relevant and irrelevant thoughts. This aspect of the brain is associated with the liver, as it is the seat of the digestive faculty in the body, where a similar division of nourishment from waste takes place. When it is out of balance we are unable to think clearly, plan, and differentiate right from wrong. An excess of the sanguine or air humour, whose seat is in the liver will fill the head with excess air and wind causing a head full of confused thoughts, obsessions and anxieties. When the midbrain is suffering from an excess of air or wind, centring and calming herbs, such as chamomile and lime blossom, are considered helpful. If an excess of cold and damp have overwhelmed the midbrain warming herbs, such as hyssop, lavender, sage, vervain, and rosemary will help.
3. The rear part of the brain is associated with the Earth or Melancholic humour, and like the earth it is where thoughts are consolidated and held as memories, it has a relationship with the retentive faculty and its seat, the spleen. When it is in excess the brain becomes slow and memories difficult to retrieve. Coldness is also the main cause of paralysis, palsy, convulsions, fainting and swooning. Coldness often

causes head pain, and is seen as one of the main causes of migraines, with herbs such as feverfew, sage, angelica, and the mints being helpful.

The eyes, ears, nose, and mouth

The eyes are associated with the luminaries; the two planets that give out light, the sun and the moon. The sun is associated with the apprehension of light by the eyes. The sun also has a specific relationship with the right eye of a man and the left eye of a woman. The moon is associated with the receptive aspect of sight, the receiving of images, and is said to reside in the watery humour within the eye. The sun apprehends the visions, which are then received by the moon.

Due to their openness to the outside world, the ears are said to be cold and dry in nature and ruled by the earth humour and the planet, Saturn. The ears are, therefore, particularly prone to cold conditions, which often cause pain and congestive conditions.

The nose and the sense of smell are associated with Mars, the planet that rules the fire element and choleric humour. When things are heated up they give off aromas, releasing their smell, making it natural to connect smelling with fire, heat, choler and Mars.

The tongue is associated with taste and the judgement of foods, which aligns the tongue with the liver, Jupiter and the sanguine humour. However, due to its association with speech and communication, the tongue itself is considered to be ruled by the planet of communication, Mercury.

The heart

The heart is the seat of the divine soul in the body, and it is where the vital spirit resides. It is governed by the sun, and in a similar way that the sun brings warmth and light to the cosmos, the heart brings warmth and light to the body. It is called the "Sol Corporalis"—the sun of the body. It holds both innate heat and radical moisture, distributing them around the body, keeping warmth and moisture in balance. The arterial and active aspect of the heart is the manifestation of the action of innate heat in the heart, with the name coming from the Latin "Ars" meaning craft or activity. The balancing and lubricating "radical" moisture manifesting in the heart is held and carried in the blue watery part of the circulation, still referred today as the venous circulation from the name of the goddess and the planet Venus, the ruler of the water element. The temperament of the heart is warm and moist, the same temperament as the blood, which of course is dependent on the heart for its movement around the body. This temperament is associated with the planet Jupiter. In the same way that Jupiter is the ruler of the planets, the heart is the ruler of the body and the organs. The heart is prone to becoming overheated and dried out by excessive and extreme emotional states and protecting it from such damage is a central concern of any physi-cian. When the innate heat in the heart is diminished, warming protective herbs, such as angelica and rosemary are helpful. When the heart is in danger of being scorched and dried out by excessive emotions the traditional protective cordial herbs are used. Culpeper lists them as rose, lemon balm, violets, borage and bugloss.

The lungs

The lungs are under the rulership of Jupiter. In particular, the expansion of the lungs and the inspiration are connected to the air element and humour. The inspiration of breath draws the divine pneuma into the body feeding the innate heat and there-fore the vital spirit, giving us the "breath of life". The temperament of the lungs is cold and moist, and phlegmatic. The lungs are considered to be the seat of the phleg-matic humour, even though the organ itself and the inspiration of breath are ruled by Jupiter, the temperament of the lungs, and the exhalation of the moist breath are phlegmatic. This makes the lungs susceptible to coldness, moisture, and conditions of excess phlegm. They are more prone to problems in the colder seasons, autumn and winter, and in the colder stages of life, especially in old age—the time when phlegm is greatest. The warmth of thyme, angelica, mint, and elecampagne all provide protec-tion from dampness and cold overwhelming the lungs.

The stomach and bowels

The stomach, intestines, and bowels are all phlegmatic organs. The stomach, however, requires heat to draw out the nutrients from food and make the chyle, but because of its phlegmatic temperament it often suffers from weakness brought on by a "cold" or "damp" stomach. The digestion of those with a phlegmatic temperament is weakest, and those with a choleric temperament strongest. The intestines and bowels are also phlegmatic in temperament, and bloating, cramping, and pain is most often a sign of excess cold and dampness in these organs. This is why warming herbs and spices are so helpful in aiding the digestive process, strengthening the stomach, intestines and bowels. Mint, thyme, hyssop, and lovage will all help to clear dampness and phlegm from the stomach and bowels.

The liver

The liver is the seat of the blood or sanguine humour. It is ruled by Jupiter, and it is where the digestive faculty resides. The natural spirit activates and sustains life in the physical body and arises in the liver. The humours are concocted in the liver and said to be passed through the veins to the rest of the body. When we look at the anatomy of the liver, we see that the nutrients that flow from digestion pass out of the liver in the hepatic vein, and from there are passed within the circulatory system around the body. This shows us that although the understanding of the circulatory system was incomplete in the time of Culpeper, they were correct that the humours—once digested into their separate parts—do pass out from the liver within the venous system, even if subsequently it is within the arterial system that the nutrients are then distributed to the rest of the body. The temperament of the liver is warm and moist and it is seen as particularly prone to the obstructive effect of cold humours emanating from the Spleen, the seat of melancholy that sits beside the liver in the top of the abdomen. Warming, opening herbs, such as angelica, lovage, and sage, can be used to clear these cold blocks and obstructions. Excess choler, or the heating effects of external toxins and infection can also damage the liver through scorching it and drying it out, in this case cooling herbs, such as dandelion root, artichoke, chicory, and thistles are recommended.

The gall bladder

The gall bladder is the seat of the choleric humour. Its temperament is hot and dry, it is the organ within which the bile is heated, refined, and concentrated. Due to its natural state of heat, the bile can become dried out causing blockage to its flow. In this case, opening and discussing remedies, such as wormwood, motherwort, hops, and gentian, are very helpful to cleanse and flush the gall bladder.

The spleen

The spleen is the seat of the earth or melancholic humour. It is also the seat of the retentive faculty, the virtue in the body that enables food to be retained by the tissues and for nutrients to be held in the blood. Its temperament is cold and dry, it is ruled by Saturn, and it is prone to becoming overwhelmed by an excess of melancholic humour. When this happens the cold vapours that arise tend to rise up to the stomach causing loss of appetite and weakening the breakdown of food. The melancholic vapours may also affect the liver but in particular may invade the heart, causing a slowing and diminishing of the vital spirit, bringing on palpitations, arrhythmia, and feelings of anxiety and depression. In this case, warming uplifting remedies to cheer the heart, such as borage, St John's wort, mistletoe, and motherwort, are helpful. To clear the melancholy from the spleen warming aromatic herbs, such as angelica, juniper, sage, hops, and elecampagne, are indicated.

The reproductive organs

The reproductive organs are ruled by the planet Venus and are moist and warm in temperament. They are the seat of the procreative spirit. The procreative spirit resides in the testes of men and in the ovaries and womb of women, it is ruled by the planet Venus and is also warm and moist in character. It is the energy of reproduction and produces in us the desire to procreate. Venus is the planet of fertility, love, romance, dreams, emotions, and of the water or phlegm humour. The procreative spirit is strengthened by Venus and the herbs that work in sympathy with her, whilst it is diminished and dulled by the cold drying effect of Saturn and the earth humour, and weakened by Mars and the choleric or fire humour. All conditions of cold affecting the womb are helped by gentle warming and cleansing herbs, such as vervain and moth-erwort, and conditions of excess phlegm by yarrow, lovage, angelica, and mugwort. Conditions of excess choler and heat effecting the womb may be treated with cooling herbs, such as violets, mallows, shepherds purse, and raspberry leaf.

The kidneys and the bladder

The kidneys and bladder are cold and moist in temperament and are ruled by the Moon. They can both suffer from hot inflammations and cold congestive problems. In conditions of heat, such as infection and inflammation, cooling softening herbs, such as mallows, violets, plantain, and oat straw, can be used. Due to their cold moist temperament the kidneys and bladder benefit from warming herbs, especially when the dampness has led to "putrefaction" and infection. Herbs such as thyme, juniper, vervain and garlic will often help to clear this damp congestion and infection. They are also prone to cold blockages, due to their cold wet temperament, and the forma-tion of stones that can consequently occur. So warming herbs that break and dissolve stones, such as vervain, cleavers, and nettles will help, with cleansing and opening herbs, such as motherwort, birch, betony, and agrimony, helping to flush them out.

The joints

The joints are ruled by the phlegmatic humour and the moon, being associated with water and flow. The medical term rheumatics comes from the ancient Greek word "rheo" meaning "to flow". The joints can be affected by both excess cold and excess heat. When there is excess cold and dampness the result is swelling, stiffness and pain. Warming herbs, such as rosemary, sage, and feverfew, are helpful, with external applications of heating and drying herbs, such as mustard, ginger, and chamomile. When the joints are affected by too much heat the natural moisture is thinned and attenuated, leaving a hard glass like vitreous humour in the joints. This stiffness then also causes pain and inflammation. Cleansing and clearing herbs for the joints are then very helpful, such as nettle, celery seed, meadowsweet, and birch leaves. Drying herbs, such as willow and meadowsweet reduce swelling and pain, whilst warming herbs such as turmeric help to bring back suppleness.

The skin, muscles, sinews, limbs, hands and feet

The skin is ruled by the moon and the phlegmatic humour, the bones and sinews by Saturn and the sanguine humour, and the hands and feet by Mercury and the etheric humour.

5. The four administering virtues

Virtue	Organ	Humour	Planet
The apprehensive virtue	Resides in gall bladder	Choleric humour	Mars
The digestive virtue	Resides in liver	Sanguine humour	Jupiter
The expulsive virtue	Resides in kidneys	Phlegmatic humour	Venus
The retentive virtue	Resides in spleen	Melancholic humour	Saturn

There are four administering virtues or faculties of the body, each of these is associated with a bodily process or function. They are the attractive faculty, the digestive faculty, the retentive faculty and the expulsive faculty.

1. The apprehensive virtue

> "The attractive virtue is hot and dry; hot by hot quality, active or principal: and that appears because the fountain of all heat is attractive, viz the Sun; dry by a quality passive, or an effect of its heat; its office is to remain in the body, and call for what nature wants." (Culpeper, 1669).[1]

It is innate heat that gives the organs their attractive quality, this quality was known as the "apprehensive" faculty, the word coming from the Greek verb apairo, meaning to take hold of or to bring an essence out of something. The apprehensive virtue is said to reside in the gall bladder and like the choleric humour, which resides there, it is ruled by the planet Mars and is hot and dry in quality, aligned with the fire element. It is the apprehensive faculty that enables the vital spirit to capture the life force from the air and foods that we eat. Its heat draws out the goodness from food in the stomach and enables the "natural" spirit in the liver to activate the digestion and separation of the four elements in food, providing the basis for the four humours that nourish the organs and tissues. Its heat enables the animal or animating spirit in the brain to apprehend ideas from our senses, and enables the "procreative" spirit to attract others to us.

2. The digestive virtue

The digestive virtue resides in the liver; it is ruled by the planet Jupiter and is hot and moist in quality and is aligned to the air element. The digestive faculty consists of four separate concoctions, which absorb, digest, process, distribute, and eliminate the waste from foods. Each of the four concoctions produces forms of nutrient and divides this from the waste that is excreted.

1. The first concoction is the heating of the food in the stomach to produce "chyle". This nutritious chyle is separated out and passes by the mesenteric and portal veins to the liver. The immediate waste from this separation is passed down the digestive tract and is excreted as faeces.

2. The second concoction takes place in the liver, where the humours are made and differentiated from the chyle. The humours are then distributed via the hepatic veins to the heart where they are then distributed around the body. Any excess of the melancholic humour is then stored in the spleen, while any excess of the choleric humour is stored in the gall bladder, excess of the phlegmatic humour is passed as waste to the kidneys and is excreted as urine.

3. During the process of the third concoction the liver passes the humours first to the noble organs; the heart and the brain, nourishing the vital and animal spirits that reside there. The humours then begin to form into the tissues and other body fluids. The waste products from the transformation of humours into vital spirit are excreted via the lungs, as the exhalation and the waste products from the transformation of humours into animal spirit are excreted as mucus from the nose.

4. In the fourth concoction the transformation of blood into tissues and substances such as breast milk and spermatic fluids is completed, with the waste products being excreted via the kidneys and through the skin as sweat. Once the humours have solidified, to become flesh and other body substances, and the waste has been excreted, any residue is kept back to replenish the radical moisture.

3. The expulsive virtue

> "The expulsive virtue casteth out, and expelleth what is superfluous by digestion … The expulsive faculty is cold and moist; cold, because that compresseth the superfluities; moist because that makes the body slippery and fit for ejection, and disposeth it to it". (Culpeper, 1669).[2]

The expulsive faculty resides in the kidneys and is associated with phlegmatic humour. It is ruled by the planet Venus, is cold and moist in quality, and aligned with the water element. The coldness helps to consolidate matter in the bowels aiding in its effective elimination, and the moistness helps to facilitate the cleansing of waste products. Excessive heat may dry waste matter making it difficult to clear leading to constipation, or in the kidneys leading to retention of urine or the formation of stones. In the bowels, excessive coldness can also slow down the movement and passage of material bringing on fermentation, bloating, wind, and pain. If the kidneys are affected by excess cold or moistness it can make them prone to stagnation and infection from putrefaction.

4. The Retentive Virtue

> "The retentive virtue is in quality cold and dry; cold, because the nature of cold is to compress, witness the ice; dry because the nature of dryness, is to keep and hold what is compressed. it is under the influence of Saturn" (Culpeper, 1669).[3]

The retentive virtue produces constriction in the stomach, enabling it to hold onto food until it has been reduced to chyle. The retentive virtue has its seat in the spleen where any excess melancholic humour is stored in the form of the thicker aspect of blood. It is ruled by Saturn, it is cold and dry in nature and is aligned with the earth element. Its action within the whole body is to ensure that nutrition, secretions, and even thoughts that need to be retained are held onto. In the brain it has an influence on the memory and retention of information, a function that takes place in the hindbrain. Excess retention leads to blockage and obstructions and is exacerbated by conditions of excess coldness and melancholy. Cold vapours can arise out of a spleen overwhelmed with melancholy leading to melancholy affecting the heart and vital spirit. These excess melancholic vapours also rise up and reduce the heat of the stomach interfering with the breakdown of foods. They will also block the flow of nutrients from the stomach to the liver, which will further reduce the digestive faculty and the concoctions, thus weakening the natural spirit.

These seven natural things work together to enable the life force to flourish, and with the aid of the correct balance of the six "unnatural" or external things; air, food, activity, sleep, retention and evacuation and mental balance, health can be kept in its optimal state.

6. The spirits of the body

Spirit	Organ it resides in	Temperament	Planet
Procreative spirit	Womb and testes	Warm and moist	Venus
Natural spirit	Liver	Warm and moist	Jupiter
Animal spirit	Head	Cold and dry	Mercury

In humans, the two life giving forces of creation and maintenance are called the procreative and the conservative virtues, whilst the third force of destruction manifests as disease, aging, and finally the death of the body. The procreative virtue arises in the body as the procreative spirit, whilst the conservative virtue arises in the body as the natural spirit and the animal spirit.

The spirits do not have a physical nature in the way that blood, bile, flesh, or mucus does, but exist as an energy that activates the necessary functions within the body to sustain life. They arise in particular organs and from there organise the function of essential bodily activities.

The spirits are dependent on the balanced provision of underlying humours for nourishment and support. Through ensuring the correct balance of the four humours, a physician can help the spirits to arise in a strong and vital way, promoting health and freedom from sickness. When we are healthy and feeling positive, we still use the expression "I'm in good spirits". Similarly, when we are feeling down we will often say that we are in low spirits.

To strengthen and maintain the spirits of the body is the main endeavour of a practitioner. The spirits arise in the body as a manifestation of the universal forces of the cosmos of creation, maintenance, and destruction. These cosmic energies have been recognised from the beginning of time as the three divine forces that imbue all existence, and have been honoured across ancient and modern traditions in the guise of the triple goddess, the three graces, and the holy trinity amongst others.

The final aspect of the natural cycle of the cosmos, destruction, comes in the form of illness and decay, eventually leading to the death of the body. It is experienced as the natural process of aging, a process brought about by the gradual loss of the natural moisture of the body as it is diminished throughout a lifetime. The destructive forces can also manifest as the effect of nature being out of balance in the body resulting in disease.

An imbalance in the humours may also lead to illness and disease through disrupting the flow of the spirits, interfering with the procreative, vital, animal, and natural spirits. This can affect the ability of the procreative spirit to produce desire and complete conception, the vital spirit to energise the heart and facilitate the flow of innate heat to the organs and tissues, the ability of the natural spirit to enable the digestion and concoctions to take place in the liver, and the ability of the animal spirit to perceive sensations and activate the body.

The fourth spirit that arises in the body is the vital spirit, It is the divine life force in the body, which is traditionally considered separately.

The two underlying internal causes of all disease are an excess of one or more humours, or anything that causes a diminution of the spirits.

The procreative virtue and the procreative spirit

This first creative virtue gives rise to the procreative spirit, which resides in the testes of men and in the ovaries and the womb of women. It is the energy of reproduction and produces in us the desire to procreate. It is considered to be under the governance of the planet Venus and is warm and moist in character. Venus is the planet of fertility, love, romance, dreams, emotions and is of the water element and phlegm humour. The procreative spirit is strengthened by Venusian pursuits and activities, as well as the herbs that work in sympathy with her. Venusian activities are those which promote sexual attraction, and moist nourishing herbs, such as orchids, were considered to promote "venery" or sexual excitement, which can also be stirred up by hot herbs, such as members of the mint family. The procreative spirit is diminished and dulled by the cold drying effect of Saturn and the earth humour and exhausted by the heat and dryness of Mars and the choleric or fire humour. As we age and enter the autumn of our lives, we too experience the coldness and contraction that takes place in that season, and it is therefore natural that sexual heat and desire will also diminish. Excess heat, often seen today in the form of overwork and high stress, is also a certain way to diminish levels of libido and desire as it has a drying and desiccating effect on the natural moistness that fortifies fertility and sexuality. Alcohol, which is also hot and dry, is a good example of a choleric influence on the body reducing the procreative spirit, the urges of attraction, and the strength of fertility.

The conservative virtue and the natural and animal spirits

The second set of virtues arises from the natural "conserving" cosmic energy. This virtue creates two further spirits, which maintain the life and energy of the body; these are the natural spirit, and the animal spirit. These spirits ensure the healthy function of the liver and the mind.

The natural spirit

The natural spirit resides in the liver. It is governed by the planet Jupiter and is warm and moist in quality. Jupiter is often called the royal planet, as it is the largest planet in the solar system and is said to be the ruler of the planets. The liver is associated with the blood or air humour, which is considered to be the "principal" humour because all the other humours are carried within it. When the natural spirit in the liver is activated by the innate heat, the digestive faculty is enabled to concoct the chyle from the stomach into the four separate humours in what is known as the second concoction. The liver is thus said to "breed the blood" from the crude humours or elements in the food we eat, and to refine them into the pure humours that are full of nourishment and clear of poisons and base residues. The natural spirit enables the sensation of taste to discern which food is congruous for the liver to make the blood and the humours. If the natural spirit and the liver are strong our ability to discern the correct foods works well, and the appetite will match the needs of the body. The natural spirit also activates the discerning part of the brain, the part which makes judgements, discerning the beneficial from the malign, and refining our thoughts and ideas from the undifferentiated perceptions that flow into the mind from the senses.

The natural spirit functions like a good ruler over the body, allowing all that is beneficial to enter and to be used, while rejecting and defending us from all that is bad and unhelpful. It is the representation of the divine in the physical body in the same way that the king and queen are the representatives of the divine on earth.

The animal spirit

The animal spirit resides in the head and the brain. It is ruled by the planet Mercury, is considered to have a cold and dry temperament, and is aligned with ether. It is divided into two virtues; the internal virtues and the external virtues. The internal virtues are concerned with thinking, intellect, and the will, and the external virtues are concerned with sensation and perception.

The three internal intellective or reasoning virtues

There are three internal virtues, which are called the intellective or reasoning virtues. These consist of apprehension, judgement, and memory. These internal virtues generate the motor functions of the body, they produce the desire and will to act, which is then executed in the material world through movement and activity.

1. Apprehension

Apprehension and imagination take place in the front of the brain, their nature is active and dynamic, and they are associated and nourished by the hot and dry choleric humour. In a similar way to heat in the stomach extracting nourishment from food, the heat in the front of the brain extracts and takes hold of the impressions entering the brain. It both transforms emotions arising as vapours from the heart into thoughts, ideas, and desires, and receives the sensations and perceptions coming from the sensory organs. If there is an excess of heat in the brain we become frenetic, overwhelmed with competing thoughts and ideas, as if we are in a state of mania, which can also lead to headaches caused by heat. It is dulled by excess coldness or melancholy, which closes down our openness and enthusiasm to new fresh ideas. When the innate heat in the vital spirit is weak it also reduces the ability of the brain to focus and apprehend ideas.

2. Judgement

Judgement takes place in the middle part of the brain, which is the seat of reason. It is associated with the air and blood humour, which reside in the liver and regulates the thoughts that have been apprehended by the front part of the brain and stops them running randomly, arranging them and refining them into rational streams of consciousness. The expansive nature of air enables this virtue of the brain to connect and combine with the apprehensive and retentive qualities in the front and rear parts of the brain, bringing thoughts and memory into creative harmony. The middle of the brain is therefore the seat of reason, where the approval of good ideas and the rejection of bad ideas takes place. When we sleep the reasoning part of the brain is inactive, and thoughts run randomly producing dreams; it is said that by looking closely at dreams we may most accurately assess the temperament or constitution of a particular person. It is only during dreaming that the unfiltered emanations of the heart, the soul of the person, freely arise, allowing us to see exactly what kind of temperament resides there.

3. Memory

The memory and the retention of ideas takes place in the rear part of the brain. Like the earth humour, which is associated with the retentive faculty of the body, this area is considered to have a cold temperament. However, if the brain becomes too cold the ideas and memories remain retained and unavailable to be brought forward into the apprehending and discerning parts of our brains. As we age and the innate heat of our bodies and brain diminishes we become less able to think quickly, and become forgetful as the heat needed to activate and to move the memories to the middle of the brain becomes weakened. Excessive melancholic or earth humour tends to make us dull-witted, closed-minded, and stuck in unhelpful thought patterns, as well as fearful of new ideas as we can no longer process them.

The five external or sensitive virtues

The external virtues are called the sensitive virtues and are aligned to the senses and organs of perception. These virtues generate the sensory function of the nervous system, the stimulation of the sensory organs generates feelings in the heart, giving rise to understanding and information in the mind.

These perceptive senses are ruled by the moon, they are known as the five particular senses of seeing, hearing, smelling, tasting, and feeling. Together the five particular senses are regulated and harmonised by the common sense. The common sense is considered to be mercurial and etheric in nature, as it can combine with all the other senses equally, knitting them together and uniting them. Each of the five particular senses has a planetary ruler and a humoral correspondence.

Sight

The sight is said to reside in the crystalline humour within the eyes, and it is produced by a combination of the cold and moist aspects of the moon and phlegmatic humour and the hot and dry aspects of light itself emanating from the sun. The sun and the moon are known as the "luminaries" and the moon was given precedence over the left eye while the sun was given precedence over the right eye. The moon is associated with the receptive aspect of sight, whilst the Sun is associated with the capturing and apprehension of the images, these planetary characteristics combining and complementing each other enabling us to perceive and apprehend the world around us.

Hearing

Hearing resides in the ears, and is ruled by Saturn. The ears are open to the outside and are considered to be cold and dry in temperament. Hearing problems are often caused by excessive cold in the head, as is vertigo, fainting, and migraines.

Smell

The sense of smell in the nose is considered to be ruled by Mars and is hot and dry in temperament. When we heat things they tend to let off vapours and smells. The nose is also close in proximity to the frontal apprehending part of the brain, which is also associated with heat.

Taste

The sense of taste resides in the palate, it is governed by Jupiter and is hot and moist in temperament. When the liver is functioning correctly our sensations of taste guide us to the correct foods that we need for nourishment. It is the sense that rejects foul and inappropriate foods and attracts us to good-tasting and nourishing foods.

Touch

The sensation of touch and feeling is under the rulership of the moon, it covers the whole body, like the waters that cover the planet. It receives all the sensations that we perceive and allows them to flow around the body. The feelings that we now differentiate as emotional feelings are also included in the sense of feeling, with emotions rising and falling like the tides, flowing and spreading like waves, and sometimes overwhelming us like floods.

7. The vital spirit

Spirit	Temperaments	Organ it resides in	Planets
The vital spirit	Innate heat and radical moisture	Emanates from the heart	Sun and moon

The vital spirit resides in the heart and is considered to be ruled by the Sun. The heart is considered to be the "sol corporalis" or the "sun of the body". It is the distributor of divine light and spirit in the body, in the same way that the sun is the source of divine light in the cosmos. The heart is seen as the celestial vehicle in the body into which the soul descends from the realm of divine light; it radiates the light of spirit to the three realms of intellect, emotions, and the physical body. The vital spirit travels around the body in the arteries activating and motivating the organs. The vapours that arise in the heart as emotions travel to the brain and become the source and initiators of thoughts.

> "The Vital spirit hath its residence in the heart, and is dispersed from it by the Arteries: and is governed by the influence of the Sun. And it is to the body, as the sun is to creation; as the heart is in the Microcosm, so is the Sun in the Mega-cosm. For the Sun gives life, light and motion to the Creation, so doth the heart to the body. Therefore it is called Sol Corporalis (The Sun of the body), as the Sun is called CorCoeli (The heart of the heaven), because their operations are similar" (Culpeper, 1652).[4]

Looking after the vital spirit through good spiritual conduct and a balanced lifestyle will produce a clean strong spirit, that is pure and divine in nature, and will bring happiness and health:

> "Callicles, that the disciplined man whom we have described, being just and brave and reverent is perfectly good: and a good man does well in his actions, and because he does well is happy and blessed, whereas the wicked man who does wrong is wretched." (Plato, Gorgias, 507c).[5]

The vital spirit itself is made up of the two complementary opposites of heat and moisture, known respectively as innate heat and radical moisture. In the same way that the sun and moon complement one another, these two aspects must always be kept in balance, and when they fall out of balance we will see patterns of disease arising. It is not usual that these aspects of warmth and flow in the vital spirit are the cause of imbalance themselves, as this imbalance can only occur through their deple-tion. It is not possible for the Vital spirit to become excessive in the body, in the same way that divine light could not overwhelm the cosmos. However, when the vital spirit is depleted it can lead to blockage, stagnation, and the diminution of the function of organs. So it becomes clear that when we see excessive heat in the body it is not caused by too much innate heat, but either by an excess of the choleric humour, or a deple-tion of the cooling radical moisture. Similarly, when we see excessive moisture in the body it is not caused by too much radical moisture, but by either an excess of phlegm humour or a depletion of the balancing innate heat.

Innate heat

The innate heat is considered to be closely associated with sun energy, giving heat to the body. Heat is movement, and it is the innate heat in the vital spirit that moves the blood. Heat defines life, it produces movement and warmth in living organisms—objects without life are static and cold. The innate heat in the vital spirit attracts the living essence within air, food, and the space around us to join the dance of life in the body. Innate heat is thus the warmth of life and resides within us as long as we are living. The vitality of the body depends on the innate heat being distributed effectively to all the body tissues and organs.

The innate heat is originally passed to the baby from the male seed in the sperm, and with the waters from the womb providing moisture, it makes up the aqua vita, or life force, given to us by our parents. This constitutes our "innate pneuma" or breath of life. This life force is also carried in the air around us as "accidental pneuma", which is used to continually supplement our innate heat via the lungs. Once received, the accidental pneuma is passed via the pulmonary vein from the lungs to the heart where it is combined with the radical moisture to create the vital spirit.

Radical moisture

The innate heat in the vital spirit is balanced and moderated by the radical moisture. In the same way that the innate heat is governed by the sun, the radical moisture is considered to be governed by the moon, in conjunction with the planet venus. Thus, the masculine active, forcing qualities of the sun are complemented, calmed, and cooled by the feminine, moist, flowing, and distributive qualities of Venus and the moon. These planets are feminine energies that embody the flow of life, and the fertility brought by water. The light of the sun alone is not enough to give life. Life can only occur where there is also water and where the opposites of hot and cold, moist and dry, light and dark are in balance. The radical moisture enables the vital spirit to move and flow around the body distributing its life force to the organs without scorching or damaging them through excessive heat.

The radical moisture originally comes from the waters of the womb in which the baby grows. It is then continually replenished throughout life by the residues of the breakdown of digested foods during the fourth concoction. Together, the radical moisture and innate heat combine to enable the aqua vitae or life force to sustain our bodies in the form of the vital spirit.

The radical moisture was likened to the oil in a lamp, and similarly to a lamp we only have a limited reservoir of that originally comes from the waters of the womb. The radical moisture is considered to be limited in quantity like the oil in the reservoir of a lamp. We commence our lives with a finite amount, and although we do supplement and replenish it throughout life, it will eventually run out leading to death. The physical manifestation of this gradual depletion, is evidenced by the drying of skin and tissues as we age.

The vital spirit itself will be diminished through any interference with the extraction of nourishment from food when the concoctions are disrupted by an excess humour. Without the provision of balanced humours, innate heat and radical moisture, which make up the vital spirit are not nourished and become depleted.

These seven aspects, or natural things, give us the complete overview of the working of the humoral body in the Galenic system. This model gives us a way of describing the internal interactions and relationships of the body. By using the planetary symbolism associated with each internal aspect we are able to further connect them to their interactions with external causes and influences. The planetary symbolism enables us to see the connections between the inner microcosm and the outer macrocosm. We can use this model to interpret any signs of internal imbalance, and to predict the most helpful external responses in the form of lifestyle, herbs, and diet to correct the disharmony.

CHAPTER EIGHT

The constitutional temperaments

All traditional systems of medicine have ways of classifying individuals. In these systems it is recognised that people are like nature, exhibiting distinct patterns, characteristic behaviours, and cycles. When living in a temperate climate as we do in Europe, North America, parts of Asia and Australasia, these natural patterns are most clearly seen in having four main seasons, each corresponding and arising out of the four basic elements.

Western humoral philosophy recognises that the characteristics that delineate each element and season will therefore also arise within people. As this balance varies within the body these differences would also be seen on the skin, through our behaviour, in our physiology, and also in one's physical appearance. People, like seasons, are similarly envisaged as having a main dominant element or humour, dividing them into four humoral groups or temperaments, with each group sharing the characteristics and properties of the season that most reflects them.

It makes sense then, that people will also manifest excesses and depletions of various properties in the same way as experienced in each particular season. For example summer/fiery people will be hot and dry, potentially lacking in moisture and likely to overheat, while winter/watery people will be cold and wet, potentially lacking in warmth and liable to become overwhelmed by damp conditions. Characterising people in this way will give an indication of how they are likely to act, respond, and behave in the world and will also be likely to indicate the ways in which they become sick.

This viewpoint is clear and simple, but allows for many variations—in the same way that no summer or winter will be the exact replica of the ones that went before or will come after. It may even be that we get an exceptionally warm winter day, or a cold wet summer day, so nothing is precluded.

The language and concepts of humoral philosophy are embedded in the Western mind-set and are quite easily re-awakened. We all understand what it means to be fiery, watery, airy, or earthy, which gives both practitioners and patients a common language with which to explore how it may be possible to move closer to wellness and balance.

Assessing people in this way means they are viewed as complex, sensitive beings, rather than merely the presentation of a pathology. It enables practitioners to respond to the person who is in front of them, rather than defining them by the disease that they have. It provides a dynamic system of interpretation that shows how to model a response that best suits the particular temperament. It makes it possible to then recognise the constitutional strengths, which can be drawn upon to aid a person in their recovery, as well as constitutional weaknesses that need support and nurture.

Illness arises when one of the humours accumulates to excess and overwhelms the others. It is usual that it is the dominant humour, and people with such an excess should therefore avoid those things which amplify that humour, whilst feeding and nourishing those humours that balance it out. Ideally we should nourish all the humours so that we remain in a balanced temperament, and in practice this often means cultivating aspects and habits that are not always the ones which seem most attractive to us. Chronic illness is always rooted in humoral imbalance and the imbalance is almost always in the direction of our dominant humour.

Each of us will have a dominant humour and we will tend to build our life around the strengths of that humour. Fiery people will usually tend to do fiery things, so will act in a hot, fast, and impetuous way and be quick and direct. Whereas watery people will be more lyrical and adaptable in the way they approach life, able to flow and adapt to people and circumstances around them although lacking the focus and momentum of the fiery types. Each temperament has its place and function in the world, and we must remember that we all have some of each temperament, and our challenge is to bring them all into the most equal, appropriate, and beneficial balance. Understanding our temperament allows us to play to our strengths, talents, and abilities, and enables practitioners to help give people a clear understanding of how best to navigate their way through the world.

The four primary temperaments

The elements, the humours, and the temperaments are all combinations of the four basic qualities; the two primary active states; hot and cold, and the two passive states; moist and dry.

The opposites hot and cold are the primary "active" qualities, while the secondary opposite qualities, dry and moist, are considered to be "passive" because they arise out of the effect that the primary qualities have on matter. Dryness comes from the effect of heat clearing moisture, while moistness follows from the effect of cold causing condensation and moisture to appear.

This gives four main temperaments, which are combinations of the primary active qualities and the passive secondary qualities;

Sanguine/air: Hot and moist
Choleric/fire: Hot and dry
Phlegmatic/water: Cold and moist
Melancholic/earth: Cold and dry

The effects of these qualities go from some very general manifestations to much more specific ones. The most general ones tend to be shared by most people of that temperament, while the more specific ones tend to only be seen in some but not all of the people of the same temperament.

We find that there are some general correspondences to each of the primary and secondary qualities:

Heat
It is found in choler (fire) and sanguine (air) types. Heat will tend to have an activating effect, so those with these "hot" complexions tend to be faster, more active, driven, focused, louder, extroverted and energised.

Its positive qualities are:
Stimulating, moving, pushing, expanding, forcing, directing, and encouraging, and it opens through warmth.

Its negative qualities are:
Its destructive nature, its ability to scorch, burn, and consume, fire will consume until there is nothing left.

Cold
It is found in phlegm (water) and melancholy (earth) types. Coldness tends to have a slowing and calming effect, so those with these "cold" complexions will tend to be slower, quieter, calmer, steadier, dreamier, more introverted and lazier.

Its positive qualities are:
Consolidating and bringing things together, it pacifies, slows, penetrates, and steadies.

Its negative qualities are:
Immobilising, crushing and flattening, being obstructive and becoming inert and fixed.

Dryness

It is found in choler (fire) and melancholy (earth). Dryness has a contracting effect, so those with these complexions will tend to be thinner, slighter, harder, coarser, drier, and sometimes smaller.

Its positive qualities are:
Focusing and refining things to their bare essentials, allowing things to form and build up. It is stabilising and connecting. It contracts, retains, and gives form and substance.

Its negative qualities are:
Friction, and therefore constriction and stasis, disconnection occurs as things turn to dust and fall apart.

Moistness

It is found in sanguine (air) and phlegm (water). Moistness tends to have a swelling effect, so those with these complexions will tend to be fatter, broader, softer, and rounder, and sometimes taller.

Its positive qualities are:
Spreading and flowing, it accommodates, connects, mixes and communicates, it clears and flushes out.

Its negative qualities are:
Flooding and overwhelming, becoming stagnant, drowning out and becoming sodden and stuck.

The eight combined temperaments

The temperament of a person may sometimes be of one type; sanguine, choleric, phlegmatic, or melancholic. However, it is very common to find that people have combined temperaments that are a mixture of two types, with one of the two being the dominant one, known as the "principal" temperament.

This means that we will not only have the sanguine temperament, but there is also the sanguine/phlegmatic, and the sanguine/melancholic temperament. For each of the other principal temperaments there will be similar combinations with secondary temperaments.

However, it is helpful to be aware that temperaments with the same primary qualities don't combine.

Choler: hot and dry, will not combine with sanguine; hot and moist.
Phlegm: cold and moist will not combine with melancholy; cold and dry.

This is because if we combine hot and dry with hot and moist the combined heat of both complexions will eventually dry up any of the moisture, and the temperament would gravitate towards just being hot and dry and eventually become choleric.

While in the case of phlegmatic and melancholic temperaments, the moisture in the phlegmatic humour would overwhelm the dry nature of the melancholy and without any heat to dry it out, the temperament would become increasingly dominated by the moistness of the phlegmatic humour and eventually also become phlegmatic.

This gives us twelve possibilities, four single temperaments and eight combined temperaments:

Complexion	Principal Temperament	Secondary Temperament
Sanguine	Hot and moist	
Sanguine/phlegmatic	Hot and moist	Cold and moist
Sanguine/melancholic	Hot and moist	Cold and dry
Choleric	Hot and dry	
Choleric/melancholic	Hot and dry	Cold and dry
Choleric/phlegmatic	Hot and dry	Cold and moist
Phlegmatic	Cold and moist	
Phlegmatic/sanguine	Cold and moist	Hot and moist
Phlegmatic/choleric	Cold and moist	Hot and dry
Melancholic	Cold and dry	
Melancholic/choleric	Cold and dry	Hot and dry
Melancholic/sanguine	Cold and dry	Hot and moist

Take note of how the "principal" temperament of each combination may be balanced or amplified by the secondary temperament.

A sanguine person is generally hot and moist, and they will always be expansive and in danger of becoming too dispersed energetically, their humours are always moving up and out in a similar way to water evaporating and expanding and dispersing when it is warmed. When the secondary temperament is phlegmatic, its added moistness makes these types especially prone to moist congestion, cooling innate heat and exacerbating conditions of stagnation and congestion. The increasing lack of heat, which should be driving out poisons, weakens their protection against infection, and the excess moistness makes them prone to what is called putrefaction. Sanguine/phlegmatic people are therefore more prone to infectious diseases, abscesses, boils and phlegmatic problems, with all sanguine types being especially prone to these kinds of problems during the winter, which is of course the cold and moist phlegmatic season.

In contrast, when a sanguine person has a melancholic secondary temperament it provides a balancing effect. The hot and moist complexion is now cooled and dried by the melancholic temperament. These sanguine types are therefore less likely to suffer from the typical swellings and inflammations that affect most other sanguines, and have less susceptibility to the infections that affect sanguine/phlegmatic types.

These combinations also affect the personality of the individual, with sanguine phlegmatics being slower, calmer, better at empathy and accommodating others, but less active and focused, while the sanguine melancholics will be steadier, more grounded and more consistent but more secretive.

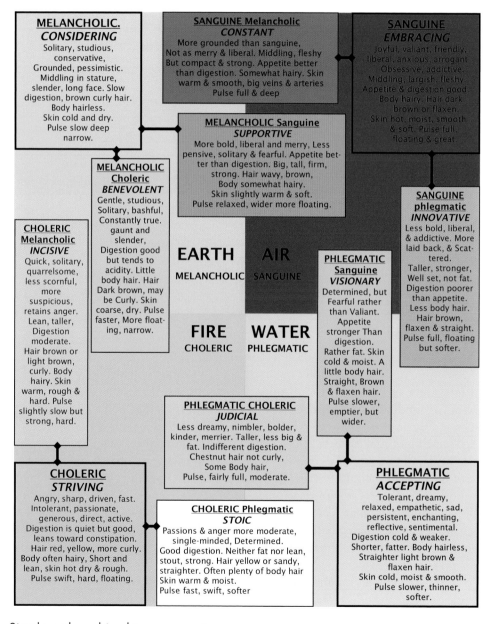

Simple and combined temperaments.

We can also use these insights to help us when recommending lifestyle and diet appropriate to each temperament. The sanguine person is most balanced when under a melancholic influence, so melancholic foods, activities, friends, seasons, herbs, will be balancing and steadying for sanguine types and vice versa.

Assessing the temperaments

When deciding a person's temperament, an intuitive sense of whether they are a "hot head", "chilled out", "well-grounded" or an "air head" can often provide a good starting point.

Traditionally, there are also certain physical aspects that we can look for which may correspond to these basic temperaments, such as the kind of digestion, body shape, hair, skin, pulse, and how their tongue looks, all pointing to the underlying temperament. However, all of these things can be influenced and changed by other external factors, such as diet, environment, genetic inheritance, stage of life, and lifestyle, meaning that it isn't always immediately obvious which temperament we should assign to someone.

It is therefore important and helpful to have a way of assessing temperaments which somehow goes to the root of things. By considering the emotional characteristics of our patients, we have a good chance of finding their dominant humour as the emotions arise directly from the heart of the person, this being where their soul or "vital" self-resides. If someone is coming to you for help and assistance they are already open to you, thus giving you an invitation to make a connection with them on an emotional level and discover these deeper things about them.

By building up a good rapport with a person we can start to get a feel of what emotional stance they take in the world. Seeing how a person reacts to situations, and how they relate to the people in their own lives can be a really helpful way of identifying their temperament, we can add to these observations of how they respond to us during a consultation.

We can explore with them the emotional correspondences of each temperament and see which emotions they feel most at ease with. The emotional state to which they seem to return to most often, and the one in which they are most at home with, will be the one most likely to be their natural temperament.

It can also be helpful to reflect on the fact that temperaments also correspond to the phases of life, how youthful, how inspirational, how considered, and how stagnant a person is will show a great deal about their underlying character.

The following lists and descriptions cover the traditional viewpoints of body type, physiological functions, and personality, but cannot be used as a rigid definition of all the possible ways each temperament manifests. It is best to use them as a guide into a deeper journey of discovery, enabling us to gain clearer insights into those around us. The physical aspects of each temperament have been included because they represent the historic viewpoint of humoral manifestation through physiology. Although this can give some guidance, it should not be adhered to dogmatically, but is best seen as observations about how the complexions may be seen in a person. Even Culpeper believed that the complexion was an emanation of the soul that resided in the heart, which was best assessed through the persons dreams, emotional state, and psychology, rather than how their body looks.

Sometimes it may take a number of encounters before we really feel sure about a patient's temperament, and it is not unusual that as we get to know someone better our assessment of their temperament changes and evolves. If we are still unsure which temperament someone has, a helpful way of clarifying things is to look for the characteristics that they lack, and through a process of elimination uncover the strongest aspects and therefore dominant aspects of their temperament. If we still are having a problem assigning a temperament, then simply asking ourselves whether they feel warm or cool can at least get us onto the right track.

The sanguine temperament

Air is hot and wet, mobile and changeable, it can be a calm breeze or a raging storm.

Watchwords
Embracing/obsessive.

Characteristics
Jovial, valiant, friendly, liberal, anxious, arrogant, addictive, creative, eccentric, artistic.

Anxiety states
Caused by frenetic and overwhelming thoughts.

Physiology
Digestion and appetite are good. Body middling in size, largish, fleshy. Body hairy. Brown, flaxen hair. Skin hot and moist, smooth and soft. Pulse full, floating, and great.

Signs of excess
Head full of confused and unquiet thoughts, hypochondria and anxiety, inflammatory conditions, abscesses and boils, skin irritation, angry and uncomfortable. Heaviness and drowsiness, stretching and yawning, mouth ulcers, easily fatigued, sweet taste in the mouth, erratic circulation and high blood pressure.

Associated diseases
All infirmities of the liver and veins, lung disease, pleurisy, excess leads to putrefaction and fever.

Pulse in excess states: floating, full, forceful, drumskin.
Tongue in excess states: swollen, thick coating, patchy.

Personality

The sanguine or air temperament is expansive and contains the energy of growth, it is the springtime energy when all the plants burst up towards the sky out of the earth. The air humour tends to dominate in infancy and strengthen in the spring. It has the energy of youthfulness, and the joyful exciting energy of childhood. Children's minds tend to be open and expanding at a rate that is never met again in later life, absorbing huge amounts of information and gaining constant new wisdom and insights. As they grow they break and dissolve boundaries, and are often able to bring others together, frequently challenging the prejudices and narrow mindedness of their parents and culture.

Like children, sanguines are quick, easily distracted and changeable, moving from one thing to another in an instant. The sanguine personality can therefore be fickle and unpredictable, but generally tends towards optimism, friendliness and playfulness. Sanguines are fun to be around, often taking the role of being the life and soul of the party, they don't like to see others sad or left out and tend to be open to others and generally inclusive. They maintain a childlike ability to take most things lightly, although this can also make them unreliable, and somewhat unpredictable.

Their natural confidence and self-assurance can make them seem rather aloof at times and can also come across as arrogant, opinionated or superficial. Like air itself they are difficult to contain, they like to expand and explore, communicate and create, they are often artists, writers, performers and poets. They like to live life to the full, leading them into excessive habits and potentially making them prone to addiction and obsession, like teenagers they can become obsessed by ideas, personalities and the desire for things—they are the archetypal consumers, perhaps this is reflected in the cult of youth, which is so dominant in consumerist Western society.

Their obsessive nature is often reflected in becoming over anxious about health issues, with small things often getting blown out of proportion. However, they respond well to authoritative direction, always liking to have a parental figure in their lives to guide and reassure them.

The liver secretes the bile, and this collects in the gall bladder, the seat of the choleric humour. Bile is the hottest of the humours, and if it builds up it causes hot irritations, both physical and emotional. When the liver energy gets blocked there is, therefore, going to be a build-up of the hot bile, and this can then cause the sanguine person to express anger and irritation, and can sometimes make them quite explosive in character. When this energy is confounded, like a child being given a boundary, frequently it elicits an indignant response. Sometimes this might cause a tantrum, sometimes they go off and sulk, hiding away for the day. However, like a child the feeling can be quickly left behind when a new exciting possibility presents itself.

> "They always get the best press in this society because they tend to do most of the writing. They tend to worry about their health and respond to authoritative direction" (Hedley, 2021).[1]

"A Man or woman in whose body heat and moisture abounds, is said to be Sanguine of Complexion. Such are usually of a middle stature, strong composed bodies, fleshy but not fat, great veins, smooth skins, hot and moist in feeling. There is a redness intermingled with white in their cheeks … Their pulse great and full. They dream of red things and merry conceits. As for their conditions, they are merry, cheerful creatures, bountiful, pitiful, merciful, courteous, bold, trusty, given to the games of Venus. A little thing will make them weep, but so soon as'tis over; no further grief sticks to their hearts" (Culpeper, 1652).[2]

Avoid
Excess of all kinds, being too dispersed and scattered. Avoid hot damp foods, such as honey and wine, avoid sugary foods, bread, and excess onions and garlic. Sanguines will get away with eating most things most of the time, they enjoy eating and tend to be at risk of eating in excess.

Take
Watery soups, pickles and vinegar, fish, wild meats, summer fruits, beer, and cider. Do regular exercise, ideally a co-operative sporting activity. Engage in singing, writing, and forms of creative expression. Eat regular meals and do not snack between meals. Find a long term partner to be committed to, or develop an enduring and all engaging interest or discipline, find earthy, dependable, solid friends.

Useful herbs
Calming and centring herbs such as chamomile, linden, oats, yarrow, elderflower.
  Milk thistle and dandelion for liver.
  Valerian, and passionflower, hawthorn, rose, and lemon balm for anxiety.

Case history

A middle aged woman, who when in her twenties had settled in Britain from abroad. Considerate, sociable, and person-centred, she had enjoyed working as a PA in a busy office, finally getting married to her boss and having a child. Having emigrated to Britain she missed her family, and since leaving the workplace she had also felt isolated. She had suffered from TB as a child and had a traumatic delivery of her own child six years previously, having post-partum complications including a severe infection and damage to her sacrum causing chronic back pain. Once home after the birth, she found herself alone, unwell, and unsupported by a husband who mainly made himself absent (isolation is especially destructive for the sanguine personality). She worried about the decline in her own health, and also worried about her child's health. After the traumatic birth experience she began suffering from chronic fatigue, severe weight loss, unexplained digestive crises, multiple allergies, migraines, and constant untreatable cystitis. She had taken numerous remedies and been to a wide range of practitioners, apart from one osteopath, none of them had managed to bring significant improvement and consequently her levels of anxiety about her ill-health had increased to an extreme level. When she came for treatment she was suffering from a continual urinary infection, chronic fatigue syndrome, premenstrual syndrome, weekly migraines, and acute coxygeal pain. Vomiting at the onset of a migraine would lessen its severity and sometimes clear it completely; this was a sign of an excess hot, moist humour needing to be purged. She suffered from inflammation of the bladder, bowels, itchy skin, weakness and at times severe anxiety. She was prone to chest infections and coughs. The damp, moist sanguine temperament is more susceptible to all of these presentations. She was emotionally and physically overwhelmed by her health problems, and she was rarely out of pain. When she came for treatment she responded well to constant authoritative re-assurance, simple herbal infusions, and a regular deep tissue massage, in the main we avoided alcoholic extracts of herbs as they seemed to exacerbate the heat and inflammation, and to potentially put more stress on the liver. She was put on a consistent herbal regime of strong infusions of a detoxifying and diuretic urinary mix containing shepherd's purse, cleavers, and horsetail, which instantly improved her urinary symptoms as long as she kept taking it. It also helped to clear the excess dampness and heat. To counter the recurrent chest infections she took regular decoctions of elecampagne root with thyme and yarrow. She took strong chamomile infusions to help with the anxiety, which also helped the pain, and used a mix of vervain, valerian root, and motherwort for panic attacks and anxiety associated with PMS. After a few years of treatment on this regime, she was able to attend sessions with a yoga therapist, and eventually started to attend a regular yoga class. This gave her both social interaction and an engaging discipline to regularly work on. She eventually managed to feel strong enough to return to France once a year for a month's holiday, which gave her something to look forward to and focus on. Her migraines lessened and became infrequent, her urinary pain receded, and her levels of energy and activity improved.

Combined sanguine temperaments

The air humour combines well with water giving sanguine/phlegmatics, and with earth, giving sanguine/melancholics. It cannot combine with fire, as the addition of more heat and dryness would mean that the moist aspect of the sanguine humour would be overwhelmed by heat and would eventually also become dry.

Sanguine/phlegmatic

Watchwords
Innovative/unfocused

Characteristics
They are less bold, liberal, and addictive. They tend to be more laid back and scattered.

Physiology
They are well-set, tallish, often fat. Their digestion is poorer than their appetite. They have less body hair, the hair may brown or flaxen and straight. The pulse is usually full, floating but softer.

As they have a secondary humour that also has a moist aspect this will amplify the moistness that is already central to their constitution. This will make them especially prone to moist congestion and eventual cooling of the innate heat due to lack of flow of the necessary nutrients around the body. This leads to a lack of heat driving out poisons and therefore a lack of protection from infection. Sanguine/phlegmatic people are therefore more prone to these infective diseases, boils, sores, sinus and catarrhal problems in the spring including hay fever. All sanguine people are more prone to these kinds of problems during the latter half of winter, which is of course the cold and moist or phlegmatic season. They can connect and flow with people and ideas making them explorative and innovative, but often lacking direction they can become unfocused.

Sanguine/melancholic

Watchwords
Constant/deceptive

Characteristics
They are more grounded than true sanguines, but not as merry and liberal.

Physiology
They are middling, fleshy, and strong. Their appetite is better than their digestion, and they may be somewhat hairy. Skin warm and smooth, big veins and arteries. Pulse full and deeper.

The secondary humour being cold and dry, tends to balance out the heat and moisture, it grounds them, making them more constant, more loyal and more able to stay on track.

They are able to see the bigger picture whilst not getting carried away by fantasy and grand plans. Their emotions tend to be less on display, but they still tend to have moments of loud and effusive expression and activity. They keep things more hidden than sanguines being more secretive and sometimes deceptive.

The choleric temperament

Fire is hot and dry. It can warm, activate, motivate, and open, but it can also scorch and desiccate.

Watchwords
Striving/angry.

Characteristics
Angry, sharp, driven, fast, intolerant, passionate, generous, direct, active, decisive.

Anxiety states
Caused by mental tension, stress.

Physiology
Digestion is quiet but good, leans toward constipation.
Hair red, dark, curly. Body short and lean, skin hot dry and rough.
Pulse swift, hard, and floating. Tongue narrow, red, yellow coating.

Signs of excess
Feels hot, sweaty, thirsty, acidity, nausea, constipation, jaundice, irritability, skin problems, acne, carbuncles, sudden anger, fevers, shingles, frenzy, fury, poor sleep. Bladder and kidney blockage & stones.

Associated diseases
Fevers, carbuncles, shingles, skin problems, itching, frenzy, kidney and bladder problems, dry coughs and bronchitis.

Pulse in excess states
Fast, hard, narrow, strong and forceful, bowstring, long, and skipping.

Tongue in excess states
Red, narrow and thin, yellow coating.

Personality
The quality of the fire element is hot and dry, producing a focused, driven, and striving but potentially warm personality. The choleric energy is greatest in the summer, when the sun is at its fullest, and its heat is at its greatest. This corresponds to the early adulthood, when vitality, energy and drive are greatest. It is a time of focusing, finding direction, and building the foundations of the life one wants to lead. We are still welcoming and open to new things as we were in our youth, but this now has a direction, and a focus which was previously lacking. There are things that we want to achieve: finding a partner, starting a family, finding a career or life path, being able to enjoy acquiring things and becoming independent from our parents.

It is a time of getting things done, creating, and building. It produces active, focused people, who are often competitive and aspirational. Cholerics come across as clear and direct, they are incisive and determined, even single-minded, and sometimes a little self-centred. They make good leaders, rarely doubt their convictions and tend to have immovable opinions (until they change them for the next immovable opinion!). They are team leaders rather than team players, but are dependable and honourable in the main. However, they also tend to warm to others, and can be great motivators with a strong charisma. Their warmth can make them generous and open, extending light and warmth to those around them. One may sense a constant underlying tension when we are with them, as it is difficult for them to stop and to settle. Cholerics will inevitably always be at the front of the queue as they will always strive to be on top of everything.

Like Mars, their ruling planet, they can be rather militant and unbending, and have uncompromising expectations of others, especially those who they have authority over. They make strict parents, but always apply their rules in the belief that they will benefit those who are forced to follow them.

It is easy to work them up into a state of anger or frustration, and they will tend to be judgemental and a little narrow-minded. When they are challenged, they may quickly become angered. They will refuse to give in to illness, seeing it as a weakness, they will often work to excess, and get strongly attached to fixed ideas and desires. They can also be self-righteous, dogmatic, short-tempered and self-serving. Without the benefit of water they find it difficult to go with the flow, or to accommodate the beliefs, feelings, or ideas of others.

The choleric temperament is characterised by the top athlete who sacrifices everything to achieve their goal, then falls from grace being seen leaving a nightclub in the early morning having taken too many intoxicants and in the arms of an illicit one night stand.

> "I don't see many sick Choleric people. They notably hate being ill, are dreadful patients and cut out the memory of previous illnesses. They respond to discipline, direction and clearly stated, short term goals." (Hedley, 2021)[3]

> "Such persons are usually short of stature, and not fat, it may be because the heat and dryness of their bodies consumes radical moisture. They are naturally quick witted, bold, no way shame faced, furious, hasty, quarrelsome, fraudulent, eloquent, courageous, stout-hearted creatures, not given to sleep much but much given to jesting, mocking and lying." (Culpeper, 1652)[4]

Avoid

The choleric should avoid fatty and spicy foods, fatty meat, salty and dried foods, stimulants, alcoholic spirits or excess wine, and indulging excessively in competitive activities and sports.

However, forced inactivity will cause a build up of internal heat leading to burnt choler developing, this then obstructs the vital spirit, causing depression and agitation. Commonly this can happen in retirement, or in cholerics with sedentary occupations.

Take
Fish and wild meats, beer and cider, soups with barley, summer fruits, sufficient water, regular exercise. Regular short cleansing regimes or episodes of fasting. Choleric people appreciate discipline and make good soldiers, they feel secure when they can develop respect for an authoritative figure.

It is always good for them to have a project on the go that has clear short-term goals.

Useful herbs
Cooling and softening herbs: rose, violets, plantain, mallows, hibiscus.
Herbs that clear heat from the liver and digestive system: hops, meadowsweet, dandelion, dock, and rhubarb.
Herbs that clear heat from the skin: burdock root, melissa, echinacea.
Herbs that clear heat from the blood: nettle, cleavers, dock, echinacea.
Tempering herbs for heat: linden, elder, betony, feverfew, vervain.

Case history

A choleric patient presenting with intermittent fever, chest pain, a pleural rub, exhaustion, night sweats, with a history of suffering from a bout of severe bronchitis as a child. Self-employed, would work through the exhaustion and pain, found that warming herbs, such as echinacea and thyme, would "bring out" and exacerbate the symptoms. Eventually, a strong infusion of lime blossom taken twice daily improved symptoms over time. The soothing and moistening effects helped to calm and cool the lung irritation, the calming nervine effects helped to reduce the excessive stress and drive that continually exhausted the patient and undermined his capacity to rest enough to recuperate. Nettle was also used whenever the fatigue and low energy returned and regular infusions of nettle tea kept the lungs clearer and free from infections.

The combined choleric temperaments

The choleric personality also often combines with water or with earth, it cannot combine with air as the combined heat in both would eventually dry out all the moisture in the air temperament. The combinations are:

Choleric/phlegmatic

Watchwords
Stoic/self-righteous

Characteristics
Passions and anger are more moderate, they are single-minded, determined.

Physiology
Stout and strong, neither fat nor lean. Hair is yellower, straighter, skin warm and moist. Pulse is fast, swift, softer, not floating or deep.

The addition of water to the fire personality moderates some of the choleric excesses. They are more accommodating and adaptable, the water element gives them more stamina and makes them less likely to burn themselves out. They can become immune to the opinions of others as they will often become swept away in their own flow of ideas and opinions.

Choleric/melancholic

Watchwords
Incisive/suspicious

Characteristics
They are quick, more solitary, loyal, clear-thinking and able to stick with things to the very end. They can be quarrelsome, less scornful, more suspicious, but can retain anger.

Physiology
They often have lean, sharp angular bony features, they may be taller, with moderate digestion. Hair is dark or brown, often curly. Skin is warm, rough and hard. Pulse is slightly slow but strong, narrow and hard, middle to floating.

The addition of earth to fire makes them more incisive, more determined, and less likely to give up or change tack. It also brings loyalty and an ability to make clear and fair judgements, showing a determination to get to the bottom of things. They make good, fair, judges and don't hold back with often harsh but true observations.

The melancholic temperament

Earth is cold and dry, it steadies, retains, is dependable and delves deep, but is prone to get stuck.

Watchwords
Considerate/fearful.

Characteristics
Solitary, studious, conservative, grounded, fearful and careful.

Anxiety states
Caused by pessimism, worry.

Physiology
Middling in stature slender, long face. Slow digestion, weaker appetite. Brown or dark curly hair. Body hairless, Skin cold and dry. Pulse is slow, deep, narrow. Tongue is bluish or purple.

Signs of excess
Anxiety, fatigue, poor appetite and digestion, cravings (especially chocolate and sweet cakes, biscuits) cold sweats, irregular heartbeat, anxiety and cold extremities. Liver congestion, feelings of fullness around the solar plexus. Bitter belching, stiff painful joints, aching back and hips, itchy skin.

Associated diseases
Chronic disease. All diseases of melancholy, cold and dryness; madness caused by fear and grief. Bone pains, gout, toothache, deafness. Obstructive nature of melancholy can cause palsies, migraines, impotence, haemorrhoids, and hernias.

Pulse in excess states
Narrow, short, confined and deep and sometimes hidden. It may be weak, forceless and varying in rate and rhythm, all of these are signs of coldness effecting the blood.

Tongue
The tongue will be flaccid, short, pale or purplish, have a thin white coating or no coating, and possibly a few red spots. The lack of heat will often also show in the tongue looking wet. If excess melancholy has caused the vital spirit to become very diminished then there will be a pale wet tongue, often with swollen edges marked by teeth marks.

The melancholic personality

The melancholic humour is strongest in middle age and in the autumn and early winter. Melancholics tend to be middling in stature, and sometimes quite thin, although with a solidity to them. The face is usually longer, thinner and gaunter. Remember that this corresponds to the middle-aged period in our life, when lines begin to show, and the bones are covered less by a soft fleshiness and we become stiffer, more rigid, and more angular. The melancholic has an appetite greater than their ability to digest. The coldness in their temperament decreases the amount of body hair, while head hair is usually dark or brown, their dryness often makes it curly. The skin is generally rough, dry, and cold, and may have a yellowish hue. The voice may have a singing quality. They are often studious, enjoy their own company, and are quiet.

Melancholics tend to be loyal. They are deep thinkers, considering and studious, and are able to see things from many angles and to be receptive to all points of view. They tend to bury themselves in study and books, and are not happy until they have got to the very bottom of things. They tend to avoid crowds and social occasions preferring their own company. They are like Earth herself who allows the many varieties of creatures to inhabit her creation, and although boundaries may be set as to what should and shouldn't be done, she tends to look benignly on all of her creation. This manifests in the earth person as a feeling of compassion and understanding towards others, they are often loyal and entirely trustworthy people. They can therefore be counted on to keep secrets, and will remember promises they have made to others, even many years later, these things will be of great importance to them. The Romani people used to consider the earth to be our grandmother, the one who has seen the passing of many cycles, and the repository of wisdom gained from experience. She is gently protective, supportive, and grounded, emanating a sense of security and acceptance, a trustworthy anchor when we feel unsure, vulnerable, and insecure.

Although others may find melancholics a bit quiet and reserved, they are often the ones who keep their head when everyone else around them is losing theirs, providing measured and considered advice when everyone else is in a panic or a state of confusion. As well as being investigative and deep thinking, they are often also able to take the long view of things, making them wise and considering, if they choose to speak at all, they choose their words carefully, unlike the sanguine personality, often speaking before thinking.

Melancholics may be found taking great pleasure in pursuits such as reading, and creative projects that require patience and perseverance, such as artistic endeavours requiring great skill. They often benefit from having long-term projects that give them direction, while also making the best use of their stamina and desire to see things done thoroughly and properly. In the current culture with so much in our lives being fast, fleeting, and superficial, the melancholic viewpoint may seem to be a bit dull, but it may also be the antidote to much of the stress and worry we find ourselves suffering from today.

The melancholic temperament can tend towards negativity, fearfulness, pessimism and grief, and sometimes those with this temperament may seem to expect the worse. They are prone to hang onto thoughts and feelings, meaning that they can get stuck focusing on the heavier emotions, such as fear and grief. When out of balance they can become jealous and covetous, and overly worried about not having enough. They can often worry about the future, feeling insecure about change and impermanence, wanting things to stay just as they are. However, while this negative manifestation of the earth temperament is often the one that is most commented on nowadays, it is by no means the only or even the main way that melancholy may manifest in those who have an earth constitution.

> "They are prone to getting blocked and stuck, but at least they will hang in there" (Hedley, 2021).[5]

> "Superfluous melancholy causes care, fear, sadness, despair, envy, and many evils besides" (Culpeper, 1652).[6]

Avoid
Excess food, heavy foods (beef), drying foods such as lentils, eating too late in day, lack of activity, thinking too much, and getting caught in introspection.

Take
Light nourishing foods; soft cheeses, shellfish, eggs, lamb, olive oil, root vegetables, squash, dried fruit. Cleansing foods; asparagus, celery, fennel. Take gentle exercise, long walks, gardening. Have regular baths with relaxing herbs such as lavender, rosemary, or bay. Have a productive long term project, find exuberant "sanguine" friends.

Useful herbs
Gently warming:
Fennel, angelica, lovage, black pepper, sage, cardamom, coriander.

For the heart:
Lemon balm, motherwort, borage.

For anxiety:
Valerian, linden, cowslip, rose.

Case history

An older man, of a solitary nature, had worked throughout his life as a self-employed electrician. He had always been valued for his thoroughness, tidiness, reliability, attention to detail, and for being able to quietly get on with the work in hand, making very little demands on his clients. He worried continually about his health, though he was a very active retiree; regularly walking up to ten miles over the South Downs, a solitary pastime that he found gave him great pleasure and relaxation. His pulse tended to be slow, forceful, tight, and floating. His strong vital spirit being blocked by cold obstructions the blood cannot flow forwards so the pulse is pushed up and out.

His digestion had always troubled him, usually it was fine during the day until he ate his main meal. After the main meal he would start to suffer from bloating, belching, and painful trapped wind. He would eventually pass a lot of wind and then loose stools. It often went on for the rest of the day. The pattern would occasionally change and instead of the loose stool he would be prone to constipation, which might continue for a number of days. Using digestive bitters before food helped somewhat, as did having changed a difficult to digest breakfast of muesli, for a cooked apple and oat and buckwheat porridge. However, it was simply the addition of peppermint tea after the main meal that solved the decades of digestive discomfort. As long as he came every couple of months for reassurance about his health concerns, he managed to get along fine.

Combined melancholic temperaments

The melancholic earth temperament combines well with the sanguine air tempera-ment and also combines well with the choleric fire temperament, it cannot combine with water as the moistness in water would overcome the dryness of the earth. The combinations are:

Melacholic/sanguine

Watchwords
Supportive/detached.

Characteristics
More bold, merry, and liberal. Less pensive, solitary and fearful. Appetite is better than digestion.

Physiology
Big and often tall and thin. May also be more firm, strong and only slightly fleshy. Hair wavy, light brown. Skin slightly warm and soft. Pulse is wider and more relaxed.

The addition of the air element adds warmth and moisture, This makes them less rigid, more outgoing, often able to take a wider perspective. They are reserved but enjoy being surrounded by good company, they often make good teachers. They can see the potential in others and encourage upward growth. Their melancholic intro-spection with their sanguine propensity to be dispersed and distant can make them seem detached and difficult to connect with. They can be prone to poor circulation and sudden changes in health.

Melancholic/choleric

Watchwords
Benevolent/Dogmatic

Characteristics
They are gentle and studious, solitary and bashful but constantly true.

Physiology
They may also be tall, and are usually slender. Digestion good but tends to acidity. Little body hair. Hair is dark brown and may be curly. Skin is coarse and dry. Pulse is faster, more floating, narrow.

The addition of fire makes them more outwardly focused, and gives a generally warmer personality. They are considerate people, who tend to have a clear focus, and an ability to hold strong and unshakable beliefs. They may often be inclined to take a dogmatic stance, and feel more secure having fixed ideas. They excel when able to follow a life of discipline, especially if it involves developing a lifelong mastery of a subject or activity.

The phlegmatic temperament

Water is cold and wet, passive, slow and accommodating, without heat it has poor digestion leading to stagnation.

Watchwords
Accepting/anxious

Characteristics
Tolerant, dreamy, relaxed, empathetic, sad, persistent, enchanting, reflective, senti-mental, emotional, poetic, accepting, distant, unrealistic.

Anxiety states
Caused by overwhelming emotions.

Physiology
Digestion is colder and weaker. They tend to be shorter, fatter and fleshier, have a round face and nose, and straight, light brown or flaxen hair. Skin is cold, moist and smooth. Circulation is slow, with cold extremities. Pulse is soft, middling or deep, thinner, slow. Tongue is pale, wet, with white coating.

Signs of excess
Lethargy, anxiety, poor digestion, bloating, weight gain, especially around the thighs, buttocks, and stomach leading to the traditional pear shape. They may suffer palsy and convulsions from phlegm obstructing the animal spirit, excess mucous, coughs, blocked sinuses, pelvic & urinary congestion.

All cold and rheumatic diseases: fluid retention, dropsies, oedema, discharges and abscesses. Cold also causes cramps and colic.

Associated diseases
Kidney infections, cystitis, ovarian and uterine problems, fibroids. venereal diseases, rheumatism, coughs, congested sinuses and ears, I.B.S. diverticulitis, inflammatory bowel conditions. M.E.

Pulse in excess states
Thin, soft, slow, short, forceless. It may be floating but weak, as the excess phlegm pushes the pulse upwards.

Tongue in excess states
Pale, purple or blue, swollen, thick white greasy coating.

The phlegmatic personality

The phlegmatic season is the latter half of winter, when moisture abounds and we begin to see its transformation into the first new green shoots of spring. The phlegmatic humour is strongest in old age, the winter of our lives.

Water is the medium of flow, governed by the moon. In Romani spirituality the moon is known as the goddess Shon, the enchanting goddess of fertility. It is said that she can be found in all things that shimmer and glisten: the morning dew, the light reflected off water, the silvery leaves of the willows as they blow in the wind. She is connected to song, poetry, romance, and dreams. She is the movement of emotion in our hearts, the cleansing release found in tears of joy and sorrow. She is the muse, lover, and creatress, giving birth to new growth. She is the fertile spring goddess, Freya, Olwen, and Persephone. Water is the element associated with divination, having the ability to be receptive and open to things that others might not notice. This helps water people to be good and attentive friends, able to listen and acknowledge others. The water aspect enables phlegmatics to adapt and to go with the flow, they are tolerant and accepting of others. The coldness in their constitutions can make them slower, dreamier, slow to break down and digest things, and less motivated to act. They will generally tolerate rather than confront, they are polite and self-effacing, often suffering from a sense of poor esteem and low self-worth. They love the poetic and romantic, they like sensual experiences, beautiful clothes and decoration, they enjoy being moved by music as it resonates deep within them. They are most strongly motivated by deep feelings, even though they may not be the most emotionally demonstrative, their hidden feelings run strong but deep.

Water can, however, easily build up when emotions are not allowed to flow. Without movement, stimulation and activity the water element becomes stagnant, bringing on feelings of being overwhelmed, making the phlegmatic vulnerable to sadness, grief, worry and anxiety.

They are not particularly good at promoting themselves, finding it hard to throw themselves fully into things. They can be timid, shy, and anxious, unsure of how to move forward. However, their great strength is that they can easily empathise and accept others, often holding their judgement back, preferring to understand rather than condemn. Although this makes them good carers it can also mean that they can be taken advantage of and deceived. They warm to praise and being appreciated, so much so that they can be manipulated by the unscrupulous, and especially by those who have an innate sense of entitlement.

The phlegmatic can find it difficult to find a direction in which to flow, so may present as indecisive and dreamy, but once focused and motivated will keep flowing forward and will always find a way through or past any obstacles that life may present.

"They are prone to poor digestion [on all levels] mucus accumulation and lethargy. Water is cold and wet, passive, pale and practical. The classic 'English Tempera-ment' is Phlegmatic—from living in a cold and damp place." (Hedley, 2021)[7]

"They are dull, heavy and slothful … Not usually very tall, appetite and digestion is very weak in them, veins and arteries are small, their bodies usually without hair, their pulse little and low." (Culpeper, 1652)[8]

Avoid
Excess sleep, eating too much, dairy products, sweet foods, fish, (except with warming herbs), raw foods, salads, except with spicy dressings or pickles. Spending long times in the same place, avoid getting emotionally caught up and overwhelmed, or allow-ing emotions to build up without releasing them through crying, shouting, laughing, creative activities or any other thoroughly cathartic activity.

Take
Warming foods, artichokes, root vegetables, onions and garlic, spices, pickles. Fast at the change of seasons and get into the habit of adding gentle spices to foods. Regular exer-cise always helps, find creative emotional expression. Engage in group activities with peer group. Find people to help and support, and practice having a warm open heart.

Useful herbs
Warm dry herbs, such as thyme, sage, rosemary. Gentle spices, especially cinna-mon, cardamom, coriander, fennel, and ginger. Warming and activating herbs, such as elderflowers, cleavers, mint and nettles. Cleanse with nettles and cleavers in the spring, take warm herbs, such as thyme, sage, and elderberries in the winter.

Case history

A 40 yr old phlegmatic female patient with long term gynaecological problems, recurrent ovarian cysts, and pelvic congestion. Sensitive and compassionate, she had trained as a nurse and then developed a practice as a therapist. Her kind, caring nature suited the work she had chosen and she was well known for her gentle but powerful healing abilities. She had not been able to conceive, and continued to have difficult premenstrual symptoms with pain, bloating, and exhaustion. When endome-trial pain struck a strong infusion with mugwort often helped. When there were signs of the ovarian cysts developing again, a hand bath containing rosemary and hawthorn could immediately clear the pain. Also, by using nettle and cleavers as a fresh juice the build up of stagnation would clear, enabling everything to quickly return to normal. She benefited from the long term use of angelica, vitex agnus castus, chamomile and yarrow in a daily herbal mix. Spasmodic pain associated with coldness and abdomi-nal congestion could be relieved with cramp bark and angelica root decoctions drank in small doses throughout the day.

Combined phlegmatic temperaments

The phlegmatic constitution also combines well with air and fire. Water cannot combine with earth as the cold moisture of the water humour would overwhelm the dry earth making it also wet. The combinations are:

Phlegmatic/sanguine

Watchwords
Visionary/dispersed.

Characteristics
Determined, but often fearful rather than valiant.

Physiology
Appetite stronger than digestion, rather on the fatter, fleshier side. Only a little body hair, hair straighter, flaxen or brownish. Skin cold and moist. Pulse slower, emptier, but wider.

By adding the expansive aspects of air, people with phlegmatic/sanguine temperaments are more outspoken, active, and engaging, producing good diplomats and mediators. They tend to have a better opinion of themselves and have more lightness and joviality. They like to socialise and mix, but will not be the loudest in the room. They enjoy group activity and are good contributors liking everyone to be have a fair hearing. They may still be rather dreamy and with the air element added can often lose all connection with the ground, becoming easily carried away by fantasy and imaginings, making them dispersed and prone to indecision.

Phlegmatic/choleric

Watchwords
Judicial/contrary

Characteristics
Less dreamy, nimbler, bolder, kinder and merrier.

Physiology
Indifferent digestion, need to avoid large meals, but generally will cope well with most foods as long as they don't overdo it. Taller, less fat, chestnut hair, which is less curly, some body hair. Skin moist and slightly warm. Pulse fairly full, moderate in width, strength and rate.

The addition of fire makes them warmer, more generous, and encouraging to others. They are much better at getting projects off the ground, making them good people to have in a team, they are often happy to support when they see the wisdom of others, and help to keep the momentum going in a steady, productive fashion. Although the fire gives them clarity and direction, the underlying water element can make them changeable and contrary.

CHAPTER NINE

The humours

U nlike the blood, the fluids, the organs, and the tissues, the humours are not in themselves distinct and separate entities within the body. They are that which everything we encounter in the body is made from. Each humour has a special relationship with a certain organ, which is called its "seat", and each humour activates a particular faculty or "virtue"; choler sits in the gall bladder and activates the apprehensive faculty, sanguine sits in the liver and activates the digestive faculty, phlegm sits in the lungs and actives the expulsive faculty and melancholy sits in the spleen and activates the retentive faculty.

When there is a good balance of the humours or "eucrasia", a good state of health will be apparent in the body. When that balance is lost it is usual that one of the humours will have become excessive and will have overwhelmed the others, in this case it is described as being "plethoric" and one will attempt to rectify the situation by cleansing the body of the excess of that humour.

Each organ has a natural affinity with a particular humour, so it is also usual to see any humoral imbalance also reflected in those particular organs. We will look at each humour in the body, the organs and faculties that it is associated with, what the likely causes of excess are and what signs and symptoms of that excess are commonly found.

The sanguine humour, blood

"Blood is made of meat perfectly concocted, in quality hot and moist, governed by Jupiter: it is by a third concoction transmuted into flesh, the superfluity of it into seed, and its receptacle is the veins, by which it is dispersed through the body" (Culpeper, 1652).[1]

The sanguine humour is hot and wet and manifests as the blood itself. It is associated with air, as it carries the breath of life, or pneuma from the lungs around the body. Due to it being the medium in which all the other humours are contained, the blood humour is called the "principal" humour. However, this isn't meant to indicate that it has any kind of superior quality, or that it is on the top of a hierarchy of humours, as they are all deemed equal parts making up the whole.

> "Of all these humours blood is the chief, all the rest are superfluities of blood; yet they are necessary superfluities, for without any of them, man cannot live" (Culpeper, 1652).

The sanguine humour is under the rulership of the planet Jupiter, it activates and energises the two cold humours, phlegm and melancholy, helping to bring movement and flow. The spring is when the sanguine humour is at its greatest, when the warmth of the strengthening sun replaces the cold moisture of the winter with warmth, making the spring warm and moist. This is also the time of germination of seeds and the birth of young animals, connecting the sanguine humour with youth. Like young creatures it is fast, active, changeable, explorative and expanding.

It is associated with the liver, the lungs, the ribs, and the sides, with the inhalation and expansion of the lungs and the veins within which the humours are carried out of the liver.

Its seat is in the liver and it provides us with the digestive faculty, which breaks down food into their constituent elements. The first concoction of foods takes place in the stomach where they are cooked and broken down into their constituent parts, and the second concoction is in the liver producing the individual humours that provide nourishment for the body and organs.

The blood humour can become abnormal in two ways, either when it is overwhelmed by an excess of any of the other three humours, or when its own moisture increases so much that its own heat is diminished. When the heat in the blood lessens in this way it becomes very prone to infection, traditionally called putrefaction, leading to fevers and inflammatory conditions.

When the sanguine humour is in excess, the signs are: the head full of confused thoughts, obsession and anxiety, inflammatory conditions, hot and itchy skin, allergies, mouth ulcers, boils, red swollen face, heavy body, and easily getting tired.

The choleric humour, fire

> "Choler is made of meat more than perfectly concocted; and it is the spume or froth of blood; it clarifies all the humours, heats the body, nourishes the apprehension, as blood doth the judgement. It is in quality hot and dry; fortifies the attractive faculty as blood doth the digestive; moves man to activity and valour; its receptacle is the gall and it is under the influence of Mars" (Culpeper, 1652).

The choleric humour is hot and dry, and is the thinnest part of the blood, rising to produce the froth on the top when it is stirred up. It is stored in the Gall bladder as bile, and small amounts are passed into the blood to thin it and enable it to pass through the smaller passages to the organs and tissues. The rest of the bile stored in the gall bladder is passed into the intestines in small amounts to cleanse the gut wall, and to warm and stimulate the bowel to enable it to move and clear waste products through defecation. This corresponds to the warming action of digestive herbs, such as fennel, rosemary, mint, and thyme, which also stimulate the bowel, increasing peristalsis and aiding digestion and elimination.

It is ruled by the hot, dry, planet Mars, which is associated with heat, fire, action, war, and the acquisition of things. It is associated with the sense of smell, the emotion of anger and the attractive or apprehensive faculty in the body, which draws things out and attracts nourishment.

The choleric humour can become abnormal when the digestive process becomes too hot, and the chyle from the stomach is charred and burned producing toxic forms of choler. Hot foods like garlic and watercress can contribute to overheated choler, forming darker "leek green" bile. The hotter the choler, the darker it becomes, eventually leaving a residue rather like charred wood, which is called black bile, addust choler, or atribilis. This forms a hard cold residue, blocking the organs and passages and eventually if it is not purged from the system leads to chronic illness, tumours, and madness.

The signs of excess choler are: feeling hot, sweaty, thirsty, having acidity, nausea, constipation, irritability, skin problems, acne, carbuncles, sudden bursts of anger, fevers, shingles, migraines from excess heat, frenzy, fury, poor sleep. Choler is antipathetic to the bladder and kidneys causing blockage and stones.

The melancholic humour, earth

"Melancholy is the sediment of the blood, cold and dry in quality, fortifying the retentive faculty, and memory; makes men sober, solid and staid, fit for study; stays the unbridled toys of lustful blood, stays the wandering thoughts, and reduces them home to the centre: its receptacle is the spleen, and it is governed by Saturn" (Culpeper, 1652).

The melancholic humour is cold and dry, and it is considered to be the natural sediment of the blood, which remains when the other humours have been concocted in the liver. It has its seat in the spleen, which sits under the heart and is next to the stomach.

A small amount of the black bile held in the spleen enters the blood where it gives it density and consistency, providing physical strength and stamina, it passes in the blood to give the hardness found in bones, hair, and nails.

It is under the rulership of the planet Saturn, and is anti-pathetical to Jupiter and Venus, cooling passions and drying moistness. The melancholic time of the year is the autumn, when coldness and dryness combine after the hot dry season of the summer. In the stages of life, it corresponds to middle age, when we are nourished by all that we have learnt and attained in the first two stages of life from our growth and our activity.

It is associated with the bones, the tissues, the teeth, the ears, the sense of hearing, and the memory.

The melancholic humour is also connected to the retentive faculty or virtue and transforming nourishment into tissues as part of the fourth concoction in the liver.

The seat of the melancholic humour is the spleen which sits beneath the heart and is adjacent to the stomach. When melancholy is in excess it brings on fatigue because its cold vapours affect the heart and the emanation of innate heat. It weakens the appetite and digestion because of its proximity to the stomach and its consequent cooling and blocking effect on the activity of the stomach. When there is unnatural heat in the body this changes melancholy into a toxic burnt substance, giving us black bile or atribilis. This abnormal melancholy can be produced by:

1. Excess heat in the liver, burning the chyle from the stomach.
2. Weakness of the spleen meaning that the melancholy isn't properly contained.
3. Excess cold in the body, which congeals and solidifies excretions and waste products allowing them to build up.
4. Prolonged stagnation, congestion, and lack of flow and elimination.
5. Chronic disease, causing overheating and burning of the humours.

Excess melancholy is liable to leave residues between the stomach and liver, compromising the assimilation of food and digestion, and interfering with the production of blood leading to weakness and also anaemia.

Signs of an excess include: cold sweats, irregular heartbeat, anxiety, cold extremities, liver congestion, bitter belching, stiff painful joints, aching back and hips, and itchy skin.

The phlegmatic humour, water

"Flegm is made of meat not perfectly digested; it fortifies the virtue expulsive, makes the body slippery, fit for ejection; it fortifies the brain by its consimilitude with it; yet it spoils Apprehension by its antipathy to it. It qualifies Choler, cools and moistens the heart, thereby sustaining it, and the whole body from the fiery effects, which continual motion would produce: its receptacle is the lungs, and is governed by Venus, some say the Moon, perhaps it may be governed by them both, it is cold and moist in quality" (Culpeper, 1652).

The phlegmatic humour is cold and moist, it is the lymph fluid, and a watery aspect of the blood that is not fully made into blood itself but can mature into it. Its seat is the lungs. It is associated with the winter, when moisture abounds and we are liable to be overwhelmed by dampness, floods, and stagnation. It is also the humour that predominates in old age. The body cools and dries during the middle years meaning that movement and clearance of fluid slows so that the body becomes more swollen and cold, and therefore likely to suffer from damp, stagnation, and stasis as we enter old age.

It governs the expulsive virtue, helping the body to eliminative waste products through urination and defecation. It nourishes the phlegmatic tissues and organs, which include the brain, the senses, the stomach, bowels, bladder, eyes, especially the left eye, the skin, and the joints. It also produces saliva and mucus throughout the body.

Phlegm can harden when affected by either extreme heat or cold. Cold makes it thick and sticky causing the blockage of flow through passages and within organs. While heat will make it split into a thin watery "serous" discharge and a thick residue that will build up causing pain and inflammation, as well producing the hard nodules associated with arthritis.

Signs of excess include: lethargy, palsy, convulsions, and epilepsy from phlegm obstructing the animal spirit. Weight gain, poor digestion, bloating, excess mucous, coughs, blocked sinuses, pelvic and urinary congestion. All cold and rheumatic diseases, fluid retention, dropsies, oedema, discharges, and abscesses. Cold also causes cramps and colic.

Working with the humours

When the natural balance of the humours is lost, it is due to one or more of the humours becoming excessive. This initially just affects the function of that humour itself and the organs that are connected to it and then leads onto it overwhelming the other humours and interfering with their function. These two states are called dyscrasias, and when the humour is just in excess of itself it is referred to as a qualitive dyscrasia, and when this goes onto overwhelm other humours it is referred to as a quantitive dyscrasia.

Clearing excess through catharsis and protecting the vital spirit

Responses to the various humoral excesses, whether in an organ, a system, or the whole body will be similar.

Primarily we must identify the underlying cause of the humour itself becoming excessive and ensure that the excess is cleared.

Secondly, we must protect the body and organs by correcting or mollifying the imbalance, usually by using a herb or intervention that promotes the opposite temperament to the imbalance.

We are therefore always looking initially for what is excessive in the body and then attempting to identify which humour it is that has lead to the excess. Whether the offending humour has affected just a particular organ or system, as in a qualitative dyscrasia, or the whole body, as in the state of a quantative dyscrasia, through a process of catharsis the offending humour will need to be ripened and cleared from the body. The ripening is achieved through a process of heating or making mobile the excess humour in an appropriate way so it may then be cleared through defecation, diuresis, sweating, or vomiting.

As each humour is also associated with an emotional and mental state, and may have become excessive because of an overwhelming experience of that emotional state, we may also need to consider emotional and mental catharsis as part of the treatment. This may be simply by allowing a sanguine patient to share their feelings of anxiety or obsession, the choleric to release feelings of anger through shouting, the melancholic to let go of fear and be encouraged to move on emotionally, and the phlegmatic to release feelings of being overwhelmed or full of sorrow by crying.

This rebalancing and releasing of humours is sympathetic in nature, so that one is strengthening the functions of the body or mind through which the natural balance of humours is usually maintained.

The protective response will usually be antipathetic in nature, for instance using cooling strategies to counter excess heat, or drying strategies for excess moisture. Each organ has its own temperament, and maintaining the balance of its temperament is important to keep it in a state of optimal function.

Each of the spirits in the body also have a natural temperament, so we may also need to use remedies that will encourage the return of the spirit to its correct temperament.

When the vital spirit becomes overwhelmed by heat, such as when we are over-whelmed by anger, we can use cooling cordial herbs (rose, lemon balm, violet and borage) and when it is overwhelmed by cold, such as with melancholic vapours rising up from the spleen, we can use warming protective herbs (angelica, rosemary, juniper, St John's wort).

When the cold and dry animal spirit in the head becomes too cold, for instance due to excess phlegm or melancholy, we can use warming cephalics, such as vervain, cowslips, lavender, and feverfew. When it becomes overheated due to excess choler or phrensy and excess air we will use cooling herbs for the head, such as rose, violets, willow, or lettuce.

When the warm and wet natural spirit in the liver becomes too moist we will use the cleansing bitter herbs such as wormwood, angelica, and wood avens. If it has become too hot and dry then the cooling moistening remedies, such as dandelion and milk thistle, are beneficial.

The procreative spirit is also warm and moist, so coldness causing loss of libido is helped by warming herbs, such as the mints, and if over strong it is calmed by cooling herbs, such as willow.

Depletion is a characteristic of the spirits, excess is a characteristic of the humours

There are often times when apparent signs of excess are actually caused by a depletion in the body of the opposite quality; for instance, excess damp and cold can be due to the loss of innate heat, rather than an excess of phlegm humour, and excess dryness and heat can be due to the loss of radical moisture rather than an excess of the choleric humour.

These situations occur due to the depletion of one of the spirits, either the vital, natural, animal, or procreative. The spirits also have a balance of temperament, and if they lose this balance then the organs associated with them will suffer. For instance, if the vital spirit becomes depleted in innate heat we will see problems such as heart weakness, coldness, lethargy, congestion and a general weakness in the function of all organs because the activating effect of innate heat is lacking. If the vital spirit loses its balance of radical moisture, then the heart can also suffer, causing agitation, fear, a rapid or erratic heart rate, heart pains, and angina.

When the animal spirit loses its heat this can lead to conditions of cold effecting the head and nerves, often causing pain, migraines, confusion, vertigo, and numbness.

In this case, warming cephalic herbs, such as betony, rosemary, vervain and cowslip, might be chosen.

Although the depletion of heat or moisture is not directly caused by the lack of a humour, such as choler (heat) or phlegm (moisture), it may be that an underlying humoral imbalance has caused the depletion to occur. We may still need to strengthen the spirit with a warming or cooling herb even though the imbalance itself may have been caused by an excess of a hot or cold humour. For instance, one may still use a hot and dry herb like St John's wort to strengthen the innate heat, even when it is excess choler that is the underlying temperamental imbalance. One may conversely use a moistening and cooling herb, such as sweet violet, to support the radical moisture even when the underlying imbalance has been brought about by excess phlegm blocking the digestion and the concoction of the humours.

In these situations, it is important to remember that the excess heat or dampness we see is due to a loss of radical moisture or innate heat, rather than it being due to excess phlegm or choler. We therefore need strategies to strengthen the innate heat or radical moisture alongside purging the excess humour and also mollifying the symptoms arising from the imbalance.

A simple rule of thumb is to always look at the tongue as part of the diagnosis; a tongue that lacks a coating is always a sign of depletion of one of the spirits. So a red tongue without a coating is likely to be showing that excess heat (red) is present because of a lack of radical moisture to cool the temperament, and a bluish wet tongue without a coating will indicate the lack of innate heat (blue and wet) to activate the liver, the organs, the digestion and the concoctions.

Clear the humours, balance temperament of the organs

There are also situations where we must treat an underlying humoral imbalance in an opposite way to the response that is needed to improve the temperament of an organ. For instance, we may find that excess choler has overheated the liver and dried its passages leading to a blockage. As the liver is the organ that produces the blood, and it is the blood that carries the innate heat, we can find that this could be causing head pain associated with coldness. We then may use a cooling remedy, such as dandelion, to reduce and clear the heat in the liver and clear the excess choler by opening the passages of the liver, alongside using a heating remedy, such as rosemary or feverfew to treat the coldness in the head. We may find that we can also use a single herb that both clears heat from the liver while at the same time warms the head; vervain would be a good example of such a herb.

In the following chapters on the individual humours we will look at each of the humours, identifying what it is that;

1. Causes the humour to become excessive
2. The effects and the signs of that excess on the body
3. The responses and solutions that will return the humour into balance

Excess states of blood

Causes

Sanguine temperament

Over-indulgent lifestyle	Excessive mental and physical activity

Excess Blood

Blood is wet= Excess moisture

Moisture causes congestion and dampness, which cools and congests the liver, blocking flow of the Vital Spirits and Innate Heat

Slows digestion & Concoctions, increases excess phlegm and moisture	Lowered Innate Heat ceases to drive out & cleanse the body of external heat so poisons invade

Also-Excess choler	Putrefaction and Infection

Causes excess heat in blood

Blood heats, expands and thins into vapours, causes Heat, Fever, and Inflammation, vapours distil and separate into watery discharges of mucous

Signs

Confused, anxious, unquiet thoughts, heaviness, hypochondria, bloating, drowsiness, depression.

Tongue Swollen, thick coating, patchy	**Pulse** Floating, forceful, drumskin, surging

Excess Blood Causes a Congested State

Tongue Swollen, pale, blue, wet.	Pulse Thin, deep, soft

Develops into:

Hot Damp State

Red swollen face, boils, Mouth ulcers, Heavy feeling. Fevers, inflammation. Skin problems, urinary infections, Angry & uncomfortable

Tongue Red, purple, yellow greasy coating	**Pulse** Tight, full, hard, Floating, surging.

Solutions

Eat less food. Eat more fruits, vegetables, fish, wild meat, vinegars & pickles	Cultivate A life purpose, a committed relationship, a garden, Express emotions- sing, dance

Purge moisture diuretics; Dandelion leaf, Vervain, Yarrow, Horsetail, Nettle.	Calm over-excited spirits Passionflower, Skullcap, Tilia, Hawthorn,

Clear blockages of liver

Warming, opening herbs: Fennel, Aniseed, Angelica, Elecampagne, Lovage root, Chamomile.	Strengthen with liver tonics: Linden, Betony, Agrimony, Oats, Motherwort, Borage.

Nourish Liver:
Burdock, Milk thistle,

Cool with condensing & Contracting remedies.
Willow, Meadowsweet, Agrimony, Roses.

Purge heat: Yellow Dock.
Dandelion, Artichoke leaf, Wormwood, Echinacea.

Expel excess heat with diaphoretics:
Elder, Yarrow, Mint, Linden, Catmint, Clary.

CHAPTER TEN

Excess of the sanguine humour

Causes of excess

The sanguine humour corresponds to the blood and the element of air. The main cause of excess sanguine humour is overindulgence, whether that is from overeating, overthinking, or over-worrying. All of these will lead to the blood humour becoming excessive.

The spring is the season of the rising blood humour. It was considered particularly important to cleanse the blood of any cold, crude, unrefined humours that may be left in the system after the winter, when the digestive process and concoctions have been at their weakest. The winter is a time when dampness abounds, meaning that as spring is also wet and warm in temperament there is a risk of this leading to an excess of moisture in the blood. It was therefore often recommended to take a diuretic tonic containing herbs like cleavers, nettles, and dandelion to cleanse the blood in the spring, especially for those with a sanguine constitution.

Blood is wet, so excess causes damp congestion

The excess dampness will overwhelm the liver, the seat of the blood humour, and lead to congestion, blockage, and cooling of the liver. It will slow the concoction and digestion of foods and the digestive faculty, which also resides there. The excess moistness will block the uptake of the nutrients from food, and will block the absorption of the heat within foods into the innate heat, and will thus weaken the vital spirit.

When the vital heat is lessened in this way, the other faculties cannot function, reducing uptake, digestion, retention of nutrients, and elimination of wastes. It also reduces the body's innate ability to resist poisons and infection, and external heat and poisons are then able to invade the body.

The signs of excess blood

"Phrensy" or a head full of confused and unquiet thoughts is often accompanied by hypochrondria and anxiety. There are likely to be inflammatory conditions, abscesses and boils, skin irritation, and bursts of anger and discomfort. Feelings of heaviness and drowsiness, stretching and yawning, with the patient being easily fatigued. Mouth ulcers and a sweet taste in the mouth, along with erratic circulation and high blood pressure. Excess blood is also associated with all infirmities of the liver and veins, lung disease, and pleurisy.

The tongue will usually be swollen, coated, patchy, and the pulse full, floating, and surging.

The excess of moisture in the blood leads to a congested state, this worsens the feelings of heaviness, depression, fatigue, anxiety, and confusion. The tongue becomes wetter due the stagnant fluids building up overwhelming the heat and movement of blood—a wet tongue is a sign of low heat. The pulse becomes thinner and deeper due to the diminished heat and the blockage to the flow of blood as it tries to pass through the excess moisture.

Responding to excess blood humour

Those with a sanguine temperament should avoid excesses of all kinds and avoid being too dispersed and scattered. They must eat regular meals and not snack between meals and avoid hot damp foods, such as honey, wine, sugary foods, bread, and excess onions and garlic. They will benefit from eating watery soups, pickles and vinegar, fish, wild meats, summer fruits, beer, and cider. Sanguines will get away with eating most things most of the time, they enjoy eating and tend to be at risk of eating in excess.

Regular exercise, dancing, or a team building sporting activity is very beneficial as it clears excess dampness and moves any build up of heat in the body.

It is good for them to engage in creative expression, such as singing, performing, writing, or other artistic endeavours. They should find a long term partner to be committed to, or at least develop an enduring and all engaging interest or discipline, it helps if they can find earthy, dependable, solid friends, and also to do some gardening.

Purging and cleansing

To purge and clear the excess moisture, they should take diuretics, such as dandelion, nettle, and cleavers in the spring, yarrow, vervain and celery in the summer, and fennel and sage in the winter. They should calm their overactive mind, emotions, and spirits with centring herbs, such as lime blossom and chamomile, and use cooling nerviness such as scullcap and passionflower.

With excess moisture it is also helpful to strengthen the digestion with warming aromatic herbs, such as hyssop, fennel, aniseed, angelica, lovage, and elecampagne. These herbs also ripen and prepare the excess humour for evacuation via diuresis and sweating

Nourish and protect the liver

If the liver has become overwhelmed and exhausted due to the excess dampness and the loss of vital spirit, the natural spirit which resides there will also become diminished. To nourish the liver, dandelion root and milk thistle seeds are very helpful, as are artichokes and burdock root. It is important to warm and protect the liver; when borage, agrimony, oats, lime flower, wood avens and betony can be used.

Putrefaction and invasion of poisons

With excess damp heat accompanying the build up of excess blood, infection and putrefaction can occur. Putrefaction excessively warms the bloodand hot vapours arise, this may lead to excess heat, fevers, and inflammation. The hot vapours will also distil causing excess mucus, watery discharges, and eventually pus.

This hot damp state may be seen in the following ways: a red swollen face, boils, mouth ulcers, feeling heavy and uncomfortable, fevers, inflammations, skin problems, urinary infections, and sudden bursts of anger.

The tongue is likely to look red, swollen with thick yellow greasy coating, and the pulse is likely to be full, tight, hard, surging and floating.

Purging infection, heat and dampness

The response is to cool the blood with condensing and contracting remedies: willow, meadowsweet, birch, bramble or raspberry tops, borage, agrimony, and roses.

We may purge the heat from the blood and the liver with: yellow dock, dandelion, wormwood, artichoke leaf, echinacea, and clear excess and dampness with diaphoretics, such as elder, mint and catmint, lime blossom, eupatorium, yarrow, and clary.

Case history

An outgoing woman in her mid-forties, largish in stature, enjoys playing music, walking and swimming. She had developed a successful career in the creative industries and had reached the pinnacle of her career in her early thirties, becoming the head of design in a large company. She tended to overwork, oversocialise, and eventually became addicted to stimulants (cocaine) to keep up with her fast metropolitan lifestyle. At the same time, she also began suffering from depression and started to take antidepressants, which for some time seemed to help. After ten years she decided to have a fresh start; she left the highly stressed job and became freelance, moved out of the city, and stopped taking drugs. Two years on she presented with feelings of bloating, heaviness, depression, drowsiness and an unquiet and overactive mind. She often felt panicked, and sleep was often disturbed. Her diet was low in fresh vegetables, fruit, fibre, and nuts, but high in refined carbohydrates, caffeine and sweet snacks, her bowel motions were erratic, and could vary from hard to loose.

She had a swollen, wet, pale purple tongue, with a thick white to grey coating. There was an excess of moisture making it swollen, and pale; the moisture has blocked the flow of innate heat, making the tongue appear wet and the excess moisture and coldness affecting the bowels has produced the thick white coating. Her pulse was thin and deep, soft and forceless. In this case an excess of moisture has made the pulse thin, like the flow of a river being obstructed by a flood.

She was given a mixture of wormwood, vervain, motherwort and angelica root to take three times a day. The wormwood to purge and cleanse the excess moisture and to get the digestion working well again. Vervain to help cleanse the excess moisture and calm the unquiet thoughts. Motherwort to lift the spirits, calm the heart, and release mental tension. Angelica to strengthen the heart and the spirits and clear dampness. She was also given Roman chamomile aromatic water to take whenever she felt panicked and to take if she woke in the night and couldn't calm her mind.

The initial impact was a big improvement in her energy, her bloating and heaviness improved, her bowel motions became more regular, and she felt much more focused and clear. The improved motivation this gave her meant that she managed to improve her diet, rejoin her music group, and prioritise her wellbeing above her work. She managed to stop her antidepressants within the first month and soon was feeling more grounded and happy. Like children, people with a sanguine constitution can bounce back very quickly, the danger is that once well again they forget what they need to do to moderate their behaviour and fall back into old patterns of excess.

Excess states of Choler

Causes

Choleric Temperament

External heat, stress, anger, excitement, overwork, heating foods, stimulants.

Excess heat causes dryness

Leads to constriction, reducing flow and stagnating vitality

Dries Radical moisture reducing flow

Causes build-up of Heat in Organs and blood

Atribilis
Excess heat burns up bile Leaves hard, cold addust residues of atribilis. Forming blocks

Produces obstructions & stoppings especially in Liver and Urinary passages

Blocked flow of Humours and Blood

Signs

Heat

Feels hot, sweaty, thirsty, constipated, irritable, skin problems.

Pulse	Tongue
Fast, hard, narrow, strong, bowstring, skipping & Forceful, long	Narrow, red, thin, yellow, coating

Deficient moisture:

Feels restless, agitated, night sweats, wringing hands

Pulse	Tongue
Surging- comes on strong, leaves weak, heat gives force, low moisture gives emptiness. Becomes scattered, vacuous	narrow, red, dryness causes cracks, little or no coating

STAGNATION

Stressed, depressed, easily upset, emotionally unstable, P.M.T. irritable.

Pulse	Tongue
Floating fast, forceful, bowstring/ drumskin.	Thin, red tip, and sides, thin white coating

Blocked

Chronic illness, madness, hard swellings, tumours

Pulse	Tongue
Weak, Hidden, narrow, skipping choppy	Purple, black spots, dry & cracked

Solutions

Find a life focus, learn a discipline

Short regular fasts, less sugar, caffeine, alcohol, release anger

Expel heat use bitters
Wormwood, Century, Gentian, Berberis, Vervain.

Cool Blood
Yellow dock, Lettuce, Chicory, Red clover
Protect heart
Motherwort, Juniper, Hawthorn, Mistletoe.

Nourish moisture
Rose, Borage, Balm, Violets, Cowslips, Asparagus root.

Strengthen vital flow & Etheric force
Fennel, Lavender, vervain, St Johns wort, Mugwort, Cowslip, Lily of the valley, Motherwort, Broom.

Open stoppings
In Liver
With bitter stimulants:
Wormwood, Gentian, Dock.
With soft moist remedies
Burdock, Dock, Dandelion, Milk thistle,
In Kidneys with cleansers:
Nettle, Cleavers, Dandelion leaf.

Clear Atribilis blocks
Ripen with
Elecampagne, Lovage root, Echinacea, Cimicifuga, Thuja. Burdock, Celandine
Purge with
Wormwood, Yellow dock, Dandelion,

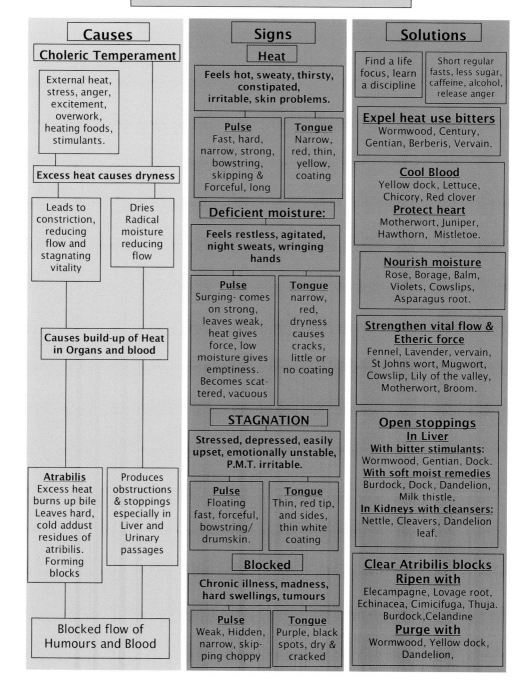

CHAPTER ELEVEN

Excess of the choleric humour

Causes of excess

The choleric humour corresponds to bile and the fire element, it is hot and dry in temperament. The main cause of excess is overheating from internal causes, such as anger, stress, and overworking, or external causes, such as an over hot environment, too much hot dry food, too much alcohol or intoxicants, or the effects of fevers and illness.

Choler is hot so excess leads to dryness, constriction, and blockage

The choleric humour makes up the thinnest part of the blood, and rises up to produce the froth on the top of blood. It is stored in the gall bladder as bile and small amounts are passed into the blood thinning it, enabling it to flow through the smaller passages and to reach the organs and tissues. The rest of the bile stored in the gall bladder is passed into the intestines in small amounts to cleanse the gut wall, and to warm and stimulate the bowel, increasing peristalsis and aiding digestion and elimination through defecation.

The choleric humour can become abnormal when the digestive process becomes too hot, and the chyle from the stomach is charred and burned producing toxic forms of choler. Hot foods like garlic and watercress can contribute to overheated choler, forming darker "leek green" bile. The hotter the choler, the darker it becomes, eventually leaving a residue rather like charred wood called black bile, addust choler, or atribilis. This forms a hard cold residue blocking the organs and passages, leading to constriction, tightness, and dryness, reducing flow and stagnating vitality.

These hard blocks can lead to the formation of tumours and swellings producing obstructions and "stoppings", especially in the liver, intestines, and urinary system. They are also likely to cause nodules, hard swellings, and tumours, and to be the foundation of chronic illness, nervous debility, dementia, tremors, and in some cases madness.

Excess heat will scorch and dry radical moisture reducing the cooling effects of its flow, causing a build-up of heat in organs and localised areas.

Signs of excess choler

The patient will feel hot, sweaty, thirsty, suffer constipation, acidity and nausea, and may suffer from jaundice. They will commonly be irritable, suffer from fits of sudden anger, fury, and frenzy. They may suffer skin problems, such as acne and eczema, as well as carbuncles and shingles. It may be the cause of fevers and also poor sleep. The heat and dryness can affect the bladder and kidneys, causing blockage and stones.

Signs of excess choler in the tongue and pulse; the pulse will be fast, long, and strong, with the heat making the pulse hard and tight like a bowstring. Sometimes the heat can make the heart rapid and even a bit erratic, with the beat skipping ahead. There is likely to be a yellow coating, denoting heat on the tongue, it is likely to be narrow and red, and often be thin, showing the drying out of the tissues. If the tip is red it always indicates excess heat in the heart either because of stress or due to emotional upset. When there has been a long term state of dryness we will also expect the tongue to have a cracked surface. Red spots indicate stagnant blood, and red prickles heat in the lungs.

Signs of heat being caused by loss of radical moisture

A depletion of the radical moisture contained in the vital spirit can also lead to the appearance of excess heat.

When the cooling radical moisture is depleted the friction that then arises in the body also causes the appearance of excess heat. In this case, the pulse is likely to be surging, coming on strongly, but leaving with weakness. This is caused by the heat in the blood giving the pulse strength, but the lack of moisture then making the following pulse feel weak and empty. If the depletion of the radical moisture is of long standing, then the pulse may become scattered and vacuous as the heat in the blood becomes dispersed without the moisture being there to allow it to flow. The tongue will be likely to look red, narrow and have no coating. It is red because if coldness was the cause, the tongue would look blue. It is also likely to be narrow as the lack of moisture means that the tongue is not plumped up, and as moisture is replenished by the residue of the concoctions and the coating is also a residue of concoctions the lack of any coating is a clear indication of depletion.

When the radical moisture is low there are often symptoms of restlessness, agitation, night sweats and the patient may often be prone to wring their hands.

Stagnation

As an excess of bile and heat may lead to blockages, which then produce signs of stagnation of blood and fluids. The patient is likely to become stressed, depressed, easily upset, emotionally unstable, suffer from PMT and irritability.

The pulse will be floating as the heat pushes it up, fast and forceful, with the blockage from the stagnation making it hard or like a drum skin. As the blockage increases, the pulse will become weak and deep or hidden. With the heat thinning the blood the pulse becomes soft, fine and forceless, however it will remain long showing that there is still heat present, with it possibly being interrupted and skipping.

With stagnation of the blood the tongue becomes thin, often with a red tip and sides, and may have a thin white or yellow coating.

If the excess choler has lead to cold hard atribilis blocks, the tongue will become darker purple, there may even be black spots, and it will be dry, cracked, and narrow.

Responding to excess choler

Choleric people benefit from finding a life focus, learning a skill, and developing a talent. They appreciate discipline and make good soldiers, feeling secure when they can develop respect for an authoritative figure. It is always good for them to have a project on the go that has clear short-term goals.

It is good for cholerics to do short regular fasts, especially at the change of season. Having a regular exercise regime that includes short intensive sessions helps to clear excess heat and any burnt choler from the system. Although they do well in competitive sports they shouldn't do them excessively. However, forced inactivity will cause a build up of internal heat leading to burnt choler developing, this then obstructs the vital spirit, causing depression and agitation. Commonly this can happen in retirement, or in cholerics with sedentary occupations. Excess emotional heat can be cleared through releasing anger by shouting, screaming, dancing, playing drums, or any other strongly cathartic activity.

Cholerics do better on fish and wild meats rather than fatty meats, such as beef, and pork. They must limit dairy products and too many hot spicy foods. They should also avoid salty and dried foods, stimulants such as caffeine and cocaine, have little or no sugar and only small amounts of alcoholic spirits or wine. They should eat plenty of light salads and vegetables, with nuts and seeds, soups with barley, summer fruits, and it is better if they stick to beer, cider, caffeine-free herbal teas and always take sufficient water.

Herbs used to expel excess heat

Bitter herbs, such as wormwood, century, gentian, berberis, vervain, and gipsywort will open passages and flush out the heat from the liver. To open the passages of the liver and enable ripening of the blockages, soft moist remedies, such as burdock, dock, dandelion, and milk thistle, will help.

Herbs traditionally used to cool the blood are: yellow dock, chicory, wild lettuce, meadowsweet, and red clover flowers.

To protect the heart from excess choler, the cooling cordial herbs are used: rose, violets, balm, and borage. When the heart has become affected by burnt choler lily of the valley, motherwort, and broom will all strengthen and protect the heart and the vital spirit.

To strengthen the vital and etheric force when affected by atribilis we can use fennel, lavender, vervain, yarrow, mugwort, and cowslip flowers. These herbs will also ensure that any blockages that are also affecting the stomach, spleen, and liver are warmed and cleared.

To cool and cleanse the kidneys of excess choler we can use nettles, cleavers, shepherds purse, yarrow, dandelion leaf, and asparagus root. Especially cooling are mallows, oat straw, and couch grass.

If the body has become overwhelmed by cold blockages of burnt choler, then they are ripened with elecampagne, angelica, avens, echinacea, cimicifuga, thuja, and celandine. To then purge them from the system gentle laxatives, such as wormwood, dandelion, burdock, yellow dock, and fenugreek, will all be effective.

Case study

A middle aged woman presented with chronic hypertension. She had been treated for a number of years with conventional antihypertensive drugs, but they had failed to bring her blood pressure down. The ongoing raised blood pressure had caused enlargement of her heart muscle (cardio hypertrophy), which could make her short of breath, caused chest pain, and could make her more vulnerable to future heart problems. She was an active and driven choleric, and otherwise in good health. She was responsible for an adult disabled son, who she had to be an advocate for, and generally felt emotionally tense and stressed.

We had tried a wide range of relaxant antihypertensive herbs, such as hawthorn, lime flowers and lemon balm, without having any success in lowering her blood pressure. It was by chance that the patient found that her blood pressure dropped to a more normal level when she had been prescribed a herbal combination for gut parasites by a naturopath. When she reported the improvement we trialled each of the herbs in the mixture individually and discovered that it was wormwood that was having the antihypertensive effect. She then started using the tincture of wormwood at a dose of 10 ml once a day and found that it maintained her blood pressure at an acceptable level. She also found that her mood was much better, she felt in better spirits generally, and was less tense and stressed.

Wormwood is ruled by Mars, the planet of fire, heat, and war. It is hot and dry in the first degree, and is cleansing and opening. It was particularly revered for its ability to both clear phlegm and choler. In this case it helped to purge the excess heat from the system allowing the blood pressure to normalise. Melancholy is often the result of chronic excess heat leaving behind cold burnt choler that blocks the flow of vital spirit. Wormwood not only helps to cleanse the excess heat from the system, but also will clear these cold melancholic blocks and improve the spirits.

Excess Melancholy

Cause

Excess Melancholy

External cold	Lack of nourishing warming foods, excess cold food
Lack of activity	

All lead to:

Cold obstructions

Liver
Blood cools & blocks passages.
Less concoction of Humours and blood

Spleen
Sits beneath stomach and stops free flow of nutrients to liver

Bowels
Cold, sluggish, blocked

Less heat in stomach,
Weaker digestion.
Less concoction of humours.
Blood concoction diminished
Vital spirit less nourished
Vital heat depleted.

Leads to Lower innate heat

Reduction in attractive, digestive, and expulsive faculties.

Melancholic vapours
Spleen obstructed, vapours rise up & overwhelm the heart, reduce Vital Spirit and Innate heat.

Signs

Fatigue, poor appetite & digestion, cold sweats, pessimism, anxiety.

Pulse	**Tongue**
Narrow, short, deep, weak, hidden, fine, confined	Pale, blue, swollen, especially swollen on sides.

Reduced concoction of blood increases coldness and moistness, leading to dropsies & cold swellings.

Bitter belching, fullness, constipation, heartburn, itchy skin, stiff painful joints, stinking breath, weariness, anxiety, negativity and dark thoughts, dull witted.

Blood deficient tongue
Pale, dry, narrow, little or no coating.

Vital spirit deficient tongue
Flaccid, teeth marks, bluish, broad, thin white coating, a few red spots.

Anxiety, palpitations, fearfulness, depression, nightmares, headaches.

Solutions

Nourish body with easily digested foods, Soups, stews, root veg, cooked grains, squash, dried fruit, lamb, soft cheese, fish. **Reduce** refined sugars, red meats, wheat.	Increase activity. Take on a long-term project. Mix with sanguine types. Seek excitement.

Use aperient herbs to warm & activate stomach & liver
Angelica, Lovage, Black pepper. Fennel, Sage, Hyssop, Thyme, Cardamom, Mints

Clear blocks in liver, spleen
Wormwood, Chicory, Hops, Elecampagne, Vervain, Centuary, Rhubarb rt

Nourish liver
Artichokes, Burdock root, Dandelion root, Milk Thistle
Temperate liver herbs
Avens, Betony, Tilia, Valerian. Agrimony,

Warm and protect heart, head & Vital Spirit
Angelica, Bay, Basil, Hyssop, Rosemary, Hypericum Motherwort, borage, Valerian

Assuage Melancholic Vapours
Fragrant smells, spices & incense: Rose, Lavender, Chamomile, Cardamom, Orange blossom, Frankincense.

CHAPTER TWELVE

Excess of the melancholic humour

The melancholic humour corresponds to the sediment of the blood and the earth element. The main causes of excess are those things that increase coldness and stagnation within the body. Internal causes include having a strongly melancholic temperament, spending too much time in introversion, and being on one's own for too long. Because melancholics are often solitary and studious by nature, it can be easy for them to become isolated and starved of the warmth brought by the company of others.

They are not easily moved to be active, so often will spend much of their time following sedentary occupations and activities. If they are not eating warm nourishing foods, or have too many cold foods, or are exposed to cold environments, melancholy becomes excessive. It is most prevalent in the autumn and winter, especially during the colder, darker months, becoming more common in middle and old age, making us more susceptible to its effects as we get older.

Excess melancholy

The melancholic humour is cold and dry, and governs the retentive faculty in the body. When it is in excess, too much retention occurs. This causes blockages of the passages, reducing the movement of fluids, blood, and nutritious humours to the organs. It reduces the movement of the innate heat to the organs reducing their activity and the function of the main faculties of the body.

This reduction of heat in the stomach causes a weakening of the digestion, a loss of appetite, a feeling of heaviness in the stomach, bitter belching, heartburn, and constipation. Excess melancholy will also block and reduce the flow of the hot bile from the gall bladder, which is needed to activate the intestines and bowels, to cleanse the bowels of waste, and to aid in elimination.

The slowing of the digestion and the blocking of the passages in the liver means that the concoctions are reduced, depleting the production of healthy blood. The blood becomes further stagnated by the blockage of the flow of choler from the gall bladder, which is needed to thin the blood enough to enable it to flow through the smaller vessels.

As the seat of melancholy, the spleen frequently becomes blocked with excess melancholy. The spleen sits between the liver and the stomach and the cold melancholic vapours that arise from it interfere with the movement of the chyle from the stomach to the liver and also rise up and overwhelm the heart. This blocks the flow of innate heat and reduces the transformation of the humours during the concoctions. These vapours also interfere with pnuema from the air that we breathe being passed from the lungs to the heart, further reducing the innate heat and vital spirit, which the pneuma strengthens.

Signs of excess melancholy

Initially we will see symptoms of fatigue, malaise, and tiredness. The depletion of digestive heat due to cold blockages in the stomach causes loss of appetite, weakened digestion, fullness, heartburn, colic, constipation and stinking breath.

The blockages in the liver will cause abdominal pains, or "stitches" in the sides, and will lead to jaundice, irritability, and hot itchy conditions of the skin due to the retention of toxins in the blood.

In the head, the lessening of the innate heat causes dullness, forgetfulness, confusion and may also be the underlying cause of migraines, shaking, tremors, numbness, fainting, nightmares, and headaches. Coldness affecting the joints will make them stiffer and more painful and will also be the cause of cramps and spasm in muscles.

As the melancholic vapours rise and overwhelm the heart, we are likely to see anxiety, pessimism and depression increase, with physical symptoms, such as palpitations, irregular heartbeat, chest pains, and variations of rhythm. The loss of movement and flow from the reduced innate heat may also cause conditions of water retention, swellings and "dropsies" to occur. The reduction in elimination of waste products leads to dry and itchy skin problems.

Initially we are likely to see a pale or bluish tongue, with swollen sides, signifying the blockage in the spleen. Eventually it will become purple, indicating that there is stagnation. It may well have a thick coating, often this is white, but sometimes it will become yellow when there is fermentation in the stomach or intestines. The pulse is usually deep, fine, soft, and narrow. When the blood becomes deficient we see a pale tongue, which is frequently narrow, and having little or no coating. The blood is needed to distribute fluids, so we often see a dry surface. If the vital spirit has become depleted, we are more likely to see a lack of coating or a patchy coating; a wet tongue indicating low heat, with it being broader, flaccid with teeth marks, and some red spots, showing the stagnation of the blood.

Responding to excess melancholy

Increasing activity and engaging in expressive, active, and joyful pastimes will greatly help to clear melancholy, as does cultivating relationships with outgoing sanguine types. Long walks and taking on long-term projects all help to gently clear and balance excess melancholy.

The diet benefits from not eating excessively large meals or too late in the day. Including easily digestible foods; soups and stews in the winter, soft cheeses, lamb, shell fish, squash, parsnips and sweet potatoes, well-cooked grains, such as barley, quinoa, and buckwheat. Olive oil, dried fruit, and cleansing foods, such as asparagus, celery, celeriac and fennel are also helpful. Warming gentle herbs and spices, such as thyme, basil, oregano, cardamom, coriander, and cinnamon, can be added to foods along with black pepper to warm the stomach. These warming herbs also assuage the cold vapours arising from a spleen blocked with melancholy.

When the stomach needs extra assistance, herbs like angelica, lovage root, hyssop, and sage are all very beneficial. They also help to warm and protect the heart and the vital spirit.

If there are signs of blood stagnation and the liver being blocked, then warming, opening herbs such as wormwood, elecampagne root, vervain and yarrow may be used.

To clear blocks in the liver and spleen, bitter herbs such as wormwood, dock, elecampagne, dandelion, hops, chicory, vervain, centuary, and gentian should be used. To nourish the liver and enable it to regain its warm moist temperament, one should take artichokes, burdock root, dandelion root, and milk thistle. To help maintain the correct humoral balance of the liver, temperate liver herbs, such as wood avens, betony, lime blossom, and agrimony, are useful.

The cold nature of melancholy blocks and diminishes innate heat and the melancholic vapours, which rise up from the spleen cool and damage the heart. This calls for warming and protective herbs for the heart, such as angelica, rosemary, bay, juniper, and hyssop.

Case history

A reasonably active male in his early seventies who had lived in a rugged and beautiful part of the country for most of his adult life, and had always enjoyed walking in the hills, presented with fatigue and loss of stamina with various heart problems including erratic blood pressure. His overriding love of walking had been frustrated for much of his adulthood, as he had invested his life energy in setting up a community based project, which had been his focus for the last 30 years. Having set it up and managed it himself he found it difficult to let go of it, and after all the years still spent very long hours on the computer ensuring that it was always administered correctly and ran smoothly. He consequently felt a big responsibility to both the project and to all those involved. This is a typical presentation of a melancholic; they are loyal, dependable, and trustworthy—even to the detriment of their own health.

He had been concerned about his blood pressure for over twenty years, which seemed to be unstable. It was sometimes very high and at other times quite normal without any obvious explanation. Investigations had shown some scarring in one of his neck arteries, possibly from an accident in his youth. He worried about his blood pressure and when he had recently experienced shoulder and arm pain (probably due to his very sedentary work) he feared that it was related to his heart. Recent numbness in his legs had caused further anxiety. He had a minor transient stroke some months previous and was very anxious and fearful for the future. He had been for many inconclusive medical tests over the years and had been prescribed many different blood pressure medications and blood thinners.

When he presented he complained that there was a significant reduction in his walking capacity, general stamina, flexibility, and balance. His worry about not having any way forward and no definite answers to his problems was making him feel depressed and exhausted. He had written an in depth medical history, which focused on his physical worries but gave no mention of his emotional or spiritual life—typically for a melancholic, he mainly focused on the material world easily forgetting the more fluid and spiritual aspects of himself.

His sedentary lifestyle, due to his solitary and studious nature, had compounded his poor circulation, tight muscles, and poor posture. His tongue was a blue pink with little coating and was wet. The blue colour showed a constitutional state of coldness, the wetness showing low innate heat. His pulse was slightly fast, narrow, fine and short, quite tight and middle to floating. The shortness showed a slight heart weakness, with the narrowness and tightness showing cold constriction of the pulse, and the cold blockage pushing the pulse upwards as it can't freely and fluidly move forwards.

The lack of exercise, and the long hours spent sitting on the computer, had over a period of time exacerbated his cold dry melancholic temperament. The lack of a clear medical diagnosis had increased his fearfulness, frustrating his typically melancholic need to get to the bottom of things and feeding his worry and pessimism about his declining health. His long-term life project setting up the retreat centre had given him motivation and meaning, but as he was getting to a stage where he was needing to hand over responsibility for it, he was finding it difficult to develop new interests and passions and to remain positive and enthusiastic.

Giving him plenty of reassurance that over-worrying about the blood pressure was neither necessary nor beneficial was immediately helpful, and giving him hope by suggesting a gentle strengthening regime for the heart through more activity and taking supportive herbs gave him something positive to focus and to work on.

Physical investigation of his neck and shoulders showed that much of his numbness was likely to be due to long-term muscular tension, rather than the result of strokes and neurological problems. If he could do more exercise, spend less time on the computer, and get some regular massage he would be likely to see an improvement in the symptoms fairly quickly.

A warming herbal tonic was given that contained angelica, thyme, elecampagne and elder berry to help with the heart and the circulation, with motherwort (specifically recommended by Culpeper to strengthen the heart and to warm and digest cold humours). A mixture of dried lime flowers, chamomile, vervain, lemon balm, and violet, was also recommended as a regular daily tea to calm, balance, and soothe the nerves and emotions.

After a month of this regime he felt that his energy was improving and he was feeling more positive generally, he was worrying less about blood pressure and finding that the readings were generally lower and sometimes dropping quite low. He felt confident enough to reduce some of the stronger medications with the agreement of his doctor, and had felt a lot better for it. A capsule of valerian root morning and evening was added to the regime to further strengthen the heart, release muscular tension, and to help overcome the nervous and emotional exhaustion. We found that a specific cardiac tonic mix of herbs including lily of the valley and broom flowers also helped, it stabilised his blood pressure and improved his stamina. He responded well to the herbal strategy and to the support and reassurance he was given, making him feel less anxious and more able to let go of his attachment to the project. He had more time and energy to once again develop wider interactions and put more energy into his friends and to make a plan for a future beyond the project that he was now gradually letting go of. He started to walk every day and soon felt fitter and happier. He began to get regular massages for his back and neck and gradually noticed improvement.

Excess Phlegm

Causes

Excess Cold & Damp

External factors

Internal factors

Diet: Cold foods

Lifestyle: Inactivity

Climate: Damp, cold

Phlegmatic temperament, poor digestion, deficient innate heat

All lead to excess moisture

Excess moisture cools Innate heat- weakens digestive virtue- so unconcocted "Crude " humours fill the blood

Congest the Blood

Choke the Spirits

Further cools Innate Heat

Low internal heat no longer able to push out external poisons, putrefaction and infection follows

SIGNS

Lethargy, dullness forgetfulness, sadness, bloating, weak digestion, colic, fullness in chest, catarrh, phlegm.
Skin pale, cold and smooth.

Pulse Thin, soft, slow, short, forceless.

Tongue Pale, swollen, white greasy coating.

Deficient Vital heat

Emotionally low, needs warmth, panicky, low back pain.

Pulse Short, deep, forceless, hidden

Tongue Pale, blue swollen, wet.

When cold & congested:

Kidney infections, cystitis, ovarian and uterine problems, fibroids. Rheumatism, coughs, migraines, fainting, dizziness, cramps, lethargy, palsy, paralysis, and epilepsy

Pulse Slow, choppy, bound, slippery, fine, soft. Variable rate, rhythm, & force

Tongue Dark purple, black spots, usually wet, thin white coating

SOLUTIONS

Warm blood & Digestion
Gentle spices; Fennel, Mint, Thyme, Lovage Rt, Angelica, Rosemary, Hyssop, Aniseed, Juniper.

Eat fermented foods, pickles & vinegars.
Avoid: dairy, sugar, raw food, beef, ice cream.

Cleanse Liver: Wormwood Chicory, Gentian, Century

Set life goals, get active, be with choleric types, find passions

Balance Phlegm Humour: Valerian, Cicely, Aniseed, Cowslip, Sage, Feverfew, Bay, Garlic, Ginger, Cardamom.

Cleanse crudities

Diuretics
Nettles, Cleavers, Birch, Horsetail, Shepherds purse, Dandelion leaf, Yarrow
Diaphoretics
Limeflower, Elder, Yarrow, Feverfew, Eyebright
Steam with
Thyme, Chamomile, Sage.
Cleanse with
Mugwort, Sage, Marigold, Thyme, Thuja, Onion syrup.

Purge Blood
Burdock, Yellow dock. Echinacea, Avens, Elecampagne root, Betony, Nettle.

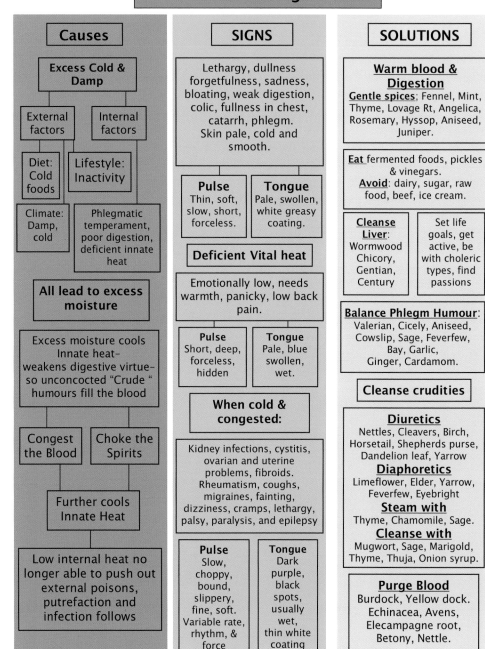

CHAPTER THIRTEEN

Excess of the phlegmatic humour

The phlegmatic humour is cold and damp, its seat is in the lungs, it is held in the watery part of the blood, and it is associated with the expulsive virtue, helping the body to eliminative waste products through urination and defecation. It tends to bring on congestion and stagnation when in excess.

It is strongest in the later part of winter and predominates in old age. The body cools and dries during the middle years meaning that movement and clearance of fluid slows. Consequently, the body becomes more swollen and cold, and therefore likely to suffer from damp, stagnation, and stasis as we enter old age.

Excess of the phlegmatic humour

Inactivity, a cold environment, eating cold foods, and having a phlegmatic temperament can all be the cause of excess phlegm.

The stomach is an organ with a phlegmatic temperament, and so it is easily affected by any increase in coldness and dampness. The reduction of heat in the stomach reduces the appetite and the secretion of gastric juices therefore impeding the breakdown of foods into their constituent parts. This becomes evident in poor digestion, bloating, distension, and colic. When there is excess phlegm in the bowels and intestines this is likely to cause a thick white coating on the tongue, however, this is also present when there is excess phlegm affecting the lungs.

The excess phlegm tends to obstruct the passages of the liver causing blockage and reduces the digestive activity of the liver. By interfering with the concoction of food into humours, blood, tissues, and fluids, this blockage brings on fatigue and lethargy.

As the excess phlegm begins to overwhelm other organs it is most likely to also have the greatest impact on organs that are already cold and damp in temperament such as the lungs, brain, bowels, and joints.

The signs of excess are therefore likely to include excess phlegm and catarrh in the respiratory system, causing blocked sinuses and ears, excess mucous, and coughs. Coldness in the head tends to dull the senses, and may be the cause of migraine, vertigo, palsy, convulsions, and epilepsy. Swollen joints, fluid retention, stiffness of muscles, and cramps may also be apparent. Pelvic congestion may have an impact on both the urinary system and the reproductive system, being the cause of irregular periods, infertility, urinary infections, kidney problems and pelvic inflammation due to stasis. Phlegmatic congestion in the blood reduces the activity of the immune system and the protective innate heat within the vital spirit, allowing infections, discharges, abscesses and a state of putrefaction to take over the body.

The blocking of the vital spirit will bring on sadness and lack of motivation, there will be increased feelings of anxiety due to emotions building up and overwhelming the heart and mind. Passions will be diminished, with the procreative spirit being reduced and dulled. Fatigue, lethargy, sleepiness and listlessness are all common signs of excess phlegm affecting the heart, the spirit, and the brain. It is common for those suffering from excess phlegm to want to avoid difficult and challenging situations and people, literally "not having the stomach for it".

Excess phlegm will show in the skin tending to be cool and damp, a weaker circulation to the extremities, with the pulse being fine, softer, and shorter, and the tongue being pale or bluish. The tongue is likely to have a white greasy coating unless the excess phlegm has reduced the concoctions, meaning that we see a tongue without a coating due to deficiency of innate heat needed to enable digestion.

If the excess phlegm has lead to deficient vital heat we are likely to see the pulse being deeper, shorter, weaker, and slower and the tongue becoming blue or purple, wet and swollen and without a coating. When the vital spirit is reduced in this way the patient is likely to be emotionally low, panicky, suffer lower back pain, and crave warmth.

When the excess phlegm has overwhelmed the body the pulse will become slow, short and irregular and often weak and deep, the tongue is likely to look purple, have dark spots, and only have a thin white coating.

Responding to excess phlegm

Warming the blood and activating the spirit through increasing physical activity, setting life goals, finding choleric, motivated people to spend time with, and developing one's passions will all help. Phlegmatics should eat light, nourishing and warming foods, such as aromatic soups and stews, smaller meals, and include pickles, fermented foods and drinks. It helps to use gentle warming herbs and spices, such as fennel, mint, thyme, lovage, angelica, rosemary, hyssop, aniseed, and juniper. Adding black pepper to meals, not eating late, and avoiding excess diary, sugar, raw foods, and heavy meats, such as beef and pork, is helpful for their weaker digestion.

We can improve the digestion by cleansing and opening the liver with warming bitters, such as wormwood, centaury, gentian, elecampagne, and chicory.

Phlegmatic organs, such as the brain, can be returned to a balanced temperament with the aid of valerian, sage, cowslip, and feverfew, all of which warm the brain and return it to a balanced temperament. The stomach and bowels, which are also phlegmatic, can be warmed with aniseed, sweet cicely, bay, ginger, cardamom and garlic.

We can cleanse the crude humours left behind from poor digestion with diuretics, such as nettles, birch leaf, cleavers, horsetail, shepherd's purse, dandelion leaf, and yarrow. Traditional blood cleansing herbs which also have a diaphoretic effect, such as limeflower, elder, yarrow, feverfew, and eyebright, can be taken. If we need a stronger purging effect to clear the dampness we can use a steam of: thyme, chamomile, sage and juniper. The steams are particularly helpful for clearing phlegm from the lungs, when they can be used as an inhalation mix twice daily. Taking an inhalation of thyme and chamomile when we have a virus clears the head and stops it aching, and cleanses and soothes the respiratory system. If taken before bed it effectively relieves night time coughing. A full body steam will help to clear excess phlegm from the whole system and is very helpful for situations where there is chronic dampness and congestion in any of the organs. It is helpful to include warming and cleansing herbs, such as mugwort, marigold, and sage, in regimes for treating excess phlegm and adding expectorants, such as onion syrup, thyme, and pines such as thuja to help to cut through and clear phlegm from the lungs.

For chronic phlegmatic blockages and the putrefaction which ensues, we can cleanse and purge the blood with nettles, burdock root, yellow dock root, echinaceaelecampagne root, angelica, wood avens, and wood betony.

Case history

A 65-year-old woman presented with pelvic pain, and a long term tendency to cystitis. Her current urinary problem had started two years ago when she had woken in the middle of the night with excruciating lower abdominal pain. She became cold, shivery and was passing urine containing blood and leucocytes. An ultrasound scan showed the possible passing of a kidney stone.

She had continued to experience constant but variable pain, especially in the pelvic region, which was often stabbing in nature, including vaginal and pubic pain and painful urination. There had been repeated tests showing signs of urinary infection, and she had taken four courses of antibiotics over the last three months. She was also prone to coughs, catarrh, and sore throats, and when given antibiotics for respiratory problems she always got a worsening of her urinary symptoms. She had a long term problem with IBS and bloating and had her gall bladder removed five years previously in an attempt to improve things.

Seven years previously, she had a mesh inserted to support the vagina to treat incontinence and has since had generalised pain, which has been diagnosed as fibromyalgia thought to be associated with an immune reaction to the mesh. After a suspected cardiac event five years previously, she was put onto beta blockers and blood pressure pills. However, due to problems with consistent low blood pressure she had begun to reduce them on the doctor's advice. She was generally anxious and depressed, had difficulty sleeping and was always worried that things would get worse, making her feel emotionally overwhelmed all of the time.

She was taking antidepressants, occasional sleeping pills, and had also taken large doses of a sweetened cranberry juice for a long time for the cystitis. She also had a strong cup of peppermint tea three times a day for the last few years as the doctor said it would help her IBS. When she came there was no sign of urinary infection, but a trace of white blood cells in her urine.

Her pulse was soft, weak, short, neither floating nor deep, and slow, all indicating excess phlegm. This was also indicated by a pale, flaccid, broad, and lumpy tongue, which was also without a coating, pointing to the digestive issues, including the loss of the gall bladder reducing the digestive heat and concoctions and leading to a depleted state of the innate heat and vital spirit. Her skin was cold, dampish, and flaccid, which we would also expect in a person with excess phlegm. All of her symptoms were manifesting in phlegmatic organs—the bladder, kidneys, stomach, bowels, throat, and the reproductive organs. Her emotionally overwhelmed and anxious state was also typical of excess phlegm.

To clear the dampness from the urinary system she was given a strong infusion made with 20g of herbs a day, containing cleavers, horsetail, shepherd's purse and oat straw, this was infused and steeped overnight in 500 ml of water. These herbs were given to clear and cleanse the phlegm from the urinary system, with the oat straw included to soothe and soften the membranes. The infusion was backed up by using 20 ml birch juice twice a day; it is warm and dry in the first degree, bringing back the flow and movement of fluids, it clears and dries excess phlegm, dries swellings especially in the bladder, kidneys and joints, and is also antiseptic and pain relieving. A pain tonic made up of a rosehip and willow bark syrup with the addition of guelder rose was given to take in teaspoonful doses up to three times a day. The gentle warmth of the guelder rose helps the digestion, as its gentle bitter properties activate the digestive organs and release spasm. This makes it a useful remedy for colic, indigestion, and IBS. Its anti-inflammatory effects and relaxant properties have lead it to be recommended to help with urinary stones and bladder pain. Willow relieves the pain and heat that arises due to putrefaction and infection, it also dries the excess phlegm and dampness within the tissues. Cider vinegar was also recommended before main meals to aid digestion, and the patient was advised not to take the sweetened cranberry juice but to use a capsule of the powder instead.

Her symptoms improved within a couple of weeks, and when things were going well she had reduced the birch juice to 10 ml twice daily, and the pain tonic to only occasionally as needed. The herbal regime was continued over the following year and a half, by then all the urinary symptoms had cleared, and there was no pelvic pain, although the back and legs sometimes ached and on those days she would still use a single 10 ml dose of the birch juice. She believed that the years of taking large doses of cranberry juice and peppermint tea had been exacerbating the urinary symptoms, and now having followed my advice to stop taking them in that way found that the occasional sip of peppermint tea was adequate to deal with the IBS symptoms when they arose.

She had not needed to take antibiotics for the urinary system for ten months, although she had taken a few doses some months before after having stabbing pains in the vagina after a two week cold/virus. I had advised her to use the urinary system medicinal infusion for a few days and the problems had then resolved. She was generally happier and less anxious and although she still took an antidepressant, she had lowered the dose and hoped to come off of it entirely at some point.

CHAPTER FOURTEEN

Astrology and planetary symbolism

Nicholas Culpeper was an astrologer; his preferred form of diagnosis was to use an astrological decumbiture chart that showed the celestial correspondences at the time of the patient falling ill. The chart's name deriving from the Latin word "decumbere", meaning to lie down.

In classical times there was no division between astronomy and astrology, they were considered two complementary aspects of the same science. They were included in the seven medieval "liberal" arts of grammar, rhetoric, logic, geometry, arithmetic, music and astronomy. By gaining mastery of these disciplines one would gain liberation from ignorance and be led to freedom, and by being conversant in the seven liberal arts one would be equipped to engage fully in civil society.

The philosophical system underpinning Culpeper's astrology had evolved out of the ideas contained in Hermetic philosophy, and it was the cosmological description within this system that provided the language through which he believed the world could best be described. The central concepts within Hermeticism were that the macrocosm of the greater universe is reflected in the microcosm of the world we live in, and that the divine force of god created all the realms of existence. The cosmos was seen as an interconnected system with the earth at its centre, the planets or celestial bodies surrounding it, the angelic realms encircling that, and all of this engulfed in the realm of divine light.

This viewpoint divided the realms created by divine light into these three distinct worlds, each corresponding to an elemental aspect. The divine light corresponds to fire, and each of the three worlds to the three remaining elements; the angelic or "intellectual" realm to air, the "celestial" realm to water and the worldly realm of matter

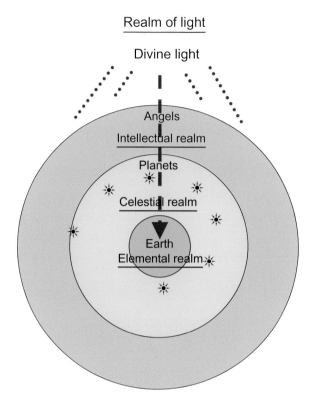

The three worlds

Divine light passes in the ether through the intellectual and celestial realms to the Earth.

1. The Angels exist between the divine realm and the planets, manifesting in the intellectual realm.
2. The Planets exist as celestial bodies that orbit the earth manifesting in the Celestial realm.
3. The Earth exists as the microcosm in the centre, manifesting in the Elemental realm of matter.

The macrocosm/microcosm.

to the earth element. The divine spirit creates, animates, and activates all of the other realms travelling within the medium of ether, the fifth elemental aspect.

Each of the realms govern a variety of cosmological aspects and qualities. The intellectual realm comprises the angels and governs the spirit, mind, and ideas. The celestial realm comprises the planets and governs the soul, the will, and the emotions. The elemental realm comprises the earth itself, and governs the physical body, matter, and sensations.

The planets are the objects that are closest to the divine realm, which can be seen from the earth, and it is therefore by studying them that we can gain the best insight into the activities and intentions of the divine creator. The planets correspond to all the aspects of the earth below, and therefore become a symbolic language that can be used to communicate complex inter-relationships in a simple way. In a time when

Creation

Fire	Ether	Divine light	Realm of light

Air	↓	Angels	World of Spirit	Intellectual Realm
				Mind Ideas
Water	↓	Planets	World of Will	Celestial Realm
				Heart Emotions
Earth	⬇	Earth	World of Matter	Elemental Realm
				Body Sensations

The governance of the three worlds

The Fire element governs the realm of light, and manifests as the source of divine creation.

The Etheric aspect governs the distribution of divine light and holy spirit to all the worlds.

The Air element governs the realm of intellect, and manifests as Spirit, Mind and Ideas.

The Water element governs the realm of celestial bodies, and manifests as Will, Heart and Emotions.

The Earth element governs the realm of the physical elements, and manifests as Matter, Body, and Sensations.

The three worlds.

few people were literate and access to books was limited, such a symbolic language could communicate complex concepts in a way that most people could immediately comprehend. Telling someone that a plant was ruled by a particular planet would indicate the seasons, organs, bodily functions, foods, diseases, and emotions that a plant had a correspondence or alignment with.

By placing the traditional planetary glyphs within the three realms of the three worlds described above, we can symbolically elucidate the relationship of the planet to divine light, and to the three realms of intellect, will, and matter. This shows how their influence is manifested through ideas and the mind, through emotions and the heart, and through the humours in the body.

Through looking at the construction of each of the planetary glyphs we can appreciate the concepts, correspondences and the symbolic meanings of each of the planets and begin to use them for ourselves as a powerful symbolic language that will bring light and understanding into the many ways that the cosmos manifests within and

Mercury

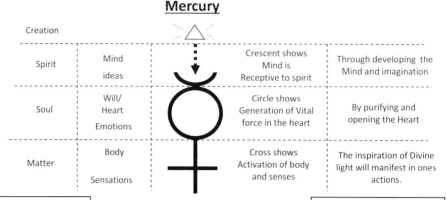

Creation			
Spirit	Mind ideas	Crescent shows Mind is Receptive to spirit	Through developing the Mind and imagination
Soul	Will/ Heart Emotions	Circle shows Generation of Vital force in the heart	By purifying and opening the Heart
Matter	Body Sensations	Cross shows Activation of body and senses	The inspiration of Divine light will manifest in ones actions.

Mercury is cold and dry and governs Ether

This planetary glyph signifies divine spirit moving through Ether, awakening the mind, generating emotions and stimulating actions of the body

Mercurial aspects
The Animal spirit resides in the head, Strengthens the brain, combines the senses (the common sense). Activates the pulse rate and physical movement.

The Animal Spirit is governed by Mercury

Internal virtues of the Animal spirit or the "Intellective and reasoning virtues" Apprehension, Judgement, Memory, Motor functions.
These are called the intellective or reasoning virtues. These consist of the imagination and apprehensions, the discernments and judgements, and the retention and memory of ideas.
This generates the motor functions of the mind, which generate the will or desire to act, and then are executed in the material world through movement and action.

External virtues of the Animal spirit or "The five particular senses": Sight, Smell, Taste, Hearing, Feeling.

The external virtues are called the sensitive virtues, and are aligned to the senses and organs of perception.
These virtues generate the sensory function of the nervous system, through the stimulation of the sense organs, giving rise to Perception and understanding in the mind and generating feelings in the heart.

Associated Diseases
Diseases of the brain, vertigo, madness, stupidity, simplicity.
Antipathetic to Jupiter and the lungs; Asthma, coughs, Hoarseness. T.B.
Diseases of the tongue, stammering, lisps.

Parts of the body
The intellect,
The tongue,
hands and feet.

Symbolic associations
Mind, intellect, reason, common sense.
Hermes, The Muses, Oracles, the Norns, Initiation, prophesy, divination, mysticism, Communication, language, wit, belief, Magic, imagination, stories, invention.
Hypnogogic insights.

Herbs ruled by Mercury
Elecampagne, Fennel, Lavender, Lily of the Valley, liquorice, Senna, Valerian, White horehound, wild carrot.
Sweet smelling herbs refresh animal spirits.

around us. The glyph for Mercury is a good starting point as it transits all three realms and represents the movement of ether from the realm of divine light to the realm of matter. By studying it we can become familiar with the connections and correspondences between the realms and the planets.

Mercury

Mercury is symbolic of divine enlightenment coming into manifestation in the world of matter, showing that by developing our minds, opening and purifying the heart we will become divinely inspired and guided.

The glyph for mercury transits all of the three worlds, showing how it is the etheric elemental aspect that connects and provides communication and continuity between all the cosmic realms. It shows how the divine force travels through ether to activate and give life to the mind, the heart, and the body.

Mercury is cold and dry and governs the animal spirit, which resides in the head. It governs the five external virtues or senses of sight, smell, taste, hearing, and feeling, while also governing the internal virtues or intellective and reasoning virtues of apprehension, judgement, memory, and the bodily motor functions. Anatomically, Mercury is associated with the tongue, the intellect, the hands and feet.

When out of balance Mercury is associated with diseases of the brain, vertigo, madness, stupidity, and simplicity. It is generally anti-pathetical to Jupiter and the lungs; therefore potentially causes asthma, coughs, hoarseness, afflictions of the tongue, stammering, and lisps.

Symbolic associations for mercury

Mind, intellect, reason, common sense, the god Hermes, the muses, the ancient oracles, the Norns. Mercury also governs initiation, prophesy, divination, mysticism, communication, language, wit, belief, magic, imagination, stories, invention, and hypnogogic insights.

Herbs ruled by mercury

Elecampagne, fennel, lavender, lily of the valley, liquorice, senna, valerian, white horehound, wild carrot, sweet smelling herbs and aromatic waters that refresh and revive the animal spirits.

The sun

The planetary glyph for the sun shows the descent of divine light to the heart, travelling within the ether. Divine light travels through the realm of spirit into the realm of the soul where it manifests in the heart as will. It then emanates as emotions, which in

Sun

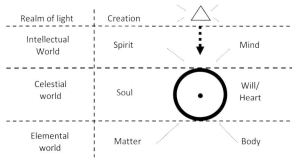

Realm of light	Creation	
Intellectual World	Spirit	Mind
Celestial world	Soul	Will/ Heart
Elemental world	Matter	Body

Descent of soul from realm of light, through intellectual world

Into the celestial vehicle of the heart,
Radiates light of spirit to all three worlds/realms.

Innate heat, desires, apprehensive faculty.

The glyph shows the descent of soul from the realm of light into the celestial vehicle of the heart.

Sun is Hot and Dry and governs the Choleric Humour with Mars

Associated Diseases
When the heat of the Sun or Mars disperses the Vital spirit, it can be the cause of infection, fever and fainting. Also heartburn, sore eyes.
N.Culpeper:
The Sun causes "all diseases of the Heart and Brain...and the nerves and arteries".

Nicholas Culpeper:
"The Vital spirit hath its residence in the heart, and is dispersed from it by the Arteries: and is governed by the influence of the Sun. And it is to the body, as the sun is to creation; as the heart is in the Microcosm, so is the Sun in the Megacosm. For the Sun gives life, light and motion to the Creation, so doth the heart to the body. Therefore it is called Sol Corporalis (The Sun of the body), as the Sun is called Cor Coeli (The heart of the heaven), because their opera-tions are similar,"
- N. Culpeper, Complete Herbal and English physician enlarged, 1843, p.212

Vital Spirit/Innate heat
Resides in heart

The Innate heat.
The vital spirit travels around the body in the arteries activating and motivating the organs. The vapours that arise in the heart as emotions travel to the brain and become the source and initiators of thoughts. It is the Innate heat in the vital Spirit which moves the Blood. Heat defines life, it produces movement and warmth in living organisms, objects without life are static and cold. The Innate heat in the vital spirit attracts and apprehends the living essence within air, food, and the space around us to join the dance of life in the body. Innate heat is thus the warmth of life, and resides within us as long as we are living. The innate heat is originally passed to the baby in the sperm, and is fed by pneuma in the air.

Herbs ruled by the Sun
Angelica, Ash, Bay, Centaury, Chamomile,
Cinnamon, Eyebright, Juniper, Marigold, St Johns Wort, Rosemary, Tormentil.
Spices refresh Vital spirits

Sun aspects
The Vital Spirit, the Innate heat, the distribution of Pneuma/ life force, the sight, it moves blood, it activates the Digestive, retentive, expulsive and apprehensive faculties.
It is Inner illumination, the dot is the source of light/God, that has descended from the realm of light through the intellectual realm into the celestial realm and the Celestial vehicle of the heart and the emotional body. It resides there as the Soul, holding the potential for continual inner illumination.

Parts of the body
The heart The eyes, esp the right eye. The pulse strength/ length. A short weak pulse, indicates weak Innate heat, weak heart or lungs.

Symbolic associations
Summer, adulthood, love, singing, soul, heart, charisma, strength, creativity originality, generosity, glory, authority, gold, Father.
Fire, heat, energy, maleness. Dominance, pride, vanity, drought, exhaustion.
In certain circumstances the Sun is considered a minor malefic planet.

the realm of intellect manifest as ideas, and in the elemental realm of matter manifest as the motivating factor behind actions.

The heart is shown as manifesting at the level of the celestial world, indicating its role as the celestial vehicle of the soul. The circle is the heart, and the dot is the sun representing the divine light within us. The heart is the seat of the will and it is from where emotions emanate. Emotions are thus the most direct connection that we have with the soul of a person, expressed most strongly through the emotion of love.

The sun is hot and dry in quality and it governs the vital spirit, providing the warmth of life and the activating energy of the innate heat. The innate heat gives life to the organs and provides life energy for the bodily virtues or spirits and the faculties of apprehension, digestion and elimination.

The sun rules the heart and the eyes, in particular the right eye in men, and the left eye in women. The sun can be a minor malefic planet when it causes excess heat in the body, leading to the vital spirit becoming too dispersed and refined and therefore weakening its strength. Excess heat can also lead to fevers, rage, anger, inflammations, itching and agitation, heartburn, and fainting. Culpeper says that the sun "causes all diseases of the heart and brain and the nerves and arteries" (Tobyn, 1997).[1]

Symbolic associations for the sun

Summer, adulthood, soul, heart, love, gold, fire, father, heat, energy, authority, charisma, strength, creativity, singing, originality, generosity, glory, maleness, dominance, pride, vanity, drought, exhaustion.

Herbs ruled by the sun

Angelica, ash, bay, centaury, chamomile, cinnamon, eyebright, juniper, marigold, St John's wort, rosemary, tormentil. Spices refresh vital spirits.

The moon

The planetary glyph shows divine light being received into the crescent of the moon in the realm of intellect, entering the mind as ideas, inspirations, intuitions, and dreams. The crescent of the moon is open to the heavenly realms, showing it as the receptacle of divine waters in a similar way to the heart being the container of the divine light. The divine waters provide the medium of flow for the emotions, helping to distribute the innate heat of the sun around the body, cooling its potentially scorching impact and balancing its heat. This allows divine motivation to flow to the realm of intellect and manifest as ideas, and to flow into the elemental realm of matter as the emotional motivation for action.

Moon

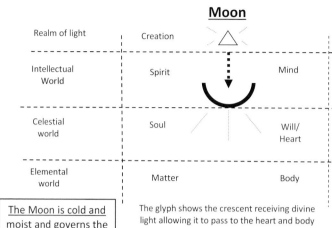

Realm of light	Creation		
Intellectual World	Spirit	Mind	Reception by the mind of Ideas descending from the realm of light, and the Soul.
Celestial world	Soul	Will/ Heart	The reception of ideas into the mind pass to the celestial vehicle of the heart, causing the movement of emotions.
Elemental world	Matter	Body	The Emotions influence and move the humours

The glyph shows the crescent receiving divine light allowing it to pass to the heart and body causing the arising of emotions.

The Moon is cold and moist and governs the phlegmatic humour with Venus

Parts of the body
The Brain, the senses, the stomach, bowels, bladder, the eyes, esp left eye, the skin, the "Rheumatics".

Associated Diseases
All cold and rheumatic diseases, Fluid retention, dropsies, oedema, discharges and abscesses. Coughs, Excess mucous from lungs. Lethargy, Palsy, convulsions and epilepsy from phlegm obstructing the Animal spirit. Cold causes Cramps and Colic. The Moon causes excess and absent menstruation, cyclical, and recurrent diseases. Fevers due to cold and moist diminishing Innate heat and

Herbs ruled by the Moon
Cleavers, chaste tree, chickweed, Lettuce, Willow, Moonwort.

Vital Spirit/Radical Moisture
Resides in heart

The Radical Moisture.
The Radical Moisture originally comes from the waters of the womb in which the baby grows, it is then continually replenished throughout life by the breakdown of foods in what is known as the third concoction during digestion. The Innate heat in the vital spirit is balanced and moderated by the Radical moisture. In the same way that the innate heat is governed by the Sun, the Radical moisture is governed by the Moon, in conjunction with the planet Venus. Thus the masculine active, forcing, qualities of the Sun are complemented, calmed and cooled by the feminine, moist, flowing and distributive qualities of Venus and the Moon. These planets are feminine energies that embody the flow of life, and the fertility brought by water. The light of the sun alone is not enough to give life, life can only occur where there is also water, and also where the opposites of hot and cold, moist and dry, light and dark are in balance. The radical moisture enables the vital spirit to move and flow around the body, distributing its life force to the organs without scorching or damaging them through excessive heat.

Nicholas Culpeper:
"As the water moistens the Earth, that so it might not be burnt up by the scorching of heat of the Celestial Sun, so the Microcosmical Moon adds moisture to the conception from the very beginning of the embrion, even to the utmost term of life. And this is what they call Radical Moisture, a term familiar enough amongst all Physitians, yet understood by few."Culpeper's Midwife Enlarged (1676) bk2 sect2.

Attributes
The Radical moisture, the physical senses and emotions. The Expulsive faculty.

The Expulsive Faculty
The Expulsive faculty resides in the kidneys, bowels and the lungs. Heat digests, and cool condenses, moves, and expels waste.
Nicholas Culpeper:
"The Expulsive virtue casteth out, and expelleth what is superflouous by digestion... The Expulsive faculty is cold and moist; cold, because that compresseth the superfluities; moist because that makes the body slippery and fit for ejection, and disposeth it to it."

Symbolic associations
Receptivity, emotions, sadness, softness, water, adaption, tolerance, cleansing, catharsis, flow, dreams, visions, night-time, sluggishness, laziness, reflection, feelings, moods. Mother, feminine, fertility, cycles, affection, sentiment, divination, physic, premonition, myth, poetry, rhythm, glamour, magic spells, witches, wisdom, aging.

The moon is cold and moist in quality and governs the radical moisture within the body, which balances and facilitates the flow of the innate heat in the vital spirit. The radical moisture has been received by the embryo in the waters of the womb, and it is replenished by the residues of the third concoction of the digestive faculty.

The moon governs the expulsive faculty, which resides in the kidneys, bowels and the lungs, bringing together and making smooth all that is superfluous to digestion so that it can be expelled. The moon governs the brain, the senses, the stomach, the bowels and the bladder, as well as the left eye, the skin, and the rheumatics. The moon also shares governance of the phlegmatic humour with Venus as both are associated with the water element.

Diseases associated with the moon

All cold and rheumatic diseases, fluid retention, dropsies, oedema, discharges, and abscesses. Coughs, excess mucous from lungs, lethargy, palsy, convulsions and epilepsy from phlegm obstructing the animal spirit in the brain and nerves. Cold causes cramps and colic. The moon causes excess and absent menstruation, cyclical, and recurrent diseases, and may lead to the development of fevers due to cold and moist diminishing the innate heat and the vital spirit, thus allowing external poisons to enter.

Symbolic associations for the moon

Receptivity, emotions, sadness, softness, water, flow, cleansing, adaption, tolerance, catharsis, dreams, visions, night-time, sluggishness, laziness, reflection, feelings, moods. Mother, feminine, fertility, cycles, affection, sentiment, divination, psychic, premonition, myth, poetry, rhythm, glamour, magic spells, witches, wisdom, and aging.

Herbs ruled by the moon

Cleavers, chaste tree, chickweed, lettuce, willow, moonwort.

Jupiter

The glyph for Jupiter shows the heart as a crescent, open to the light of divine inspiration. This open crescent sits in the celestial realm of the heart, will, and the emotions, and transforms this direct experience of the divine entering the heart into action. This is indicated by the cross of the elements, which is depicted in the lower elemental realm of matter. This corresponds with the observation that people with a sanguine temperament, which is ruled by Jupiter, will commonly act directly out of their

Jupiter

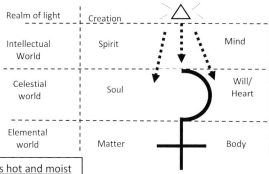

| Realm of light | Creation | |
| Intellectual World | Spirit | Mind |

Divine inspiration goes straight to the heart, they feel before they think.

| Celestial world | Soul | Will/ Heart |

Soul open to intuitions from the intellectual world, the sky gods, ancestors, Angels.

| Elemental world | Matter | Body |

Inspiration brought into the Material World, causing growth and expansion.

This planetary glyph signifies divine wisdom entering the heart bringing divine guidance into the material world.

Jupiter is hot and moist and Governs the Sanguine humour and the Natural Spirit

---

Sanguine Temperament
EMBRACING
Joyful, valiant, friendly, liberal, anxious. Arrogant, addictive. Middling, largish, fleshy. Appetite & digestion good. Body hairy, hair brown/flaxen.
Skin hot, moist, smooth, soft. Pulse full, floating & great.

Nicholas Culpeper:
"A Man or woman in whose body heat and moisture abounds, is said to be Sanguine of Complexion. Such are usually of a middle stature, strong composed bodies, fleshy but not fat, great veins, smooth skins, hot and moist in feeling... There is a redness intermingled with white in their cheeks,... Their pulse great and full. They dream of red things and merry conceits. As for their conditions, they are merry, cheerful creatures, bountiful, pitiful, merciful, courteous, bold, trusty, given to the games of Venus. A little thing will make them weep, but so soon as'tis over; no fur-thergrief sticks to their hearts"
Culpeper; Art of Physic, C.59

Christopher Hedley:
"They always get the best press in this society because they tend to do most of the writing. They tend to worry about their health and respond to authoritative direction."

Natural Spirit/Digestive Virtue Resides in Liver

The Natural Spirit
In the presence of innate heat the natural spirit in the liver activates the digestive virtue making the four humours from the chyle in the 2nd concoction. The liver "breeds blood" from the crude humours or elements in the food we eat, refining them into pure humours that are full of nourishment and clear of poisons and base residues. The natural spirit enables the sensation of taste to discern which food is congruous for the liver to make the blood and the humours. If the natural spirit and the liver are strong our ability to discern the correct foods works well, when the appetite will match the needs of the body. The Natural Spirit also activates the discerning part of the brain, the part which makes judgements, discerning the beneficial from the malign, refining our thoughts and ideas from the undifferentiated perceptions which flow into the mind from the senses.

Avoid;
Excess of all kinds, being too dispersed and scattered.
Take;
Beer and cider, Watery soups, Pickles, Fish, wild meats, summer fruits. Regular exercise, co-operative sporting activity. Singing, writing creative expression. Regular meals, Find long term partner and friends.
Useful Herbs:
Chamomile, Linden, Oats, Yarrow, Elderflower. -Milk thistle,
Dandelion for liver.

Jupiter aspects
The Natural Spirit, the digestive virtue, taste, the liver, lungs and ribs, the veins, inhalation, Judgement.

Signs of Excess
Head full of confused thoughts, obsession and anxiety, inflammatory conditions, skin hot and itchy, allergies, Mouth ulcers, boils, red swollen face, heavy body, easily tired.

Associated Diseases
All infirmities of the Liver and veins, Lung disease, pleurisy. Leads to putrefaction, Spring fevers, quinsy's.

Symbolic associations
Youth, Spring, Aspiration, justice, judgement, initiative, expansion, faith, confidence, spirituality, prophesy, vision, belief, communication, Optimism, tolerance, vanity, obsession, addiction, thunder, altruism, compassion, gluttony, Joy.

Herbs ruled by Jupiter
Agrimony, Asparagus, Avens, Balm, Borage, Chestnuts, Dandelion, Dock, Lime tree, Lovage, Hyssop, Meadowsweet, Red Roses, Sage.
Milk thistle.

emotions, and usually do so before they think about the consequences of what they are saying or doing. However, when in alignment with the divine light these emanations from the heart will bring divine guidance into the elemental world of matter, leading to growth, expansion, and the spread of enlightenment.

Jupiter is thus referred to as the "royal" planet, as like royalty it represents the divine guidance placed in the heart of the nation, directing the activity of its citizens. It is the planet of protection, judgement, and expansion, its rulership extends over the liver, the seat of the natural spirit. It rules the chest, lungs, and ribs, having a particular connection to the expansion of the lungs, which enables the inspiration of life-giving pneuma into the body, thus feeding the innate heat and vital spirit. Jupiter rules the liver and the digestive faculty, which transforms the chyle from the stomach into its four constituent humours during the concoctions. The humours themselves are then transported in the hepatic veins to the heart where they are then distributed to the organs.

Jupiter is associated with the sanguine temperament, youthfulness, spring, and growth. When in excess it causes a head full of confused thoughts, obsession and anxiety, inflammatory conditions, hot and itchy skin, allergies, mouth ulcers, boils, red swollen face, a heavy feeling in the body, and makes one prone to fatigue.

It is associated with diseases of the lungs, liver, and veins, also fevers; especially in the spring, quinsy and sore throats, it can lead to states of excess damp heat and putrefaction leading to infections and epidemics.

The sanguine personality should avoid excess of all kinds and being too dispersed and scattered. They benefit from taking watery soups, pickles, fish, wild meats, summer fruits and eating regular meals. It is better for them to drink beer and cider rather than wine and spirits. They should follow a regime of regular exercise, ideally including a co-operative sporting activity, which they will enjoy immensely. It is good for them to sing, have forms of creative expression, such as writing or painting, and to commit to a long term partner and also to find dependable, sensible, and solid melancholic friends. Useful herbs are calming and centring herbs such as chamomile, lime flower, and oats. They benefit from cleansing and drying herbs, such as yarrow and elderflower in the spring and summer, and to use cleansing blood tonics such as nettles, chicory, and cleavers at the end of the winter. They benefit from nourishing the liver with herbs such as milk thistle, dandelion and artichokes.

Symbolic associations for jupiter

Youth, spring, aspiration, justice, judgement, initiative, expansion, faith, confidence, spirituality, prophesy, vision, belief, communication, optimism, tolerance, vanity, obsession, addiction, compassion, gluttony, joyfulness, thunder, altruism.

Herbs ruled by jupiter

Agrimony, asparagus, avens, balm, borage, chestnuts, dandelion, dock, lime tree, lovage, hyssop, meadowsweet, red roses, sages, milk thistle.

Mars

The planetary glyph shows the cross of matter residing in the intellectual realm, and the circle of the heart beneath it in the celestial realm. The cross of matter in this position blocks the direct light of divine wisdom from the heart, meaning that the heart is shut off from divine love and vision. The circle of the heart is shown in the realm of the will and emotions. This indicates that without divine guidance the will drives the ideas and the intellect, and the cross of matter extending upwards into the realm of intellect shows that there is a pursuit of worldly ideals and objectives above all else. Without any connection to the elemental realm beneath, Mars is insulated from the influences of others in the worldly realm indicating a primary focus on the self. Mars therefore challenges spirituality, blocks divine inspiration, and puts the worldly elemental realm at the top and in the position of control and influence.

Mars is hot and dry in quality and governs the choleric humour that has its seat in the gall bladder. It also governs the attractive or apprehensive virtue in the body, which has the role of drawing out the essence from food, air, and water. It is also that which enables us to perceive sensory information and ideas, apprehending them and manifesting them as visions and thoughts in the brain.

Those ruled by the choleric humour are striving, fast, quick-witted, impetuous, and often quarrelsome. They make good soldiers responding well to discipline and benefit from having short-term goals and respond well to authority.

Excess choler manifests as feeling hot, sweaty, thirsty, having acidity, nausea, being constipated, experiencing skin problems, acne, carbuncles, shingles, fevers, being irritable, having sudden anger, frenzy, fury, poor sleep, migraines, sudden pain, bladder and kidney blockage and stones.

The choleric should avoid fatty and spicy foods, fatty meat, salty and dry foods, stimulants, alcoholic spirits, excess wine and excess competitive activities, but avoid forced inactivity as that may cause them to become depressed. They should take fish and wild meats, beer and cider, soups with barley, summer fruits, sufficient water, regular exercise and do regular short cleansing regimes or fasts. Cholerics appreciate discipline, benefit from having clear short-term projects and working towards achievable goals.

Useful herbs for the choleric include cooling and softening herbs, such as rose, violets, plantain, mallows, and hibiscus. Herbs that clear heat from the liver and digestion, such as hops, wormwood, meadowsweet, dandelion, dock, and rhubarb. Herbs that clear heat from the skin, such as burdock root, melissa, violets and echinacea.

Mars

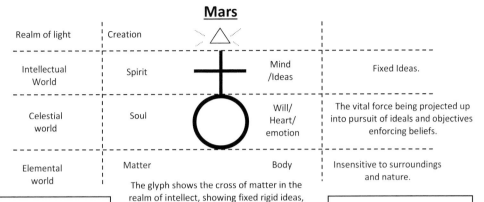

Realm of light	Creation			
Intellectual World	Spirit		Mind /Ideas	Fixed Ideas.
Celestial world	Soul		Will/ Heart/ emotion	The vital force being projected up into pursuit of ideals and objectives enforcing beliefs.
Elemental world	Matter		Body	Insensitive to surroundings and nature.

The glyph shows the cross of matter in the realm of intellect, showing fixed rigid ideas, which block the reception by the heart of the divine inspiration.

Mars is hot and dry and governs the Choleric Humour and the attractive virtue

Choleric Temperament
STRIVING
Angry, sharp, driven, fast. Intolerant, passionate, generous, direct, active. Digestion is quiet but good, leans toward constipation. Hair red, yellow, more curly.
Body often hairy, Short and lean, skin hot dry & rough. Pulse swift, hard, floating.

Nicholas Culpeper:
"Such persons are usually short of stature, and not fat, it may be because the heat and dryness of their bodies consumes radical moisture... They are naturally quick witted, bold, no way shame faced, furious, hasty, quarrelsome, fraudulent, eloquent, courageous, stout-hearted creatures, not given to sleep much but much given to jesting, mocking and lying."
N Culpeper, The Art of Physic, ch. 59

Christopher Hedley:
"I don't see many sick Choleric people. They notably hate being ill, are dreadful patients and cut out the memory of previous illnesses. They respond to discipline, direction and clearly stated, short term goals."

Attractive/ apprehensive virtue
Resides in Gall Bladder

The attractive/apprehensive virtue
The Apprehensive virtue, the word coming from the Greek verb Apairo, meaning to take hold of or to bring an essence out of something. This attractive or apprehensive quality is what enables the Vital spirit to capture the life force from the air and foods we eat. It enables the "Natural" spirit in the liver to digest the four elements in food, providing the basis for the four humours which nourish the organs and tissues. It enables the Animating spirit in the brain to apprehend ideas from the senses and from the emotions, and to retrieve memories. It gives heat and passion to the procreative force, producing and lust, attraction and desire.

Avoid; Fatty and spicy foods, fatty meat, salty and dry foods, stimulants, alcoholic spirits, excess wine and excess competitive activities, but avoid forced inactivity– will cause depression.
Take; Fish and wild meats, beer and cider, soups with barley, summer fruits, sufficient water, regular exercise. Regular short cleansing regimes/fasts. Cholerics appreciate discipline, benefit from having clear short term projects.
Useful Herbs: Cooling and softening herbs; Rose, Violets, Plantain, Mallows, hibiscus.
Herbs that clear heat from Liver/digestion; Hops, wormwood, meadowsweet, dandelion, dock, rhubarb.
Herbs that clear heat from the skin; Burdock Rt, Melissa, Echinacea.
Herbs that clear heat from the Blood: Nettle, cleavers, dock, boneset, clover.

Mars aspects
The Attractive faculty.
The Choleric humour, resides in the gall bladder. Mars governs the sense of smell.

Signs of Excess
Feels hot, sweaty, thirsty, acidity, nausea, constipated, irritable, skin problems, acne, carbuncles, sudden anger, fevers, shingles, frenzy, fury, poor sleep, bladder & kidney blockage & stones.

Associated Diseases
All diseases of choler; fevers, carbuncles, shingles, anger, affects the brain by antipathy, frenzy, fury, sudden pain/ migraine from heat. Also antipathetic to kidneys and bladder, causing inflammation, pain, blockage.

Symbolic associations
Adulthood, Summer, Power, force, valour, action, drive, masculinity, resistance, argument, brutality, war, murder, aggression, attack, stubbornness, sport, muscles, assertion, argument, fever, rashes, bile.

Herbs ruled by Mars
Broom, basil, garlic, gentian, ginger, hawthorn, hops, mustard, nettle, rocket, rhubarb, wormwood, Vitex agnus castus, blessed thistle, thistles in general.

Herbs that clear heat from the blood, such as nettle, cleavers, dock, boneset, and red clover.

Symbolic associations for mars

Adulthood, summer, power, force, valour, action, drive, masculinity, resistance, argument, brutality, war, murder, aggression, attack, stubbornness, sport, muscles, assertion, argument, fever, rashes, bile.

Herbs ruled by mars

Broom, basil, garlic, gentian, ginger, hawthorn, hops, mustard, nettle, rocket, rhubarb, wormwood, blessed thistle, thistles in general.

Venus

The planetary glyph shows divine light passing straight to the heart, stimulating emotion and becoming the driving force of actions. Without being processed in the realm of ideas, and unadulterated by thoughts or doubts, the goddess Venus fills the heart with love, compassion, and divine wisdom. The cross of matter well founded in the elemental world shows the possibility of that love being manifested in the creation of new life on earth, and also shows the powerful influence love and compassion can have in the material world. However, without the influence of the intellectual realm, the powerful emotions stirred up by love can also result in blind and unconsidered actions—"love is blind".

Venus rules the kidneys, throat, breasts, the reproductive and urinary system. She governs the phlegmatic humour and the procreative spirit. The procreative spirit requires both warmth and moisture to bring about new life, the warmth giving passion and the moistness enabling fertility. The phlegmatic humour is flowing, accepting, connecting and moving. However, phlegmatics can also be slow and lazy, anxious and fearful, and become overwhelmed by emotions unable to fully digest and absorb life situations. They can be reticent, and often indecisive, rather like the classic English temperament.

Signs of excess phlegmatic humour include; lethargy, palsy, convulsions and epilepsy from phlegm obstructing the animal spirit, weight gain, poor digestion, bloating, excess mucous, coughs, blocked sinuses, pelvic and urinary congestion, kidney infections, cystitis, ovarian and uterine problems, fibroids, venereal diseases. All cold and rheumatic diseases, fluid retention, dropsies, oedema, discharges and abscesses, cold may be the cause of cramps and colic.

Phlegmatics should avoid excess sleep, eating too much, a diet rich in dairy products, sweet foods, fish, (except with warming herbs), raw foods, salads, except with

Venus

Realm of light	Creation		
Intellectual World	Spirit	Mind / Ideas	Lack of reception of ideas; "Love is blind!"
Celestial world	Soul	Will/ Heart emotion	The vital force being held in the heart passing down to the realm of matter.
Elemental world	Matter	Body	From Love all is created, Emotions become manifested in action.

The glyph shows divine light passing straight to the heart, activating emotions without thought, love directly motivating actions.

Venus is cold and moist and rules the phlegmatic Humour

Phlegmatic Temperament
ACCEPTING
Tolerant, dreamy, relaxed, empathetic, sad, persistent, enchanting, reflective, sentimental. Digestion cold & weaker. Shorter, fatter. Body hairless, Straighter light brown /flaxen hair. Skin cold, moist & smooth. Pulse slower, thinner, softer.

Nicholas Culpeper:
" They are dull, heavy and sloth-ful... Not usually very tall, appetite and digestion is very weak in them, veins and arteries are small, their bodies usually without hair, their pulse little and low."
N Culpeper, "Art of Physic" p59

Christopher Hedley:
"They are prone to poor digestion [on all levels] mucus accumulation and lethargy. Water is cold and wet, passive, pale and practical. The classic "English Temperament" is Phlegmatic– from living in a cold and damp place."

Procreative Spirit
Resides in Womb/Testes

The procreative Spirit,
Resides in the testes of men and in the ovaries and the womb of women. It is the energy of reproduction, and produces in us the desire to procreate. It is under the governance of the Venus, and is warm and moist in character. Venus is the planet of fertility, love, romance, dreams, emotions. The procreative Spirit is strengthened by Venus and the herbs that work in sympathy with her, whilst it is diminished and dulled by the cold drying effect of Saturn and the earth humour, and weakened by Mars and the Choleric or fire humour.

Avoid; Excess Sleep, eating too much, dairy products, sweet foods, fish, (except with warming herbs), raw foods, salads, except with spicy dressings.
Take; Warming foods, artichokes, root vegetables, onions and Garlic, spices, pickles, Regular exercise, avoid getting emotionally caught up and overwhelmed, find creative emotional expression.
Useful Herbs: Thyme, sage, rosemary, Gentle Spices, elderflowers, cleavers, mint and Nettles. Cleanse in the spring, warm in the winter.

Venus aspects
The Kidneys, throat, breasts. The Reproductive and urinary system.

Signs of excess phlegmatic humour
Lethargy, Palsy, Convulsions and epilepsy from phlegm obstructing the Animal spirit. Weight gain, poor digestion, bloating, excess mucous.

Associated diseases
Coughs, blocked sinuses, pelvic & urinary congestion, kidney infections, cystitis, ovarian and uterine problems, fibroids, venereal diseases. All cold and rheumatic diseases, fluid retention, dropsies, oedema, discharges and abscesses, Cold causes Cramps and Colic.

Symbolic associations
Romance, dreams, poetry, attachment, tranquillity, sensuality, fertility, moistness, emotions, Pleasure, sensuality, femininity, mother, fortune, money, winter becoming spring, old age leading to rebirth.

Herbs ruled by Venus
Burdock, Cherries, Viburnums, Cow-slip, Elderflower, Feverfew, Lady's mantle, Mallows, Mints, Motherwort, Mugwort, Plantain, Roses, Vervain, Violets, Yarrow.

spicy dressings and warming foods such as watercress, rocket, and spring onions. They benefit from taking warming foods, including artichokes, root vegetables, onions and garlic, spices, pickles, and black pepper, in their meals. They should regularly exercise, especially when it includes gentle cardiovascular challenges, such as hill walking, they must avoid getting emotionally caught up and overwhelmed, and find creative ways of regularly expressing their emotions.

Useful herbs for phlegmatics include; thyme, sage, and rosemary, all gentle spices such as coriander, cardamom, and cumin, teas of elderflowers, mint, and fennel. They should cleanse in the spring with cleavers and nettles, and warm in the autumn with elderberries, hyssop, juniper, angelica, and thyme.

Symbolic associations for venus

Romance, dreams, poetry, attachment, tranquillity, sensuality, fertility, moistness, emotions, pleasure, sensuality, femininity, mother, fortune, money, winter becoming spring, old age leading to rebirth.

Herbs ruled by venus

Burdock, cherries, viburnums, cowslip, white deadnettle, elderflower, feverfew, lady's mantle, mallows, mints, motherwort, mugwort, plantain, white, yellow, and pink roses, vervain, violets, yarrow.

Saturn

The planetary glyph for Saturn shows the cross of matter in the intellectual realm. This shows that material and worldly concerns are elevated to the highest realm in Saturn and also in the melancholic people it rules. The cross of matter in this position blocks divine light and warmth from reaching the heart, suppressing passions and motivations and keeping the heart cold. In the Saturn glyph the crescent of the moon is in the celestial realm of the heart, showing that although the heart is receptive and open, it is only fed by material considerations rather than divine ones. By having the crescent moon in the central position, Saturn lacks the benefit of any heat or warmth, indicating its cool receptive and accepting nature. The Mars glyph is similar, as it also has the cross of matter in the intellectual realm, but by having the sun in the celestial realm instead of the moon the nature of Mars is the opposite of Saturn: hot, active, and forceful.

Saturn rules the melancholic humour and the retentive virtue, and the spleen is the seat of both. It also rules the bones, the teeth, the memory, and the sense of hearing. Melancholics are solitary, studious, and deep thinkers, they are dependable, loyal, and true. They tend to hold onto things, find change difficult and are therefore often fearful and pessimistic about the future. They have weaker digestions and are more likely to suffer from a colder circulation.

Saturn

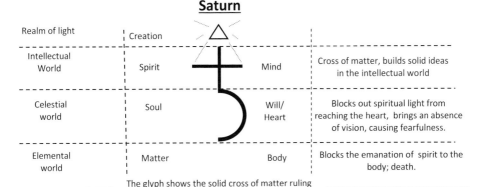

Realm of light	Creation		
Intellectual World	Spirit	Mind	Cross of matter, builds solid ideas in the intellectual world
Celestial world	Soul	Will/ Heart	Blocks out spiritual light from reaching the heart, brings an absence of vision, causing fearfulness.
Elemental world	Matter	Body	Blocks the emanation of spirit to the body; death.

The glyph shows the solid cross of matter ruling the intellectual realm, blocking divine light from the receptive crescent in the celestial realm.

Saturn is cold and dry and rules the Melancholic Humour and the retentive virtue

Melancholic Temperament
CONSIDERING
Solitary, studious, conservative, truthful, Loyal
Grounded, Fearful.
Middling in stature, slender, long face.
Slow digestion, brown, curly hair. Body hairless.
Skin cold and dry.
Pulse; slow deep narrow.
Tongue; flaccid, broad, pale or purplish, have a thin white coating or no coating.

Nicholas Culpeper:
"superfluous melancholy causes care, fear, sadness, despair, envy, and many evils besides"

Christopher Hedley:
"They are prone to getting blocked and stuck, but at least they will hang in there!"

Retentive Virtue
Resides in Spleen

The Spleen
The spleen is the seat of the melancholic humour, melancholy is the natural excrement of blood, the thick earthy part, the cold and dry residue of the fourth concoction. The spleen is also the seat of the retentive virtue, keeping all that is wholesome in the blood and tissues.
Excessive Melancholy affects the heart as melancholic vapours rise up from the blocked spleen Thus melancholy influences stopping the flow of vitality and emotion from the heart this bringing on palpitations and irregular heart beats as well as emotional upset, anxiety and fearfulness.

Avoid: Large meals, heavy foods (Beef), eating too late in day, Lack of activity, thinking too much, Introspection.
Take: Light nourishing foods; soft cheeses, shellfish, eggs, lamb, olive oil, root veg, Squash, dried fruit. Cleansing foods; Asparagus, celery, fennel. Take gentle exercise, long walks, have a productive long term project, find Exuberant "Sanguine" friends.
Useful herbs; Gently Warming:
Fennel, Angelica, Lovage, Black pepper, Sage, Cardamom, Coriander.
For the heart:
Melissa, Motherwort, Borage.
For Anxiety;
Valerian, Lime flower, Cowslip, Rose.

Saturn aspects
The Sediment of the blood, The retentive faculty, the memory, the spleen, the bones, the teeth, the ears and hearing.

Signs of Excess
Fatigue, poor appetite and digestion, cold sweats, irregular heart beat, anxiety and cold extremities. Liver congestion, bitter belching, stiff painful joints, aching back and hips, itchy skin.

Associated Diseases
Chronic disease, All diseases of melancholy, cold and dryness; madness caused by fear and grief. Bone pains, gout, toothache, deafness. Cold blocks can cause palsies, migraines, impotence,

Symbolic associations
Solidity, the development of theories, laws, science, plans, resolution, responsibility, dependability, autumn, middle age, restriction, repression, secrecy, pessimism.

Herbs ruled by Saturn
Cornflower, Comfrey, fumitory, Heartsease, Horsetail, Mullein, Shepherds purse, Melancholy thistle.

Planet	Humour	Quality	1. **Parts of the body** 2. **Attributes**
Mercury	Ether Space Animal Spirit	Cold and dry	1. The intellect. The tongue, hands and feet. 2. The Animal spirit, Strengthens the brain, The combining of the senses (the common sense). The pulse rate. Physical movement.
Sun	Choler Fire Innate heat	Hot and dry	1. The Heart, the arteries, the eyes, esp. the right eye. The pulse strength. 2. The Vital Spirit, the Innate heat, the Pneuma, the sight, moves blood, activates the Digestive, retentive, expulsive and apprehensive faculties.
Moon	Phlegm Water Radical moisture	Cold and moist	1. The Brain, the senses, the stomach, bowels, bladder, the eyes, esp left eye, The Skin. The "Rheumatics". 2. The Radical moisture, the physical senses and emotions. The Expulsive faculty.
Jupiter	Sanguine Air/Blood Natural Spirit	Hot and moist	1. The liver, lungs and ribs, the veins. Inhalation. 2. The Natural Spirit, the digestive faculty, taste, Judgement.
Mars	Choler Fire	Hot and dry	1. The Gall bladder. The Choleric humour, the sense of smell. 2. The Attractive/ Apprehensive faculty. Anger and heated emotions.
Saturn	Melancholy Earth	Cold and dry	1. The spleen, the bones, the teeth, the ears and hearing. 2. The Melancholic humour, The Retentive faculty, the memory.
Venus	Phlegm Water Procreative spirit	Cold and moist	1. The Kidneys, throat, breasts, reproductive organs. The Reproductive and urinary system, 2. The Radical moisture, the Expulsive faculty.

Table of planets.

Diseases associated with the Planet	Herbs ruled by the planet
Diseases of the Brain, vertigo, madness, stupidity, simplicity. Antipathetic to Jupiter and the lungs; Asthma, coughs, Hoarseness. T.B. Diseases of the tongue, stammering, lisps.	Elecampagne, Clover, Fennel, Lavender, Lily of the Valley, liquorice, Senna, Valerian, White horehound, wild carrot. Sweet smelling herbs refresh animal spirits.
When the heat of the Sun or Mars disperses the Vital spirit, it can be the cause of infection, fever and fainting. The Sun causes "all diseases of the Heart and Brain..and the nerves and arteries". Also; Heartburn, Sore eyes.	Angelica, Ash, Bay, Centaury, Chamomile, Cinnamon, Eyebright, Juniper, Marigold, St Johns Wort, Rosemary, Tormentil. Spices refresh Vital spirits
All cold and rheumatic diseases, Fluid retention, dropsies, Oedema. discharges and abscesses. Coughs, Excess mucous from lungs. Lethargy, Palsy, convulsions and epilepsy from phlegm obstructing the Animal spirit. Cold causes Cramps and Colic. The Moon causes excess and absent menstruation. Cyclical, and recurrent diseases. Fevers due to cold and moist diminishing Innate heat and Vital spirit, thus allowing external poisons to enter.	Cleavers, Chaste tree, Chickweed, Lettuce, Willow, Moonwort.
All infirmities of the Liver and veins, Lung disease, pleurisy. Leads to putrefaction, Spring fevers, quinsy's.	Agrimony, Asparagus, Avens, Balm, Borage, Chestnuts, Dandelion, Dock, Lime tree, Lovage, Hyssop, Meadowsweet, Red Roses, Sage. Milk thistle.
All diseases of Choler; Fevers, carbuncles, shingles, anger, affects the brain by antipathy, frenzy, fury, sudden pain/migraine from heat. Also antipathetic to kidneys and bladder, causing inflammation, pain, blockage.	Broom, Basil, Garlic, Gentian, Ginger, Hawthorn, Hops, Mustard, Nettle, Rocket, Rhubarb, Wormwood, Vitex agnus castus. Blessed thistle, thistles in general.
All diseases of melancholy, cold and dryness; madness caused by fear and grief. Chronic disease, Bone pains, gout, toothache, deafness. Obstructive nature can cause palsies, migraines, impotence, haemorrhoids, hernias.	Cornflower, Comfrey, fumitory, Heartsease, Horsetail, Mullein, Shepherds purse. Melancholy thistle.
Kidney infections, Cystitis, Ovarian and uterine problems, Fibroids. Venereal diseases.	Burdock, Cherries, Viburnums, Cowslip, Elderflower, Feverfew, Lady's mantle, Mallows, Mints, Motherwort, Mugwort, Plantain, Roses, Vervain, Violets, Yarrow.

When there is excess melancholy in the spleen, cold vapours rise up and interfere with the heart and the stomach, which both sit above it. The cold blockage this causes reduces the heat of the stomach weakening digestion, leading to heartburn and bitter belching. The heart may also suffer from weakness, affecting the strength and regularity of the heartbeat. The signs of excess melancholy include fatigue, poor appetite and digestion, cold sweats, irregular heartbeat, anxiety, cold extremities, liver congestion, bitter belching, stiff painful joints, aching back and hips, and itchy skin.

The Saturnine diseases include chronic diseases, all diseases of melancholy, cold and dryness. Madness caused by fear and grief, bone pains, gout, toothache, deafness, haemorrhoids, and hernias. Cold blocks affecting the brain can cause palsies and migraines, and cold congestion of the reproductive system will lead to impotence.

Melancholics should avoid excessively large meals, heavy foods (beef), eating too late in the day, lack of activity, thinking too much, and introspection. They should take light nourishing foods, such as soft cheeses, shellfish, eggs, lamb, olive oil, root vegetables, sprouted seeds, seaweed, squash, and dried fruit. They should also have cleansing foods, such as asparagus, celery, and fennel. They should ensure to take gentle exercise, long walks, have a productive long term project, and to find exuberant sanguine friends.

Useful herbs for melancholics are the ones that gently warm, like fennel, angelica, lovage, black pepper, sage, cardamom, coriander, and cloves. To protect the heart from melancholy one should take lemon balm, motherwort, and borage. To deal with anxiety, gentle warming nervines such as valerian, lime flower, cowslip, red rose, juniper berries, sage, and guelder rose, are all helpful.

Symbolic associations for saturn

Earth, solidity, coldness, contraction, retention, resistance, stubbornness, rigidity, foundations, studiousness, the development of theories, laws, science, plans, resolution, responsibility, dependability, autumn, middle age, restriction, repression, secrecy, pessimism.

Herbs ruled by saturn

Cornflower, comfrey, fumitory, heartsease, horsetail, mullein, shepherds purse, melancholy thistle.

ARS

CHAPTER FIFTEEN

The art of medicine: diagnosis

"Natural forces within us are the true healers of disease"

—Hippocrates.

Central to traditional medical systems is the belief that the main therapeutic tool we have in the process of healing is the body itself. The power of the natural forces within us to heal arise in two complementary ways; firstly within the patient the natural healing forces can be enabled to directly bring about a healing transformation, and secondly it is the natural forces within the practitioner that act as a guide as to how to facilitate healing within the patient. The bedrock of this idea is that we all share a divine spirit, both patient and healer, which when allowed to fully manifest will lead to harmony and balance. The patient has to believe that their body has the ultimate power to heal, and the practitioner needs to have the humility to be open to being guided from within by the divine spirit.

Application of technique, having great knowledge and a host of remembered recipes alone is not enough. Finally, the time comes for all of us when we have learnt all of the technical skills, when we have studied all of the manuals, and when we have completed periods of training with wise teachers that we must at last embrace our own creativity and inspiration to achieve our potential as healers. We must have the courage to trust our abilities and recognise that if we have great compassion for others at the centre of our practice our hearts will always provide the answers we need through connecting us to the sacred space within.

This viewpoint requires us to practice from a place of trust and confidence in our natural abilities as well as our training. As Westerners we have always been taught that wisdom is something that is outside of ourselves and that we must go outside of ourselves to find and acquire it, that it is not something that already resides within us. The ancient Greek word for education comes from "e" and "duco" meaning to draw out, pointing to the idea that the journey to wisdom is an inner one that involves us bringing to the surface that which is within us.

When we complete our learning it is often difficult to go out and practice, we most often feel that we don't "know" enough, and we continue to hanker for a wise guide to be there to reassure us. We often feel lacking and inadequate, and as if there is still something more that we need to know to be truly ready. When I was a student there was a herbalist whom I greatly admired and respected, and I had been in the fortunate position of being able to regularly observe working, so that over time he very much became my mentor. Once I had qualified, I still felt that I had so much more that I could learn from him, so I asked him if I could continue to come for observation sessions. His answer was clear and swift "no", he said, "Now it is time for you to learn by practicing, not by watching; if you continue to come it will only hold you back". I felt unsure and vulnerable, and doubted that I had what was needed to practice effectively, but he was correct, and his firm insistence that I go out and learn it for myself was the guidance I needed.

It is only when we have a patient in front of us that we truly have the opportunity to explore the experience of healing.

The consultation

So where do we start? A good point is to follow the lead of the ancient system of the seven naturals and to start with the basic "elements". These basic elements are indicated by the narrative the patient gives about their symptoms. It is time to allow the patient to start to open up, and to give us a view into their suffering. It is important to bear in mind that the telling of a story is just as important as the story itself. We soon become aware that the way someone tells us about things, how easily they speak or how reticent they are, will be very helpful indicators of the kind of the person that they are. This is probably the most important aspect of our diagnosis.

Whether they start by talking about their physical body, their feelings or their thoughts can also point to which of the temperaments they are most strongly aligned with. From what we know, it would be reasonable to expect a sanguine person to be expansive in the way that they talk about any of their symptoms, physical, emotional or mental, whereas in a melancholic it is likely for them to be more reserved, emotionally private, and considered in how they deliver their story. Cholerics often don't like to talk about their symptoms at all, they will brush aside their emotions and be very brief and succinct in what they have to say, while phlegmatics are the opposite, readily connecting with the emotional aspects of their illness and may be difficult to contain once they are in their flow.

I find that instead of having a set list of questions ready to ask the patient or a form for me or for them to fill in, I just start with a clear page. Then by letting them start their story we can allow the patient to lead us to where they feel the problem resides.

We must remember that at the heart of this approach to healing lies the process of catharsis, the cleansing of that which is at the root of the person's pain. It is quite amazing how powerful a healing effect just allowing someone to speak and to be heard is. Very often patients will say at the end of the first consultation "I feel better already, thank you for listening, it's made such a difference".

Explore the temperament

With the seven naturals, the second on the list after the elements is the temperaments. It is a great advantage to have a good feel of what kind of temperament our patient has, as the temperament of our patient shows us so many things. It will often provide the clue as to why they became sick, it will direct our gaze in the direction of what might be out of balance, and it will likely suggest the solution to their problem. We must remember that people with cold temperaments usually get sick through the underlying cold being exacerbated, and hot people get sick through heat being excessive. It is fair to say that the temperament tells all.

So how can we best find the patient's temperament? The simple answer is that we do it through observing, listening, and gently drawing out from our patient their strongest characteristics. Don't worry if at first you can't pinpoint someone's temperament, we have all learnt to adapt our behaviours to what we believe society expects, and often we may keep our true selves hidden. This is the same with our patients. I often assign a temperament to a patient on a first visit only to change my mind on later visits when they have become more relaxed, sometimes it may be because their natural disposition was subsumed by pain, sickness, or emotional distress at the beginning and only begins to show itself as they improve.

If it isn't immediately clear to you what temperament a patient has then it is very helpful to ask yourself which of the temperaments you can't see in them at all, and then start looking at which of the other three is the strongest. It often may be easier to spot a lack of fire, than to decide whether their quietness is due to them being phlegmatic or melancholic. It is reassuring to remember that simply deciding whether the cause of their suffering arises from heat or cold is the most important starting point.

Assess the humours

Once we have considered their temperament we will be able to start thinking about what kind of humoral imbalance may be playing out. The most helpful starting point is to consider their temperament and to look for the signs of the corresponding humour being in excess. It is usual that a hot person will already be in danger of the hot humours of choler and blood to be in excess rather than the cold humours of phlegm and melancholy.

The balance of the humours is usually shown by the symptoms that the patient has, so gradually as we list the symptoms we can start to see a picture forming. Remember that it is your job to investigate each of the symptoms presented, the patient will often discount or forget to tell you the things that they don't think are related to the problem that they are presenting you with. But as we are looking for the pattern behind a set of physical signs and symptoms, it is important to get the fullest possible picture. For instance, a patient may not think that a tendency to get an occasional migraine, that they had cystitis in the past, often find a cold goes to their chest in the winter, are relevant symptoms when they come to you for treatment for abdominal bloating and colicky pain. However, we will recognise that all of these symptoms relate to an underlying phlegmatic constitution and a problem with a build up of excess phlegmatic dampness in the bowels. We can confirm this by feeling their pulse, which is likely to be slow, thin, or fine and possibly erratic or "choppy". When we look at their tongue it is likely to be paler, possibly bluish, maybe wet, and to have a thick white coating. By bringing everything about the patient into consideration we can gradually form a viewpoint of what we are seeing and how to move forward with it, and it is in this way that the humoral approach is innately holistic.

As with the temperament, we are most concerned with identifying whether the patient is showing signs of a hot or cold humoral imbalance. Whatever strategies or herbs we use, and whatever the illness is, if we can recognise what the temperament is and what humour is in excess, we are likely to be able to do something that is supporting the movement back towards balance.

Examine the patient: skin, tongue, and pulse

We can start our examination even before we touch the patient. Looking at how they move, sit, speak, and breathe will all give important indicators as to what is going on both on a superficial level and deeper within their constitution. The skin colour and appearance is always helpful, assess the colour, and its appearance. We are looking for a good healthy skin colour, as well as trying to identify signs of dryness or excess moisture. When we do get to take the pulse we will have an opportunity to actually feel the surface characteristics. Be aware if it is hot or cold, moist or dry, puffy or desiccated, and then start to add these observations to your overall assessment.

Now that we have got the main narrative from the patient and spent some time observing them, it becomes possible to further extend our investigation by looking at the tongue and taking the pulse. At this point I will usually ask the patient to stick their tongue out, which for patients familiar with going to a conventional Western doctor may seem amusing, intriguing, or often confusing. However, this gives us a really good opportunity to start talking to them about what we are looking for, and how identifying their temperament and the balance of their humours will help us to address the true foundation of their illness. Patients like to hear about what we are seeing in them, and it is good to get them involved in thinking about the various ways that together we can improve their health.

I often compare looking at the tongue to feeling a single radiator in a house; if it is hot we know that the system itself is working and there's no need to check all the others. The heat in the radiator tells us that the boiler, the pipes and the pump are all working. By asking to see the tongue it is like we have got someone to stick out a radiator from their house, giving us an overall picture of how well their internal system is functioning. The tongue, like a radiator is supplied by the same system as all the other organs. It is nourished by the same blood, it is also supplied and cleansed by the same channels as all the other organs, and therefore its appearance cannot be wildly different from all of the other organs that are part of the same system. Clearly if there is a particular organ in the body that is damaged, infected, or compromised in some way that will affect its ability to function, the problem may not immediately be obvious on the tongue. However, when we look in more detail at tongue diagnosis, we will find that there are also specific correspondences to individual organs in the tongues characteristics.

It is best to start by looking at the basic tongue signs, as they are very obvious and easy to recognise. By looking at the colour, shape, and coating, we can immediately get an indication of internal harmony or disharmony. The colour is the most important of all, as it shows the deeper underlying constitutional health, it tends to only change slowly over time, and shows the underlying strengths or weaknesses. If the tongue colour is healthy, then anything else is only going to be a temporary or superficial problem. We are looking for a healthy pink hue that has a freshness to it. If the tongue is blue it indicates cold, and if red it indicates heat, if purple it indicates stasis and blockage, if it is reddish purple the blockage is caused by heat, and if bluish purple it is caused by cold. If it is narrow it indicates a lack of fluids and radical moisture, and if swollen an excess of dampness. Wet tongues show a lack of heat and dry tongues show a lack of blood to carry moisture, and cracks generally show dryness and exhaustion of the radical moisture. The coating shows the residue left behind after digestion, and it should be thin and white. Unlike the colour, it can change very quickly and is often a direct indicator in the changing course of a disease. A yellow coating is a sign of heat, and a thick white coating is a sign of dampness, usually indicating dampness in the colon or lungs. There are a vast range of variations and combinations of colour, shape, and coating, but simply knowing these basic signifiers gives us the most important information about the underlying constitution. The chapter on tongue diagnosis gives a much more detailed overview of the different tongue characteristics and their significance.

Feeling the pulse is also very helpful at this point, as it will further enlighten us as to what is going on in the body. At this point even the basic characteristics are very helpful, we can just ask the basic questions assessing strength, rate, depth, width, length and hardness. This can be a way of confirming or complementing everything that we have already noted about the patient. We can start by looking for signs of heat that will make it stronger, faster, higher, longer, harder, or signs of cold making it weaker, slower, deeper, shorter, and softer. Sometimes a pulse may not seem to match up with the other signs and symptoms we have observed, if so, don't worry, just note it down and follow your instinct. We often find that when we look back at our findings they complement each other in a way that we hadn't immediately recognised. I remember being very surprised to find a strong high pulse in an otherwise cold, older, melancholic person—I was expecting a deeper weaker pulse. I later realised that it was actually the coldness in the system that pushed the pulse up and out, and the dryness of the melancholic constitution was causing tightness and congestion, which meant that the heat also seemed greater because it didn't have open moist passages to allow it to flow forwards, also making it rise up. This constriction and blockage to flow was also confirmed by the very cold hands and feet that they also suffered from.

Assess the organs and consider the symptoms

Hopefully by this point we should be getting an idea of the person's temperament and therefore their constitutional strengths and weaknesses. So now we can turn our attention to the symptoms that they have, being aware as to whether they are general symptoms, such as lethargy, anxiety, pain or inflammation, or specific symptoms, such as a stomach ache, headache, localised pain, a urinary or digestive problem. The general symptoms may be due to a humoral imbalance, while the specific symptoms will require that we look at the organ concerned and decide whether it is too hot, cold, dry, or damp. We may then come up with a strategy to treat the specific imbalance in the organ alongside a constitutional support for the whole system.

The organs are also next on our list of the seven naturals, and in each of them we can also start by looking for any temperamental imbalance. The initial clues will come from the story that the patient is giving us, they may be reporting pain, or changes in function. It may be possible to examine an area, or to observe changes directly in the body; sometimes a change in skin colour, or swelling, or tenderness may point towards a particular problem.

The patient may themselves have a particular concern with an organ or a part of their anatomy, which we can then look at or investigate directly. Sometimes it is clear where a problem is, for instance our patient may have respiratory, digestive, nervous problems, or joint or skin problems. Wherever the problem is, it is a good idea to consider a direct response that helps the patient to feel physically better immediately, and therefore more in control. We can do this alongside an underlying constitutional approach and so offer both a short-term treatment for a symptom and a long-term strategy to address the problem at its root cause.

I have always found herbal medicine to be a very "hands on" and practical approach to healing. We can provide so many ways of easing a problem directly. It is good to try and be as adaptable as possible and always try to go straight to the place where a problem is presenting itself. It's good to think about all the different ways of using herbs as well as the many different herbs that we have available. I always enjoy reading the directions of herbalists like Nicholas Culpeper for using herbs, he will suggest using external applications, such as poultices, baths, inhalations, washes, and compresses, both in addition to internal medicines and often instead of them. I find it exciting to read some of his suggestions, such as the treatment of head pain caused by too much heat, as happens when we have been in the sun too long, by applying a tincture of the vinegar of roses as a compress to the temples. He also suggests applying fresh herbs to wounds and to swellings, using baths for pain, rubbing medicines on the body, using eye drops and ear drops, and often recommends these being made from fresh herbs or their juice.

When inspired by this kind of approach of using herbs externally applied rather than trying to give everything by mouth, I have had some of my best successes. There was a patient who spontaneously recovered from a benign lung tumour by a regular application of a mustard chest poultice, and I have seen otherwise irresolvable leg ulcers entirely heal up by using poultices made from freshly crushed herbs. Most organs can be treated from the outside as well as the inside; compresses can be placed over internal organs, such as the lungs, the kidneys, bladder, and reproductive organs. Herbs can also be absorbed through the skin into the blood stream by using foot baths or full body baths, sometimes this may be the most effective way of treating spasmodic pain by using antispasmodics, such as hawthorn as well as anti-inflammatory herbs, such as chamomile and rosemary. Some organs like the eyes, ears, mouth, and skin are naturally most easily accessible through external applications rather than by using internally absorbed herbs. I had a patient who was regularly using steroids for ever-worsening iritis, so we started using a compress made from marigold flowers daily. She had done this regularly for some time when she suddenly had an episode of eye pain come on that indicated a flare up was starting again. Unable to get to see a doctor immediately she applied a poultice of the marigold flowers and left it on for half an hour, which was much longer than usual, and to her surprise she found that the pain lessened considerably. She then repeated the poultices throughout the day and over the next few days. The pain quite quickly resolved and the eye returned to being completely normal in a short time, which enabled her to avoid going back to using steroids. Since that point she always knew what to do when things began to flare up and felt that she actually could respond to what was happening and had more control again.

It is always very good to be able to do something that is immediately helpful for a specific problem in a part of the body, even if it doesn't cure it but just relieves a pain, as this will not only help the patient, but instil confidence in them to continue with the longer-term treatments that we might also suggest. Frequently, we find that giving a simple thing changes the course of a problem almost instantly, and often the simpler the remedy the quicker that we get a result. For instance, a warming linctus with elderberry, thyme, and elecampagne will quickly clear a cough from a wet cold chest by improving expectoration and drying phlegm, while a cooling soothing combination of marshmallow root, elderflower, and lime flower will reduce coughing from a dry irritated respiratory system as with spring hay fever.

Addressing the humours

If we are detecting an excess of a humour, this is where we might think about including a strategy to cleanse the excess as part of our treatment plan. This has to be done alongside giving guidance and advice about what the patient should be avoiding to stop exacerbating or increasing the excess of the humour.

With sanguines we would be likely to use herbs that aid the clearance of excess damp heat, such as diaphoretics like elderflower, yarrow, and lime flower, and to encourage them to give up any excessive behaviour or habits. They will respond to being given some boundaries and being guided to find long term goals projects or commitments. They should be encouraged to release their exuberance in measured ways with a bit of structure rather than just through wild behaviour and excess. I will often give them herbs that centre and balance them, such as chamomile, lime flower, meadowsweet, and wood betony. The expansive sanguine temperament may greatly amplify symptoms, and sometimes this will present in extreme ways. In times of crisis it may well help to attempt to purge the excess of the sanguine humour with a vomit. This is a treatment that was formerly used frequently in Western medicine but is rarely used today. I have found it particularly helpful when the patient has extreme feelings of being emotionally overloaded, of feeling toxic inside, or of experiencing an immoveable internal heaviness, bloating, or fullness. The safest and simplest way of inducing vomiting is to get the patient to drink a large amount of slightly warm water. When I was going through initiations in Africa, vomiting was a regular feature of the process and I became very familiar with it as a treatment, and eventually lost my Western aversion to doing it. There it is done very simply and effectively by making you drink slightly warm water until you began to wretch, and at this point to trigger the vomit reflex by putting your fingers down your throat. The most important thing is to fill the stomach with copious amounts of water, this means that when the patient vomits any digestive acid or juices are too dilute to cause any damage as they are ejected through the oesophagus. It often improves symptoms instantly bringing on feelings of release and wellbeing.

The dry heat of cholerics may be cleared with opening purging remedies, such as bitter herbs, especially if the heat and dryness is causing retention and constipation; in which case one would purge with wormwood, yellow dock, and cascara. Any excess dryness may be treated with moistening herbs, such as violets, chicory, chickweed, and cooling roots such as dandelion. They often need some emotionally protective and nourishing herbs to counter their hot and fiery temperaments, so I like to use the cordial herbs, such as rose, violets, melissa and borage, as well as hawthorn to mollify and temper the heat and tension that accompanies choler. As a good calming restorative for the brain I like to use cowslip flowers. They need to be given some projects that have clear and immediate outcomes and will usually respond well to a clearly defined plan of action.

In melancholics we might think of adding warming activating herbs to clear and purge obstructions from the liver and the spleen, such as wormwood, hops, elecampagne, lovage and vervain. To raise the spirits when fearfulness and pessimism have got the better of melancholics, angelica, St John's wort, and bay are helpful. I often recommend a bath in bay leaves to cleanse the build-up of melancholy and try to encourage them to find some sanguine friends or to engage in some more exuberant activities, such as singing. They benefit from thinking less and feeling more, but should never be allowed to get stuck or to dwell on anything.

With phlegmatics we might use a hot steam of thyme and chamomile flowers to aid elimination of dampness, and to use some powerful cleansing diuretics, such as nettles, cleavers, birch leaves, and yarrow. I always advise them to avoid cold foods and to add black pepper and gentle warming herbs like thyme, basil, rosemary, fennel, and gentle spices to all meals. We must encourage them to get active, and to warm the body up every day with exercise and deep breathing. It helps to give them direction and to make them feel that their life is moving on. I always find encouraging them to plan something to look forward to always helps. They can get stuck in emotional stagnation, so try and help them to let go of troubling feelings and to let their emotions flow again, hopefully aided by a bit of laughter.

Looking after the spirits and the vital spirit

As we go through our exploration of the seven naturals we come to the spirits of the body. This is where we might be looking for depletion rather than excess as in the humours. If we have found a sign of depletion of heat, for instance shown in a poor digestion and confirmed by a wet looking tongue, it will be indicating a depletion of the innate heat. This also shows as stagnation of vitality, and often we see a lacklustre pale tongue with wet swollen edges and teeth marks.

A depleted vital spirit will affect all of the other spirits, including the natural spirit in the liver, the animal spirit in the brain, and the procreative spirit in the reproductive organs. If we have a low vital spirit the liver will not digest food nor produce healthy humours and blood, the brain will be slow, dull, and prone to nervous issues and migraines, and the levels of libido and fertility will be diminished.

Loss of innate heat will give us a narrow slow pulse that is short and deep, it will interfere with digestion and absorption as the concoctions will not work effectively. So, we will expect to see a pale tongue, with the poor digestion producing no residues able to produce a tongue coating. The lack of the coating is a clear sign that we have a depletion of innate heat, rather than just an excessive amount of phlegm humour and dampness. In these cases, we will use warming and activating remedies, such as broom, motherwort, rosemary, and juniper to strengthen the heart, with angelica and vervain being helpful for the liver. Hopefully by activating the innate heat, and therefore the spirits and organs, we will see the digestion improve, and any excess dampness that has built up will also be cleared.

In the case of excess damp and cold phlegmatic blocks being the cause of loss of heat, we would expect to see a thick white tongue coating, a clear sign of excess. In this case we will focus on warming herbs, such as mint, aniseed and hyssop for the stomach and digestion, and fenugreek for the bowels.

Herbs that strengthen the vital spirit, such as angelica, bay, juniper, motherwort, melissa, St John's wort, and rosemary can all be used to ensure that the vital spirit is protected and nourished. In fact, it is a tradition to always add at least one herb into a medicinal mixture to honour the divine spark or vital spirit in each person.

As we age, the loss of radical moisture due to long term exhaustion, anxiety, stress, and overwork will often lead to a drying out of the body. Although this is inevitable to some degree, we can still reduce its impact by using nourishing and moistening remedies, such as dandelion root, artichokes, milk thistle, liquorice, and asparagus. This is also a good opportunity to once again apply our four cordial herbs: lemon balm, violets, rose, and borage.

It is more likely that older people will be suffering from depletions of innate heat and radical moisture, and younger people from excesses of humours. It is also more likely that if we have a person with a choleric hot temperament suffering from signs of cold then it will be due to the lack of innate heat rather than an excess of phlegm, and if we have a person with a cold temperament, such as a phlegmatic showing signs of excess heat, it will be due to a depletion of radical moisture to cool through moving and clearing heat from the system rather than being due to an excess of choleric humour.

The four administering virtues and faculties of the body

Supporting the spirits will also help to activate and strengthen the natural virtues associated with them. If the spirits have the correct balance of the innate heat and radical moisture then the bodily processes that manifest as the apprehensive virtue, the digestive virtue, the retentive virtue, the expulsive virtue, and the procreative virtue should all be strengthened.

However, if any of the corresponding organs are obstructed in any way, the virtues that reside in them will also become diminished. If we wish the body to return to health we have to be sure that these four virtues are functioning well, and if it seems that there is a depletion in the activity of any of them we will need to ascertain why that is.

A depletion of vital spirit will always lessen the activity of these faculties and should always be taken into account when deciding how to respond. However, with each faculty there may be specific blockages or impediments to their correct function.

A weakening of the apprehensive virtue will show in a depleted digestive function and is likely to lead to poor breakdown of foods, which will often show in abdominal bloating, distension, and cramps. It is also likely to result in a reduced ability of the stomach to break down foods. We may well expect to see a lack of energy and motivation, a limited ability to think clearly, and a loss of libido. The tongue will often be wet, lack a coating and is likely to be thin and pale. The pulse will be fine, deep, and soft. To help improve the apprehensive virtue we may consider using warming aromatic bitter herbs, such as angelica, elecampagne, and fennel.

The digestive virtue covers all the processes of absorption and assimilation of nutrients during the processes of the concoctions. If weakened, we find that the blood itself may be diminished leading to anaemia as well as general debility. As its seat is in the liver, we will need to consider if the liver itself needs support and healing. Often the tongue will be thin, and sometimes shrunken, and likely to be pale. This is due to there being a general lack of production of humours and blood. The pulse will often be large but soft and the patient will feel heavy, weak, and irritable and suffer from signs of blockage and stagnation. Strengthening liver herbs that improve function remove blockages and improve the breeding of blood, such as sage, wood avens, hyssop, and lovage, can all be helpful.

The retentive virtue resides in the spleen, and when the spleen becomes blocked with excessive melancholic humour we find that the vapours that arise from it will diminish the function of all the organs that are in its vicinity, including the heart, the stomach, the gall bladder and the liver. The patient may well be constipated, suffer from boils and itching, be fatigued and depressed. The tongue is likely to have swollen sides, look blue or dark purple and may have red spots on it. We would expect the pulse to be deeper, shorter, and slower. We will want to expel and eliminate the cold melancholic blockages with herbs like rosemary, angelica, lovage, sage, and valerian, and purge with rhubarb root and yellow dock. Warming the stomach to overcome the melancholic vapours that may overwhelm it with gentle spices, such as cardamom, coriander, cinnamon, and ginger, is a good idea, as is using warming digestive herbs, such as basil, oregano, thyme, and rosemary.

The expulsive virtue resides in the kidneys and is responsible for the evacuation of waste products. It is cold and moist, enabling it to consolidate matter in the bowels and to smoothly and effectively clear it. If the bowels are too cold then constipation can occur, requiring warming digestive remedies and gentle laxatives, such as fenugreek. If the kidney function is diminished waste products may build up leading to gout, urinary infections, kidney stones, and if severe, swelling from kidney failure. If the expulsive virtue is weak we are likely to see a short and pale or blue tongue and a thin, weak, and deep pulse, as the build-up of waste products and dampness in the blood dilutes it making it feel thin and without body. Diuretics, such as nettles, yarrow, dandelion leaf, and birch, are all warming and aid the expulsive virtue to clear cold blockages.

Usually it is pretty clear when there is a deficiency in one of the four administering virtues, and putting it into our overall treatment approach is certainly important.

The six non-naturals

When assessing our patients we must remember that there are also a wide range of influences on health that are produced by external factors:

Air

We are aware of the effects of polluted air, but within this category it is also worth considering modern factors, such as indoor environments. Compared to historic times we probably spend much more time indoors than people did in Culpeper's and Hippocrates' days. Heating systems, air conditioning, as well as the impact of household chemicals, sprays, mould spores and dust should all be taken account of when considering external causes of air.

Diet

Everyone is becoming increasingly aware of the impact of diet, and often it really helps a patient to have some clear guidelines about how they can help themselves through adjusting their diet. I find it is best to do things in an achievable and sustainable way and not to put so many changes into a diet that the patient is set up to fail. Slow changes that become well founded are better than dramatic changes that quickly fall away. It is helpful to ask a patient to give an account of a full day's diet, telling you exactly what they ate and drank. I often ask what it is that they ate on the previous day, and then ask for some extra examples of what they may have had for lunch or dinner on other days to get a fuller picture.

Within the context of diet, I tend to include conventional medicines in this part of the assessment, asking about all the conventional medicines, supplements, and herbs that they already take. You may find that a patient is wanting to change or reduce some of their medications, and although it is not your role to tell them what they should do with the medications that a doctor or other health practitioner has prescribed, it is entirely appropriate to give them your opinion and experience in how these medicines may be affecting them both positively and negatively, after all they have come to get your viewpoint as a herbalist.

Exercise and rest

Exercise done appropriately is beneficial for everyone. It is important to encourage people to get regular daily exercise. We live in an increasingly sedentary culture and it is the cause of much of the chronic illnesses are becoming increasingly prevalent. It is important to include an assessment of the amount of exercise a person does in your consultation, and to give them achievable goals if they need to do more. When it comes to rest we need to make sure that everyone is spending time in relaxing and enjoyable ways, away from the pressures of work, and being released from the ever invasive effects of the digital virtual world.

Sleep and wakefulness

It is also common that we lack good quality sleep, and often you will find that addressing poor sleep has to be part of your guidance to help patients get back to a state of good health. It is always best to find out what lies behind poor sleep patterns and to try and address those issues rather than just trying to offer sedative and sleep inducing remedies, which after a period of time will become tolerated and lose their effectiveness.

Retention and evacuation

You may well have covered these aspects of your patient's condition in the exploration of their humours and natural virtues of the body. It is always important to include an assessment of how well the body is both absorbing and retaining nutrients and clearing waste products, and ensuring that these processes are well supported.

Perturbations of the mind and emotions

A lot of what we are working with as humoral practitioners is the inner states of mind and emotions of our patients. Finding the root causes of internal suffering and helping to find strategies to enable patients to resolve both long- and short-term causes of distress and trauma is particularly important. We may not have all the answers, and in fact it is important that every individual finds their own way of resolving inner suffering, so that they can continue to benefit from such strategies throughout their lives. The most important tool that we have is our compassion, if we can take a non-judgemental stance and support our patient's emotional journey with compassion and empathy we will be of great benefit to them. Perhaps the most important thing that we can do in this regard is to develop ourselves so that we can open our heart out to others, and through having an understanding of how to free ourselves from emotional pain and suffering we can aid others most effectively on their journey of healing.

Concluding the consultation

The moment will come when we need to come up with a strategy. Once you have absorbed all the information that you have been given by your patient, it is a good idea to step back a bit and try to get a broad overview of what you wish to achieve. Remember that you can't do everything in one go, and it is better to gradually build up a strategy over time. Always do something to attend to what the patient has asked you to help with, even if you think there are more important underlying issues.

Try not to over think your response, once you have a good feeling for the herbs that you use you will often get an intuitive feeling about which herbs and strategies will work well with your patient, and we should learn to trust the inspirations that come to us.

A good piece of advice is that the more complicated the presentation is, the simpler your response should be. In some cases this may simply be deciding on whether you are treating a disease with a cold cause or a hot cause, and suggesting strategies to help balance out the pervading excess of heat or cold. A Tibetan herbalist once told me that if you are still in doubt of the temperament of the cause then give the patient some bitters, if they then have no improvement you know that the disease isn't caused by heat!

Remember that there is always something you can do to help every patient who comes, even if you can't do everything that the patient may hope for. Always hope for the best, and always remember to trust the herbs, they are our unfailing allies.

CHAPTER SIXTEEN

Tongue diagnosis

T he tongue is the only internal organ that we can see from the outside of the body. It shares the same blood flow, nourishment, and elimination as the other internal organs. This means that when we look at its surface it is likely to reflect very closely the surface of the other organs in the body.

If there is generalised excess or depletion within the body it will be seen on the tongue, alongside clear indicators of excess heat and cold, moisture and dryness. The tongue is therefore a valuable window into the body, and becoming familiar with how it varies and changes over time as conditions progress is an endeavour that soon repays the investment in time taken to study it. As with pulse diagnosis, the most important thing is to take as many opportunities as possible to look at patients' tongues, and to develop a familiarity with the usual variations. Start with simple observations of colour, shape, and coating, and then gradually extend your knowledge to the more subtle aspects.

Tongue colour

The colour and appearance of the tongue body is the most important aspect of all the tongue characteristics to consider.

It tends to only change slowly and gives an indication of the deeper underlying constitution and health. The tongue should have a bright pink vibrant colour. A flourishing and moist tongue indicates a good supply of body fluids, and in particular shows a strong vital spirit and a good balance of innate heat and radical moisture; a dry and withered tongue indicates the exhaustion of body fluids, and depletion of innate heat and the vital spirit.

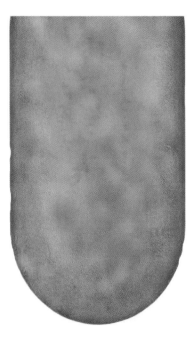

Diagram shows a normal pink, moist, tongue with a thin white coating.

The variations to colour include a pale tongue, a red tongue, a blue tongue, and purple tongue, the purple tongue may appear either as bluish or reddish purple.

Tongue shape

Tongue shape is the next most important aspect of the tongue to consider after the tongue colour. Shape reflects the relative balance of the humours indicating excess humours, as well as deficiency of innate heat, radical moisture, and blood.

However, shape is secondary to colour. If there is a bright red colour or a blue colour it indicates a hot state (red) or cold state (blue) regardless of its shape. For instance, a narrow red tongue is narrow due to a deficiency of radical moisture, the shrinkage is due to a lack of moisture to plump it up, but the redness remains because there is still blood and warmth. Whilst a narrow pale tongue is shrunken due to a deficiency of blood humour, and therefore a lack of the heat and moisture carried in the blood to plump up the tongue. Both tongues are shrunken, but one shows underlying heat and warmth, and the other shows underlying coldness and deficiency of the heat necessary to breed blood through the concoctions. Both show a shrunken tongue due to lack of moisture but the different causes of that deficiency are indicated by the tongue colour rather than its shape.

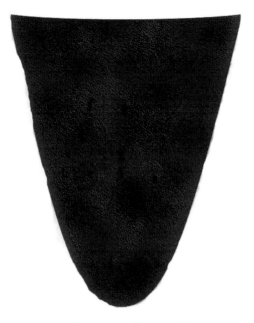

Deficient moisture: narrow short red tongue, often cracks present with little or no coating.

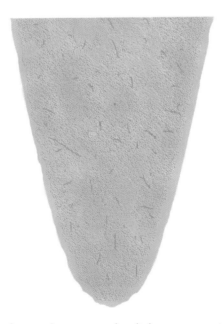

Deficient blood: narrow short pale tongue, dry, little or no coating.

Tongue coating

The coating indicates more temporary or superficial states, it can vary greatly, and can change quickly. It can also be a helpful indicator of the progress of a disease. A lack of coating always indicates a deficiency state, or the deficient activity of an organ. If the tongue lacks any sign of a coating, assume that there is a deficiency. The coating is a secretion produced when the digestive process is working well. It is a residue left behind when the concoctions are completed satisfactorily. The tongue should have a thin white coating extending over most of the tongue surface, it should look even and not have patches where it has come away from the body of the tongue. If it is in place it is called a well rooted coating, if it comes away it is called a patchy coating.

Tongue colour

- If the body is pale, it indicates deficiency of innate heat (wet) or the concoction of blood (dry).
- If the body is pale with a thick white coating it indicates excess phlegm or melancholy causing blockage.
- If the body is red, it indicates the presence of heat, excess choler/blood (coating present) or lack of cooling radical moisture (no coating).
- If the body is blue, it indicates stasis of blood due to cold.
- If the body is purple, it indicates congestion of blood, due to cold if bluish purple, or due to heat if reddish purple.

Pale tongue

A pale tongue indicates internal coldness and reduction in the flow of innate heat to the organs.

Pale tongue with a thick white coating = excess phlegm, melancholy.
- It indicates an excess of the phlegmatic humour or the melancholic humour.
- If it has a thick white coating it is indicating coldness and congestion of the colon and large intestine, or phlegm and cold damp in the lungs.
- It is indicative of excess dampness, and is often accompanied by bloating and lethargy.
- It is unusual to encounter a pale tongue with a yellow coating.

Pale tongue without a coating = deficient blood humour/innate heat.
- The lack of a coating shows a deficiency state.
- Paleness shows coldness. Warmth is produced by the innate heat in the vital spirit, and blood transports this warmth around the body, if either the heat, or the blood to move heat is lacking we will get a pale tongue.

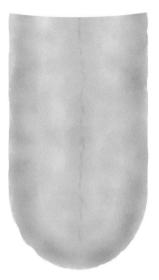

Excess phlegm; pale tongue, slightly swollen, usually thick, greasy, white coating.

Pale and wet tongue = deficient innate heat and weak vital spirit.
* Wetness always indicates deficient heat.
* Deficiency of innate heat means that fluids are not moved around the body, leading to their build up on the tongue surface. Often the tongue has teeth marks around edges if there is deficient vital spirit.
* Without a coating it indicates deficient innate heat, and if swollen it shows weak kidneys/adrenals.

Pale, flaccid, wet, thin white coating, a few red spots, shows deficient vital spirit.

If no coating and still slightly swollen but without teeth marks, shows just innate heat low rather than the vital spirit. Often if swollen with a central crack shows weak adrenals and kidneys and weak expulsive virtue.

Pale and wet tongue with a white coating = phlegmatic humour overwhelming other organs.
- Paleness indicates internal cold, the coating indicates that there is an excess of cold humours, the wetness occurs in this case because the heat is overwhelmed by the damp cold phlegm. The coating points to the primary cause being excess phlegm rather than the depletion of innate heat and vital spirit.

Pale and dry tongue = deficient blood.
- Dryness indicates deficient blood and the movement of fluids.
- Blood is the medium through which fluids are passed around the body. If there is deficient blood then fluids will not reach the organs, and it will manifest as dryness on the tongue surface. A pale tongue indicates internal coldness, and the dryness points to low blood, the liver breeds the blood. When the liver is not digesting humours and concocting them the fluid produced as a secretion at the end of the concoctions isn't available. Blood is also produced during the second concoction in the liver so lowered liver heat and energy, means deficiency of blood will follow.

Red tongue

A redder than normal tongue represents the presence of heat. This is either due to excess choler, or due to depletion of the cooling effects of radical moisture.

Red tongue with coating = excess heat/choler.
- When a red tongue has a coating of any colour it represents excess heat.

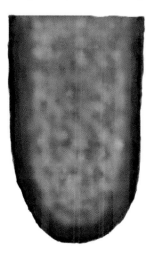

Diagram shows a red tongue, thinner and longer, with a thin yellow coating: excess choleric humour.

- A yellow coating shows excess choleric humour, or heat from an external poison or infection.
- A white coating shows that there is excess internal heat but also an excess of dampness in certain organs, usually the stomach, bowels, or lungs.

Red tongue without coating = depleted radical moisture.
- A red tongue lacking a coating shows that there is a deficiency of moisture to cool the internal organs, so that an otherwise normal level of heat will not be held in balance by the cool moisture and it will appear to be in excess, thus causing a red tongue. In this case it is also usually narrow.

Redness affecting different areas of the tongue

Looking at the location of red areas on the tongue is useful to identify the location of excess heat in the organs.

Red sides = liver/gall bladder heat. Right side only = gall bladder. Left side only = liver.
Red tip = heart heat.
Red front & tip = lung heat.
Red centre = stomach heat.
Red middle = heat in intestines and bowels.
Red back = kidney heat.

Red spots = excess heat in the blood.
- The larger the spots the more blood stasis is present. Red prickles are often signs of heat and inflammation in the lungs.

Diagram shows Vital spirit stagnation from excess heat in the heart, thin, palish, thin white coating with red tip.

Blue tongue

A blue tongue indicates cold internal blockage, either from lack of innate heat and vital spirit or cold melancholic blockage. Without heat the blood cannot be moved causing stagnation. Excess melancholy causes cold blocks and leads to a depletion of blood and distribution of heat.

Blue without a coating = cold congestion causing blood deficiency.
- The coating is absent because when the concoctions are deficient there is no residue left to provide a coating. It indicates a lack of innate heat, reducing the body's ability to complete the concoctions leading to blood deficiency.

Blue central surface, wet and greasy = excess cold affecting the stomach.
- Due to excess melancholy in the spleen impinging on the stomach or excess phlegm and dampness in the stomach, the centre of the tongue looks blue and is wet because there is a lack of digestive heat.

Blue, swollen sides = melancholic blocks in the spleen.

Blue, swollen, thick white coating = phlegm overwhelming the stomach, bowels and/ or lungs.

Purple tongue

The purple tongue is indicative of blood stagnation, congealing blood, and stasis and may present either as a blue purple or a red purple tongue.
Blue shows underlying signs of coldness, resulting in stagnation of blood.
Red shows underlying signs of heat.

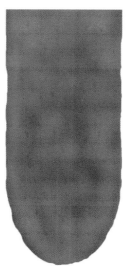

Excess melancholy and blood stagnation, purple bluish tongue with dark spots.

Bluish-purple = cold congestion.
- It evolves from a pale tongue over a period of time.
- It indicates stasis due to obstruction from internal cold. It may be accompanied by a white coating.
- Internal cold is caused by excessive melancholy or phlegm, cold congestion in the spleen and liver. This can also be due to consumption of cold and raw foods or chronic exposure to cold and damp environments.
- It will be accompanied by a lack of appetite, abdominal distension, cold limbs, and a deep weak pulse.

Bluish-purple with wet surface = deficient heat.
- If the tongue is bluish purple and is wet-looking, it indicates deficient innate heat:
- If it also lacks a coating, it is a clear indicator of low innate heat.
- Low innate heat slows movement of blood, and fluid is not moved but builds up showing on the tongue.
- It may be due to a weak heart and lungs, which is indicated by a short, narrow pulse.
- It is more commonly seen in men.

Bluish-purple with dry surface = deficient blood.
- A dry surface indicates deficient blood and an inability of the liver to make the blood humour. The blood is also the carrier of fluids and moisture around the body, when blood is deficient it produces dryness in the organs and tissues.
- Blood deficiency is closely related to deficient radical moisture, which is maintained by residues left after the concoctions have made blood. Low blood leads to low replenishment of moisture. Lack of blood or moisture causes lack of blood available and lack of flow to the tongue making it appear dry.
- Deficient blood also shows as: pale skin, dizziness, numb sensations, pale lips, scanty periods, choppy pulse varying in strength.
- It is more commonly seen in women.

Reddish purple = excess heat.
- Stagnation caused by excess heat, reducing flow. Usually producing a dry tongue surface accompanied by a yellow coating. The blood is dried out and reduced in flow.
- General signs of heat will be red face, fever, constipation, dry lips, rapid pulse.

Reddish purple with coating = excess choler/excess blood.
- If it is accompanied by a yellow coating that is well rooted it indicates excess heat and excess choler, or an excess of blood humour. If there is an excess of choler the tongue will be narrower, due to its drying and desiccating effects, while if there is an excess of blood the tongue will be broader or swollen, due to excess blood and moisture, and yellow due to the excess heat.
- It may be accompanied by the following signs of excess heat in the body: feelings of heat, sweating, thirst, acidity, nausea, constipation, jaundice, irritable, skin

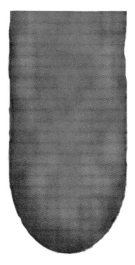

Excess Blood humour, Red purplish tongue, larger, sticky yellow coating.

problems, acne, carbuncles, sudden anger, fevers, shingles, frenzy, fury, poor sleep, bladder and kidney blockage & stones.

Associated diseases with excess choleric humour:
• Fevers, carbuncles, shingles, skin problems, itching, frenzy, kidney and bladder problems, dry coughs, and bronchitis.

Pulse in excess choleric states:
• Fast, hard, narrow, strong and forceful, strong, bowstring, long, and skipping.

Associated diseases with excess sanguine humour:
• Red swollen face, boils, mouth ulcers, heavy feeling, fevers, inflammation, skin problems, urinary infections, angry and uncomfortable.

Pulse in excess blood:
• Full, hard, tight, surging floating.

Reddish purple and lacking a coating or patchy coating = deficient moisture.
• Reddish purple shows deficient moisture. The tongue is red because without the cooling effect of moisture there are signs of heat because it is no longer being balanced by the moisture. Heat therefore appears to be in excess causing a red tongue. We can usually tell when the signs of heat are caused by deficient moisture because there is no coating, if the surface is also dry it shows a deficiency of the concoctions to produce enough blood when it is also likely that the tongue may be shrunken, narrow, or shrivelled and may also have cracks. If the tongue is lacking a coating or is

patchy, it will indicate that the blood is not being bred, and the residues which follow from that process and provide the replenishment of moisture also become absent.

Tongue shape

- If the tongue is thin in depth, it indicates deficient blood (pale) or deficient radical moisture (red body).
- If the tongue is swollen, it indicates an accumulation of fluids in the body organs, deficiency of innate heat (pale), excess choler blocking flow (red), excess blood (red) filling up the vessels.
- If the tongue is swollen, pale, and has a thick coating, it shows an excess of phlegm (white coating) or melancholic humour (swollen sides).
- If the tongue is short, it shows severe depletion of fluids. Pale due to lack of heat, red due to lack of moisture.
- If the tongue is narrow, it shows a deficiency of radical moisture (red), or deficiency of blood, (pale, dry)
- If the tongue is flaccid, it shows a depletion of nourishment and a weak heart.
- If the tongue is long it indicates presence of heat, usually excess heat in the heart. It is usually red.
- If the tongue has teeth marks it shows stagnation of vital spirit.
- If the tongue has cracks it is an indication of dryness.
- Horizontal cracks show dryness in the stomach.
- Cracks on the sides show excess melancholic humour in the spleen.
- A vertical central crack in the middle shows diminished stomach vitality.
- A long central crack from tip to root indicates heart weakness, low vital spirit.
- A long, deep central crack with smaller cracks spreading out indicates dryness in the kidneys and adrenal exhaustion.

Deficiency and depletion is indicated by the following body shapes:
- Narrow, flaccid, cracked, tooth marked.
- If deficient heat is present the tongue body colour will be pale, and if the radical moisture is deficient tongue body will be red and narrow.

Excess of humours is indicated by the following body shapes:
- Swollen, stiff, long, and moving.
- If excess heat in the form of excess choler or blood is present the tongue body will be red or purple.
- If melancholy or phlegm are in excess, the tongue body will be pale or bluish purple.

Narrow tongue

A narrow tongue points to a deficiency of moisture, either blood or radical moisture.

Narrow tongue = deficiency of radical moisture or blood.
• The fluids give the tongue body and shape. A thin, or shrunken tongue shows lack of fluids.

Narrow and pale = blood deficiency.
• A pale tongue may indicate deficient blood humour, a pale and narrow tongue indicates that the deficiency is severe, usually a dry surface.

Narrow and red = radical moisture deficiency.
• A red tongue without a coating indicates radical moisture deficiency, if it is thin and narrow it indicates that the deficiency is of long standing.

Short tongue

A short tongue is caused by fluids being depleted.

Pale and short = lack of internal innate heat.
• The tongue is pale because of the lack of heat and short because as the fluids cool they congeal and contract.

Red and short = extreme excess choler.
• The redness shows that there is extreme heat, the shortness shows that the fluids in the body have been dried, indicating heat in the liver and in the blood.

Red short and dry with no coating = deficiency of radical moisture.
• The lack of moisture makes the tongue short, and the dryness shows deficiency of blood, which will follow from the overheating of the liver that ensues from the lack of moisture.

Short and swollen = excess melancholy or atribilis blocks.
• This shows the retention of dampness behind the cold hard blocks of melancholy or burnt choler causing the swelling, and the stagnation caused by the cooling fluids means that there isn't the flow of the fluids into the organs accounting for the short-ness of the tongue.

Long tongue

If the tongue is long it indicates presence of heat, usually excess heat in the heart. It is usually red.

Swollen tongue

A swollen tongue is caused by accumulation of fluids in the body or organs.

Swollen, pale and wet = deficiency of innate heat.
- Wetness indicates a deficiency of innate heat, pale shows it is cold, swelling shows stasis and congestion.
- The deficiency of heat leads to stasis. It is the innate heat which activates all the of the natural faculties of the body; apprehension in the stomach and gall bladder, digestion in the liver, retention in the spleen, and expulsion in the kidneys and bowels. If any of these are deficient, healthy blood cannot be made, and as the blood moves fluids around the body the fluids accumulate due to stagnation.

Swollen, pale, thick white coating = excess phlegm humour.
- The swollen tongue shows retention of dampness, the paleness shows it is of a cold cause, and the thick white coating shows and excess of phlegm humour.

Swollen edges, pale = excess melancholic humour.
- A pale swollen tongue, especially if swollen on the edges indicates excess melancholy blocking the flow and movement of innate heat, blood, and fluids.

Swollen, pale and dry, little or no coating = deficient blood humour.
- Without the blood to carry the fluids the tongue becomes dry. However, because of the lack of heat and movement due to the lack of blood, there is accumulation of fluids. This shows that the liver is being overwhelmed by phlegm (white coating) or melancholy (swollen sides).

Swollen and normal colour/red, yellow coating = excess heat and moisture in the blood humour, especially in the stomach.
- Excess blood humour blocks and congests, causing the swelling, the heat makes the tongue yellow.

Swollen and normal colour, no coating = excess melancholy in the spleen.
- Excess melancholy in the spleen blocking movement of fluids from the stomach, causing swelling.
- Often accompanied by swollen sides.

Swollen and normal colour, white coating, = excess phlegm especially in the stomach and bowels.

Swollen and fresh looking red = excess choler effecting the heart and stomach.
- The heat in this case causes expansion and swelling of the tongue.

Swollen sides, on pale and/or wet tongue = excess melancholy.

Swollen sides, on red or purple tongue = excess choler and heat effecting the liver.

Swollen tip with a red tongue = excess heat affecting the heart.
• May be caused by anger, stress, upset, and heightened emotional states.

Swollen tip with a normal or pale tongue = depletion of heart energy.
• The tip corresponds to the heart, if it is swollen it shows congestion, and dampness building up in the heart, which may be caused by emotional exhaustion or physical weakness of the heart.

Flaccid tongue

All types of flaccid tongue show a depletion of nourishment, humours and flow of body fluids to the organs. It usually indicates weakness, especially of the heart.

Flaccid, pale and wet = weakness of heart and innate heat.
• Without the warmth of the heart to move the blood, nourishment of the organs becomes depleted.

Flaccid and pale with a white coating = excess melancholy or phlegm.
• The excess melancholy in the spleen blocks the flow of warmth to the heart and reduces the digestive faculty of the liver leading to a depletion of blood, which further weakens the heart making the tongue flaccid and pale. If there is a thick white coating it indicates the presence of excess phlegm. Accompanying symptoms include palpitations, insomnia, lack of appetite, lassitude, weakness, and a weak narrow deep pulse.

Flaccid, red with a coating = excess heat depleting body fluids.
• The heat is indicated by the red colour, and if accompanied by a yellow coating it further indicates excess heat.

Cracks

Horizontal cracks = shows lack of moisture in the stomach, or in the kidneys.
• If the tongue is normal in colour it shows that the stomach is lacking moisture, requiring warming aromatic bitter tonic herbs. If the tongue is red and lacking a coating, it shows that the kidneys are lacking moisture, and that loss of radical moisture is the cause, when nourishing tonic liver herbs are required.

Transverse cracks on the sides = excess melancholy in the spleen.
• Often occurs on a tongue with a normal colour.

Vertical crack in the centre = indicates poor digestion in the stomach.
• The centre of the tongue is the area that corresponds to the stomach. If the tongue is normal colour and without a coating it indicates lack of digestive function and digestive juices.

- If it is red and dry and has a yellow coating it indicates excess heat in the stomach.

Thin vertical crack extending the length of the tongue = indicates deficient heart energy.
- This is a crack which extends from the tip at the front to the root at the back. If the tongue is normal colour it reflects a constitutional weakness of the heart. If the tongue is red and has a redder tip it reflects excess heat and agitation of the heart, most commonly a sign of the heart being overwhelmed by powerful emotions. If the tongue is red and it has no coating it shows the radical moisture of the heart has been scorched and the patient needs cooling, calming, and protective heart herbs, such as the traditional cordials—lemon balm, borage, violets, and rose.

Thick deep vertical crack, with a red tongue and no coating = extreme loss of moisture in the kidneys.
- It also indicates a generalised loss of moisture throughout the body due to atrabilis building up and causing a blockage and obstruction of the kidneys, it is often associated with adrenal exhaustion, excess stress, worry, overwork and anxiety.

Tongue coating

The tongue coating is produced as a residue of the digestion and concoctions. It therefore reflects the general level of activity of the digestive organs, especially the stomach.

- The coating gives an indication of the hot or cold nature of a condition; white signifies cold, yellow signifies heat.
- Unlike the tongue shape and colour, the coating can change quickly in colour, thickness, and distribution, either as a result of treatment or pathological changes.
- The tongue coating can give an immediate indication of the deficient or excess nature of a condition; the absence of a coating always indicates deficiency of heat or moisture, and a thick coating always indicates an excess of humours.
- A slippery, greasy, or sticky coating indicates an excess of phlegm or dampness following from cold obstructions.

White coating

A white coating generally indicates cold.

White, thin, and slippery = dampness.
White, thick, and wet = excess phlegm and retention of dampness in the lungs.
White, thick, and sticky = excess phlegm and retention of dampness in the stomach or the large intestines.
White, thin, and dry on a pale tongue = deficient blood.

White, sticky, and greasy = excess melancholy in spleen, especially if swollen sides.
White and flaky = cold melancholic obstructions or black bile.
White, thick, and mouldy/patchy = putrefaction due to excess blood humour or dampness.

Yellow coating

A yellow coating generally indicates heat.
It is often associated with excess heat and choler effecting the stomach, spleen, and liver.

Yellow, thin, light = condition of heat in the lungs.
Yellow and thick = excess choler affecting the stomach and spleen.
Yellow, sticky, and greasy = heat and dampness together.
Yellow strips along the sides of the tongue = heat in the liver and gall bladder.

Grey coating

A grey coating indicates that a condition is of long standing and may evolve from either a white or a yellow coating.

Grey, wet, or slippery = dampness in the spleen, follows on from a state of excess melancholy.
Grey and dry = long standing condition of heat, depleted body fluids, and blood (pale tongue).

Black coating

A black coating is similar to that of the grey, it can represent either a hot or cold condition.

Black, wet, slippery, greasy, thick = retention of dampness and coldness in the stomach and intestines.
Black, dry, and cracked = burnt choler, exhaustion of body fluids.

CHAPTER SEVENTEEN

Pulse diagnosis

Through taking the pulse we can immediately get a feeling of the health and vitality of the whole body. Pulse diagnosis may sound like a complex and difficult skill to acquire, but it is actually a very straightforward process of assessing the variations in a small number of easy to recognise qualities.

We are simply attempting to feel the energy and life force of a person, manifested in the quality and movement of the pulse directly beneath our fingers.

The most important aspect of pulse taking is to focus on how the pulse feels, rather than what we think a pulse is telling us. This might seem to be a subtle distinction, but if we can allow ourselves to just spend a moment focusing on what we feel in the blood we quickly start to develop an ability to pick up some very helpful insights.

By keeping our assessment to some simple comparisons we can notice differences in the pulses of each individual and also how the pulse changes in an individual patient according to how they are feeling. It soon becomes clear when a pulse is strong or weak, deep or floating, fast or slow, narrow or broad, and these simple observations can directly guide us to the underlying constitutional and humoral imbalances in a patient.

It is best to start just by taking the pulse regularly and noticing these common variations of strength, speed, and quality, and seeing how the pulse changes with each patient and at each reading. Gradually we can begin to recognise when a pulse is indicating heat or cold, blockage or depletion, and by adding that to other observations about the patient, see how the pulse relates to the overall picture of the health.

The pulse is read with the first three fingers, the thumb is placed on the radial prominence, and the middle finger is placed opposite the thumb over the pulse point, the patients right pulse is felt with the left hand and the left pulse with the right hand.

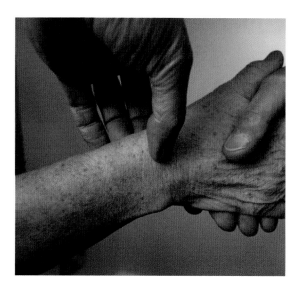

Position of the thumb.

The patients hand is held to give support, the patients arm should be relaxed and the elbow at a right angle. By using a three fingered assessment we can feel the pulse passing under the fingers, helping us to assess the overall speed, length, and strength along the whole pulse wave.

    The first three fingers are placed lightly on the skin only using as much pressure as is required to feel the pulse beating against the finger. There are some very basic qualities that can be looked for when we are first feeling the pulse: the force, the speed, and the quality. The depth of the pulse is assessed with all three fingers.

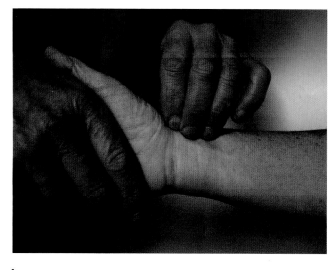

Position of the fingers.

- The floating pulse pushes up against the fingers when they are resting gently on the surface of the skin.
- The middling pulse is felt when the fingers feel the pulse wave travelling just beneath the skin surface when applying gentle pressure.
- The deep pulse is only felt when the fingers are pressed into the flesh of the wrist.

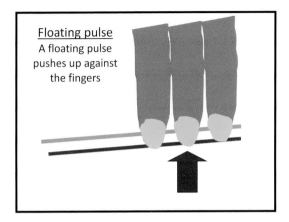

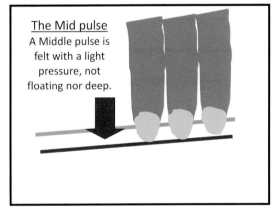

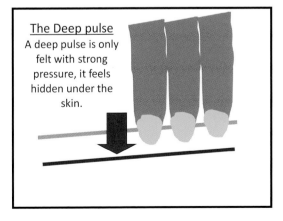

Identifying floating pulse, middle, and deep pulses.

Basic pulse diagnosis and assessment

We can start our assessment of the pulse with three basic assessments of force, speed, and quality. The quality includes the depth, length, width, and softness. Even if we never go beyond these basic assessments the pulse will immediately inform us about the state of the vital spirit, the animal spirit, the natural spirit and the balance of the humours in the blood.

- The vital spirit gives the pulse its strength. It provides its movement and the feeling of strength of the pulse as it hits the fingers. We expect a healthy strong pulse when the vital spirit is strong. Sometimes the vital spirit can be stirred up through excessive emotion, stress, or when fighting disease, and these will make the pulse feel very forceful. This excessive force can also be a sign of excess choler and heat. If the pulse is weak it shows a low level of innate heat, lack of radical moisture to help the blood to flow, a lack of healthy blood, or cold melancholic blockages.
- The animal spirit regulates the speed and rhythm of the pulse. We should expect a regular measured pulse of five beats for each complete breath. If there is mental agitation stirring up the animal spirit, or if there is excess heating of the brain, heart, or nerves the speed will increase, and if there is dullness of the animal spirit and brain, or a blockage due to coldness, it will become slower or even erratic. Causes of underlying coldness may be depletion of innate heat in the vital spirit, or excess of the phlegmatic or melancholic humours.
- The natural spirit is indicated by the balance of the four humours in the blood and can be felt in the quality of the blood itself. When any of the humours are in excess and are affecting the whole body it will be reflected in the blood and the quality of the pulse. Excess sanguine air humour will make the pulse larger, floating, longer, and faster. Excess choler fire humour will make the pulse harder, narrower, faster. Excess melancholy earth humour will make the pulse deeper, harder, slower, softer and narrower. Excess phlegm water humour will make the pulse softer, slower, shorter, thinner, and more empty.

Going into more depth when assessing the pulses

If we want to explore pulse diagnosis more fully, we can represent the different possible pulse pictures by showing where and how we might feel them in the wrist. A "pulse picture" diagram can be used to identify different characteristic pulses.

The pulse picture diagram shows the floating pulses at the top, and the deep pulses at the bottom, the middle level indicates the pulses which can either be found to be floating or deep. The left side shows the forceful pulses, and the right side shows the forceless pulses. Each of the pulses described originate from the traditional classical pulse pictures enumerated in Chinese pulse diagnosis, but have been reinterpreted to correspond to the Western humoral model of physiology.

PULSE STRENGTH	PULSE SPEED	PULSE QUALITY
Vital Spirit Its Seat is in the Heart	**Animal Spirit** Its Seat is in the head	**Natural Spirit** Its seat is in the liver
Indicates the strength of the vital Spirit	Indicates the activity of the Animal spirit	Indicates the relative amounts of each humour in the blood
Felt as the force of the blood hitting the finger	Felt as the rapidity, and rhythm of pulse waves	Felt as sense of quality of blood in artery
It has no intrinsic direction or movement, is moved by the Etheric force.	It has no body or substance apart from the movement of the pulse wave it creates.	It is the nourishing substance of the blood
The Vital spirit is the life-warmth for all the body and organs. Innate heat comes from Pneuma in the air, this heat literally keeps us warm and alive. Radical moisture lubricates the movement of this heat and provides the medium in which it flows, it prevents the heat from scorching the tissues. The Vital spirit strength is indicated by the body of the pulse wave, and the force it is able to assert on the finger.	**The Animal Spirit is the life-force that animates the whole body.** It brings all the organs and tissues together as a single living organism. It is conducted within the vital spirit to direct and move the disparate parts, animating all that it comes into contact with. It is connected to and ruled by the divine light emanating from the heavenly realm. It enters the body through the head as divine inspiration.	**The Natural spirit is the Life-blood feeding all the tissues and organs.** It is made from the concoctions of Foods in the liver, breaking them down into the constituent humours, Air, Fire, Earth, Water. Carrying them in the blood for distribution.

PULSE STRENGTH		PULSE SPEED		PULSE QUALITY
Excess	Depletion	Excess.	Depletion.	Blood: Large, floating, longer, faster.
Forceful, fast ,beats skipping ahead. Shows innate heat coming apart from moisture, extreme emotional stress, heat.	Forceless, deep, short, Shows loss of innate heat, debility, low radical moisture, low blood or cold blockages.	Rapid/racing. Agitation, fear, Extreme heat, Fast beats skipping ahead as heat separates from moisture.	Coldness, dampness Blocks the Animal spirit, Phlegm, melancholy vapours blocking the heart causing erratic beats.	Choler: Hard, floating, narrow, faster. Melancholy: Deep, narrow, hard, shorter, Slower. Phlegm: Soft, thin, short, deep, slower, empty.

Basic pulse characteristics.

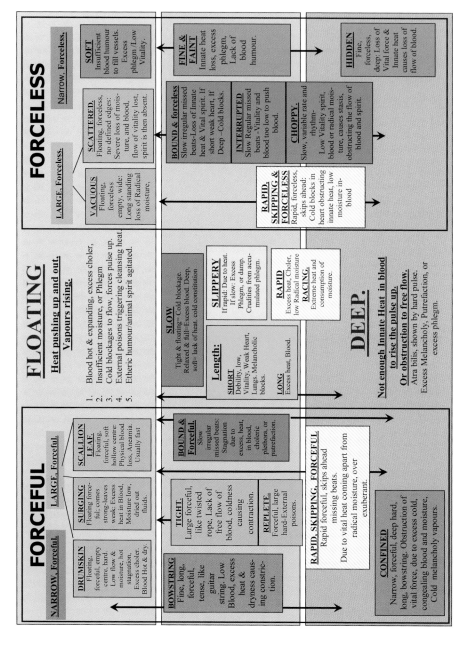

Pulse characteristics and diagnosis diagram—showing all the possible floating, deep, forceful, and forceless characters, and how to interpret them.

The following questions can be asked as a simple way of making a quick but full assessment;

Strength and speed
1. Is the pulse forceful or forceless?
2. Is the pulse fast or slow?

Quality
3. Is the pulse floating or deep?
4. Is the pulse wide or narrow?
5. Is the pulse long or short?
6. Is the pulse hard or soft?

The pulse strength and speed

1. Is the pulse forceful or forceless?

The strength of the pulse is indicative of the health of the vital spirit. The vital spirit is the activating warmth of life that animates and sustains the body and activates the organs. It is fed by the pneuma in the air taken in by the lungs, producing the innate heat. It is this heat that literally keeps us warm and alive. The radical moisture also contained in the vital spirit lubricates the movement of the innate heat and provides the medium in which it flows; its moisture and coldness prevents the heat from scorching the tissues.

The vital spirit strength is indicated by the body of the pulse wave, and the force it is able to assert on the finger. It brings with it no intrinsic direction or movement, as the blood is moved by the etheric force and the general level of heat in the body. When the Vital spirit is healthy, the forcefulness is felt throughout the pulse as it passes under the fingers, it should provide a constant feeling of force, not quickly dropping off nor conversely coming on gradually, needing time to build up to full strength. It should be of moderate length, not too short nor too long. A strong pulse can be either fast or slow, floating or deep, it may be blocked by cold, or constricted by heat. All of these things will affect the pulse's width, speed, length, and depth, but will not necessarily affect the pulse strength, as vital spirit itself may still be strong giving the pulse force.

Forceful pulses

When we assess the force, we are feeling the energy of life itself. A strong and reasonably forceful relaxed pulse will indicate good health, whilst a weak, forceless pulse will indicate sickness, ill health, and depletion. Simply through this one assessment we can immediately get a feeling of what kind of health our patient is in.

If it is excessively forceful and fast it shows innate heat coming apart from moisture. It is most often caused by extreme emotional stress agitating the heart and the vital spirit.

This excessive pulse may be felt as forceful, floating, and fast, and may have beats skipping ahead.

Forceless pulses

This shows loss of innate heat and depleted vital Spirit, general debility, low moisture, low blood, cold melancholic blocks, and excessive phlegm.

The pulse may be felt as forceless, deep, narrow, short, and even be hidden and difficult to feel, it may also have interrupted or missed beats.

2. Is the pulse fast or slow?

The speed of the pulse is indicative of the strength of the animal spirit and the level of heat or choler in the blood. It is measured by the rapidity and rhythm of the pulse waves. The animal spirit is the force that animates and activates the whole body, it is the energy within the nervous system. It can be amplified by anything that stirs up the senses or the nervous system. Anger, fear, agitation, surprise, and shock can all stimulate and heat up the animal spirit, increasing the rate of the pulse. Sadness, depression, melancholy, and grief can also slow, dull, and diminish the animal spirit, slowing and hindering the pulse.

The etheric humour that is contained within the animal spirit brings all the organs and tissues together as a single living organism. It combines with the vital spirit to direct and move the disparate parts, animating all that it comes into contact with. It is connected to and ruled by the divine light emanating from the heavenly realm, entering the body through the head in the form of divine inspiration.

Fast pulses

When the pulse is rapid or racing, it shows extreme heat in the blood or agitation of the animal spirit, which governs the nervous system, often caused by fear, anger, or heightened stress. A fast pulse may also be due to a loss of radical moisture in the blood so that it can't flow smoothly along the vessels but moves rapidly like a hot wind.

A younger person's pulse is faster: newborns, 120–140; four year olds, 110; ten year olds, 90; fourteen year olds, 75–80. A woman's pulse is generally finer, faster, and weaker, and a man's fuller, slower, and more forceful.

The speed of the pulse is assessed over the length of a normal breath, two beats on the in breath, one in the middle and two on the out breath, making a normal pulse speed five beats per breath. This roughly corresponds to 70 beats per minute.

A fast pulse is one that is 6 or more beats per breath, or 80–90 beats per minute. It generally points to there being more heat in the body.

- If fast, floating, and forceful, there is an excess of heat effecting the heart, liver, or head.
- If fast, floating, and forceless, there is a loss of moisture or a loss of blood.
- If fast, missing beats or irregular, and forceful, it indicates excess choler, if forceless, it indicates low blood or moisture.

The rapid and skipping pulse pictures

Rapid Pulse:
More than 6 beats over a complete breath, or over 90 beats per minute.
   It may be floating or deep.
   If rapid floating and forceful it is due to:

1. Excess heat effecting the heart and vital spirit, often due to an emotional crisis.
2. Excess heat in the head and the animal spirit.
3. Excess heat in the liver and the natural spirit, due to putrefaction, external toxins/infection as in a fever.

If rapid and floating and forceless it is due to:

1. Loss of radical moisture.
2. Loss of moisture in blood or low blood humour

A rapid pulse may be felt with erratic beats, and with palpitations.

Skipping pulse:
Rapid, missing beats.

1. *Forceful*: heat is keeping the pulse rapid, there may be excess heat in the heart due to emotional overload stirring up the vital spirit, or excess heat in the head and agitation of the animal spirit.
2. *Forceless*: lack of blood or exhaustion of radical moisture means that the beats skip ahead.

Slow pulses

A slow pulse is one which is four or less beats to the breath, or less than 70 beats per minute. It generally shows coldness and dampness slowing the flow of etheric force and animal spirit, often seen in colder temperaments, or in cases of excess phlegm or melancholic humour.

   It may also show a loss of innate heat. The innate heat contained in the vital spirit activates all of the organs, so if innate heat is diminished it will also lead to the weakness of the animal spirit and result in a slower pulse. The loss of innate heat may be due to debility, illness, or old age. Innate heat can also be diminished by other humours being excessive and blocking the movement of the blood and spirits.

The pulse may be felt as a slow, interrupted or erratic pulse.

- A slow, relaxed, and full pulse shows excess blood humour, and the damp heat that accompanies it.
- A slow, tight, and forceful pulse, constricted in nature indicates a cold melancholic or phlegmatic block.
- A slow and deep soft pulse shows lack of innate heat.
- A slow and floating softer pulse shows excess phlegm.
- A slow, regular, and interrupted pulse shows weakness of the heart, or melancholic blockages affecting the heart, often it will also be shorter in length showing a heart weakness.
- A slow, irregular, and interrupted pulse, shows loss of vital spirit, loss of innate heat and a weak heart.
- A slow pulse variable in rate and rhythm shows blockage caused by excess phlegm humour or melancholy humour.

The slow pulse pictures

Relaxed pulse:
Relaxed, floating, and large, shows excess air humour.
Relaxed, deep, shows dampness, excess phlegm.

Interrupted pulse:
Slow, relaxed, stops at regular intervals.
Loss of innate heat, vital force, and if the pulse is also short shows a weakness of the heart.

Bound pulse:
Slow, relaxed, stops at irregular intervals.

1. Forceful: stagnation in the body caused by excess dryness, heat, or choler.
2. Forceless: diminished vital spirit. If the pulse is also short it is a sign of weak heart or lungs.
3. Forceless, deep: indicates excess melancholy blocking the innate heat emanating from the heart.

Choppy pulse:
Slow, variable rhythm, fine, varies in force, rate, rhythm.
Low or stagnant vital force, shows cold obstructions obstructing the flow of ether/animal spirit, if pulse is deep, it shows excess melancholy, atribilis blocks, or phlegm.

The pulse quality

The sense of the quality of the blood and the pulse in the artery is indicative of the natural spirit and the balance of humours. The natural spirit is strong when there is a beneficial balance of humours produced in the liver. The humours then constitute and reside in the blood, giving the blood its body, allowing it to fill, flow, and travel through the arteries. The humours provide the nourishing substance of the blood and are transported in the blood for distribution to the organs and tissues. The pulse quality therefore indicates the relative amount of each humour in the blood, and an excess of a particular humour can be identified in the following ways:

Excess choler:
The pulse may be hard, floating, narrow, faster.

Excess blood:
The pulse may be large, floating, longer, faster.

Excess melancholy:
The pulse may be deep, narrow, hard, shorter, slower.

Excess phlegm:
The pulse may be soft, thin, short, deep, slower.

3. Is the pulse wide or narrow?

Wide pulses

The wide pulse indicates an excess of heat, or a loss of moisture. When it is excess heat, either because of excess blood humour or choler, it will usually also be floating and forceful. When it is due to a loss of moisture it means that the pulse can't move forward and becomes wide like a stagnant puddle with no flow or movement, it then is also usually forceless and often floating, such as a in the vacuous and scattered pulse picture. If, however, the innate heat hasn't yet been diminished, it may still be floating and strong, such as the drumskin pulse, surging pulse or a scallion leaf pulse picture.

Narrow pulses

The narrow pulse usually indicates a loss of blood to fill the vessels, loss of heat to make it move and expand, or some form of constriction, which may be due to excessive heat, or cold. The force and speed as well as the depth will indicate whether the cause of the narrowness is from heat or cold.

We will consider the width of each kind of pulse alongside whether it is also floating or deep.

4. Is the pulse floating or deep?

Floating pulses

A floating pulse pushes up against the finger, it becomes insufficient when pushed down. It indicates heat, if the pulse is forceful it indicates heat in the blood pushing the pulse up and out. If the pulse is forceless it usually indicates a depletion of moisture in the body allowing the heat to become dominant and that imbalance of heat will also push the pulse up. It is helpful to consider the floating pulse in relation as to whether they are also wide or narrow, forceful, or forceless.

There are four main categories of floating pulse: the floating and wide pulse either with or without force, and the floating and narrow pulses either with or without force. Remember that force generally indicates heat, and forcelessness indicates cold or loss of heat.

- Floating, large, forceful pulse indicates excess heat usually due to excess choler or blood, or a cold constriction or obstruction to flow.
- Floating, narrow, forceful indicates heat drying the blood and liver.
- Floating, large, forceless pulse indicates low radical moisture allowing heat to become dominant.
- Floating, narrow, forceless indicates low blood humour, low vital force and radical moisture, or excess phlegm.

Floating, large pulse pictures

Floating, large, forceful pulses:

Drumskin:
- This pulse is floating, forceful, hard, but empty in the centre.
- This pulse indicates excess heat and excess choler in the blood, making the blood hot and dry, leading to a loss of innate moisture, which means that the blood is left without any body and collapses in the centre.

Surging:
- This pulse is floating, forceful, it comes on strong and leaves weak.
- This pulse indicates excess blood, often accompanied by diminished moisture.
- Heat has dried out fluids, it may be due to excess choler, or excess heat in the blood humour. The excess blood and heat give the pulse its strength and the loss of the radical moisture makes it lack any body.

Scallion leaf:
- This pulse is floating, forceful, soft, with a hollow centre.
- This usually indicates a loss of blood, and is often seen in anaemia. The loss of blood means that the blood doesn't flow and is pushed up, making the pulse float. The forceful aspect comes from the vital spirit remaining active, while the hollow

centre and softness are due to the consequent lack of moisture in the blood making it unable to expand the artery.

Floating, large, forceless pulses:

Vacuous:
- This is a large, floating, forceless, wide, pulse.
- It indicates a long standing loss of radical moisture, which usually also leads to low blood humour. The heat makes it float, but the lack of moisture makes it empty.

Scattered:
- This is a large, floating, forceless, pulse with no defined edges or root.
- It shows that the vital spirit has lost its ability to flow due to a loss of moisture, or a loss of moisture within the blood humour, leaving only the heat. It is associated with a drying out of the liver or kidneys and heart of a long standing, which may have been caused by excessive heat or lack of moisture in these organs. The loss of moisture means that the pulse is no longer able to flow but disperses outwards.

Floating narrow pulse pictures

Floating narrow and forceful pulses:

Floating Bowstring Pulse:
- It is tight, thin, and hard, the bowstring pulse always indicates constriction to flow. When it is floating it indicates that heat is drying the blood and liver, reducing flow and free movement of the blood causing stagnation. When it is deep it indicates cold hard atribilis blocks constricting flow.

Floating narrow and forceless pulses:

Soft pulse:
- The pulse is fine, floating and soft. The pulse is soft due to either a lack of innate heat defining and strengthening the pulse, or a lack of blood giving the pulse a defined body. The lack of radical moisture that follows on from these two scenarios allows the heat to become dominant and then to push the pulse upwards. In the case of a lack of vital spirit and the consequent lack of innate heat, the tongue will be wet, and if a lack of blood humour it will be dry. The pulse can also be floating due to excess phlegm, which floods the tissues and pushes the pulse upwards, indicated by a swollen pale or blue tongue usually with a white or grey coating.

Deep pulses

A deep pulse cannot be detected near the surface with light pressure, but can be felt near the bone with deep pressure. The deep pulse is usually also narrow. If the pulse is deep it usually reflects a lack of heat and vital spirit, either because it is lacking, or because it is obstructed.

- Deep and forceful or hard shows constriction or obstruction.
- Deep and forceless or soft shows weakness of the heart and loss of innate heat.

Deep, narrow, forceful pulse pictures

Constricted pulse:
- It is tight, thin, hard, deep, and doesn't disappear on pressure.
- Its forcefulness shows that the vital spirit and innate heat is not lacking. However, the depth shows that the movement of the heat around the body is being blocked. This may be due to either melancholic obstruction, phlegmatic obstruction, or excess blood humour and the damp congesting heat associated with it.

Deep, narrow, forceless, pulse pictures

Fine pulse:
- Narrow, deep and forceless, it disappears on pressure.
- This pulse shows a severe loss of vital spirit and lack of blood humour.

Hidden pulse:
- Narrow, deep, and very forceless, difficult to find or absent.
- This pulse shows severe depletion on many levels including the vital, natural and animal spirits.

Floating, middle, or deep, also large and forceful pulse pictures

Replete pulse:
- Forceful, large, hard, full, usually floating, but sometimes can be middling.
- Putrefaction, infection, excess heat and moisture in the blood. Excess choler, excess blood, putrefaction, or external poisons in the blood.

Tight pulse:
- Large forceful, constricted, long, tense, constrained like rope. A thicker version of the bowstring pulse.
- Shows blockage to free flow of blood, often associated with cold obstructions, such as excess melancholy, or burnt choler. May also be present in states of extreme pain.

Floating, middle, or deep, also narrow and forceless pulse pictures

Fine and feint:
- Narrow, small, weak, disappears on pressure.
- Weak vital spirit, loss of blood humour, often caused by the low vitality and weakened digestion and production of blood.

5. Is the pulse long or short?

Long pulses

The long pulse is felt as the length of the pulse wave beneath the finger, so that the wave extends over the ends of two fingers at a time. It may be fast, slow, floating or deep. It is generally indicative of warmth, or excess choler.

- The long pulse indicates excess choler, excess blood, and heat in general.

Short pulses

The short pulse is felt like a short wave that passes quickly beneath the fingers, however it may be rapid or slow in rate or rhythm.

- The short pulse mainly indicates lack of blood or vital spirit.
- A short and forceless pulse indicates weakness of the heart or lungs and lack of innate heat.

6. Is the pulse hard or soft?

Hard pulse

A pulse becomes hard due to constriction and blockage of flow. The constriction can be due to either a cold cause or a hot cause. Assessing the other qualities of the pulse will enable one to determine a hot or cold cause.

Soft pulse

The soft pulse will indicate a lack of heat; either due to the loss of vital spirit and its innate heat, or because of a lack of healthy blood to distribute the heat around the body.

Slippery pulses

A slippery pulse is one whose arrival and departure is soft at both ends, gradually growing and fading away, making it feel like it is slipping under the fingers rather than pushing against them in a wave.

- A slippery pulse that feels full, may reflect an excess of blood humour.
- A slippery pulse that is long shows excess heat and excess blood humour.
- A slippery pulse that is slow shows excess phlegm or excess melancholy.
- A slippery pulse that is rapid shows excess phlegm blocking the lungs.
- A slippery pulse that is floating shows stagnation of vital spirit or animal spirit.

CHAPTER EIGHTEEN

Dreams and healing

W e are exploring an ancient tradition of healing, and if we can bring some of the insights we have gained about Asclepian medicine into our practice we may discover a new depth to our work as healers. We may not be able to take our patients through a period of physical and emotional preparation and cleansing, and we do not have a healing temple within which we can prepare mind, body, and spirit for a transformative healing experience. However, we may still be able to bring many of the principal aspects of the Asclepian healing journey into our work.

The first part of the Asclepian healing journey is to receive a calling to seek transformational healing. We may often find that our patients have come to herbal medicine and other forms of natural healing as a last resort. They will most likely have tried conventional approaches first and, having received only limited or no benefit, have begun to look elsewhere. In this way, many of our patients are already responding to an inner calling and are seeking a new approach to their sickness and how to find a healing resolution. They have responded by deciding to become involved in their own healing process and have taken action.

When most patients appear for their first appointment, they are setting out on a fresh journey and are looking to us as helpers on that journey. It is important to honour the call to heal that they have received, and to explore where it is coming from. We can start by simply asking the patient why they have come. I am frequently told by patients that they have been drawn to herbal medicine by reading or hearing about a particular herb that might help them. When that is the case, I will always find a way of including that herb in our treatment, as a way of acknowledging the herb that called them.

It is common that there will have been a set of serendipitous events that come together to bring a patient onto our path. I have had patients who discover one of my cards, which has lain at the bottom of their wallet for years unnoticed and suddenly seems to appear just when they are looking for some help. Sometimes people have had a chance encounter with another patient of mine, or just so happen to hear someone talking about the treatment they are getting from me.

In the ancient tradition of Asclepian medicine, dreams are considered a powerful and important medium of healing and are often also the source of the calling to be healed. We should be open to hearing about the dreams of our patients and be particularly attentive to dreams that guide patients to seek us out.

A patient who came following such a calling dream told me about it on her first visit; in the dream she had been standing at the top of a hill, in front of her she had seen a white gate in a picket fence. She had felt that she knew that she must pass through that gate, and that once she had gone through it she would never return. However, the path led into a beautiful meadow, and she felt reassured and attracted by the vista that she was now entering. Having had the dream she had a strong feeling that it was telling her to seek help and healing. She had for some time had digestive issues that she couldn't sort out for herself, and she was feeling troubled by them. When she came she told me about the dream, and said that she had worried that passing through the gate might have been a sign that she would soon die, a concern that had been heightened by the fact that her sister had recently been diagnosed with stomach cancer. Her sister had then undergone a number of unsuccessful, painful, and stressful treatments and had died not long after being diagnosed. I suggested that she have thorough investigations at the hospital to rule out any serious problems that might be causing her problems and to allay any of her fears. When all the tests came back clear, she was obviously very relieved, especially because she had always been adamant that she would never undergo any invasive treatments like her sister had. However, an extra worry for her was the knowledge that her family would not have been happy for her to refuse conventional treatment, however invasive. We commenced on a range of dietary changes and herbal supports to improve the digestive problems, and she responded to them very well. Over the next few years she continued to return for occasional guidance and to stock up on herbs. Suddenly after seven years, having enjoyed good health throughout, and with no significant recurrence of her digestive problems she became very sick and then died within a few weeks. It transpired that the original tests had missed a stomach cancer, which had spread over the years, and she had died from the effects of multiple secondarys in a number of organs. It was a terrible shock, and it was initially difficult to work out if I could have done anything differently. After taking some time to contemplate the experience, I felt that I was able to make more sense of it, especially when the dream was taken into consideration. It became clear to me that by following her calling in the dream to consult a herbalist and to look after her health naturally, she had managed to maintain an active healthy life, without undue stress or worry even though she was suffering from a life-limiting cancer. It is likely that if the oncologists had found the cancer at the outset when I first saw her she would have felt obliged to follow her family's wishes and would have undergone very invasive conventional treatments, which would have impacted on her health and quality of life, and still may not have extended her life beyond the years she lived.

In this dream the patient saw the pathway ahead leading into a meadow of wild flowers, and this was from where her decision to find a herbalist to help her resolve the sickness that she was experiencing came from. She had intuitively felt that it was also a reminder of the shortness of life and inevitability of death, but she had felt calmed by the vision she was given of the journey ahead and had enjoyed her life fully without worry.

In the ancient Asclepian tradition of temple healing, a patient would hope for a dream experience in which the healing deities might heal them directly or show them what it is that they require to progress with their healing. I have found that sometimes patients may have a revelation in a dream, or sometimes they experience a dream which seems to change them in a profound way. It also happens that either the patient, myself or even another practitioner may have a dream indicating a particular treatment or remedy. A good example of this was when my partner Zoe and I were training with African Sangoma healers; One night after returning from training in Africa, Zoe had a clear dream about a patient seeking the help of our teacher at her African house. In the dream the patient had what seemed to be a deformed leg that was twisted in a backward direction, he was unable to walk properly and needed help. In the dream Zoe saw our teacher rub red paste onto his legs and all over his body, followed by him leaving after the treatment able to walk unaided. We were in England at the time but still managed to get a message to our teacher in Africa and told her about the dream. A few days later we heard back that the dream had been accurate, and that the patient Zoe had seen in the dream had come to our teacher for healing. Not all dreams will be as literal as this, but you may often find that the dream brings up particular feelings or memories, and by discussing it with your patient new insights and inspirations about their healing journey often become clear.

We should be very attentive to the dreams that our patients have and help them to explore and interpret them. Although dream interpretation itself is a vocation and art in itself, that doesn't mean we cannot help patients to unravel signs and messages in dreams, and often a dream may also contain signs and messages for us as their practitioner.

As in ancient temple medicine, our role is to support the patient on a personal quest for healing, unlike a modern medical intervention we are not attempting to take control of a pathological process in an attempt to erase illness. We are guiding our patients on a journey to restore their best possible health, and this is likely to require them to change how they view themselves, their place in the world, their bodies, and their relationship to healing. If we can help them to once again listen to the true needs of their bodies, and help them to interpret what it is that they are being asked to change, then we can also provide them with the support they need to enable the natural healing forces within the body to bring about a resolution to their suffering. In Asclepian medicine it is the natural healing forces within the body that we are seeking to engage. This means that we must step aside, and by using our skills, experience, and compassion, attempt to provide the nurture and guidance our patients require for these natural healing forces within them to do their work.

CHAPTER NINETEEN

The herbal

Angelica

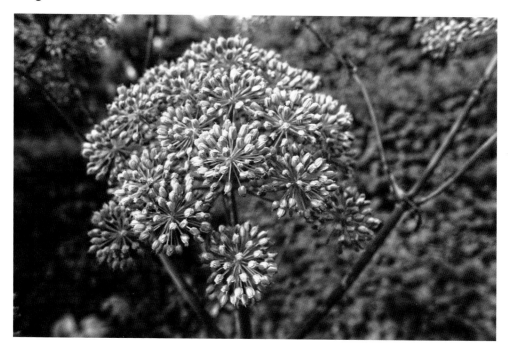

Latin:	*Angelica archangelica*
Family:	Apiaceae

Element	Fire
Planet	Sun
Humour	Choleric humour
Quality	Hot in the 3rd degree, dry in the 3rd degree. Strengthens innate heat, clears phlegm and melancholy

Organs

Lungs
Stomach
Spleen
Heart, circulation
Joints
Externally healing (fresh leaves)
Womb, reproductive passages

Actions

Expectorant
Antispasmodic
Anti-inflammatory
Carminative
Stimulant
Antifungal
Antibacterial
Diaphoretic
Diuretic

Constituents

Volatile oils
Coumarins
Phenylpropanoids: angelic and valerianic acid
Flavonoids

Traditional uses and humoral influences

Angelica is a warming, aromatic, gentle, bitter herb, considered to be hot and dry in the third degree. It is helpful in all damp, cold, and congested states. It is ruled by the sun and is under the astrological sign of Leo, the sign that rules the heart and the stomach, indicating that angelica has a particular affinity with these organs. Angelica strengthens the heart and raises the spirits bringing courage and vitality, whilst also warming and activating the stomach.

When added to any medicine angelica ensures that the remedy will travel to the desired organ as it activates the innate heat, stimulates the vital spirit, and moves blood. It is cleansing, fortifying, and protective for the blood. When the vitality is weak and the innate heat is low the body cannot maintain its resistance to the invasion of external heat and poisons. With its third degree heat, angelica has always been considered one of the main herbs for resisting pestilence and fevers. Nicholas Culpeper said "In all epidemical diseases caused by Saturn (the planet of coldness and death), that is as good a preservative as grows: It resists poison, by defending and comforting the heart, blood, and spirits".

It is considered very helpful for clearing the putrefaction that occurs when there is excess damp in any part of the body, especially from the stomach. Nicholas Culpeper added "The stalks or the roots candied, and eaten fasting, are good preservatives in time of infection; and at other times to warm and comfort a cold stomach".

Angelica has been prized as a particularly helpful herb for the elderly and the infirm, supporting the circulation, digestion, and giving protection from infections. When there is excess melancholy, cold obstructive vapours rise up from the spleen bringing on depression by overwhelming the heart, these cold vapours reduce the digestive function of the stomach by cooling its heat and by blocking the concoction of foods in the liver, this undermines the liver's ability to produce a good balance of humours and healthy blood. The warmth of angelica disperses these cold vapours, clears stagnation from the spleen, and benefits those with cold or damp constitutions, helping to rectify depletion of innate heat due to illness, old age, or exhaustion. I have often found it useful in treating conditions of weakness and depletion. I once helped a patient who had been exposed to pesticides and consequently suffered from an M.E. like illness by giving a daily decoction of angelica root, dandelion, and burdock root for a number of months.

Mythos

The archangel Michael appeared in a vision to a monk and gave him Angelica as a cure for the plague. From then onwards it was known as *Angelica archangelica*. It was considered so inimical to black magic and witchcraft that if it grew in a garden it proved the householders could not themselves be witches.

It has always been considered spiritually protective and able to exorcise evil wherever it is found in the body. The infused oil clears the body of negative spiritual influences and will confer spiritual protection.

Emotional

As expected of a sun herb in Leo, angelica strengthens, uplifts, and enlivens the heart and the spirits. It is a useful herb for melancholy, depression, exhaustion, and pessimism. It gives us hope when all seems lost, in which cases it combines well with St John's wort, rose and lemon balm. In times of severe stress and emotional shock it can be used as a rescue remedy, I suggest taking 5–10 ml of the tincture in a little water.

Digestion

Aromatic bitter herbs activate the stomach and the liver, producing improved tone throughout the digestive system, making angelica a gentle stimulant for loss of appetite, taken in drop doses before food. Nausea, bloating, feelings of fullness, distension, and cramps are all helped by taking a little angelica as a bitter tonic before meals or when the problems occur. (See angelica digestive bitters recipe below)

Nicholas Culpeper suggested it for bloating and constipation caused by a weak digestion, proclaiming that the distilled water of the root "easeth all pains and torments coming of cold and wind, so that the body be not bound" Angelica helps clear dampness from the stomach, eliminate fermentation, and its warmth will activate healthy digestion and elimination.

Spleen

The spleen is the organ of retention, the seat of the melancholic humour, and its quality is cold and dry. If there is inadequate warmth in the spleen and consequently excess coldness, the transport of nutrients and the humours themselves become obstructed; angelica warms the spleen, moves the blood, clears the excess melancholy and helps the liver to once again breed healthy blood.

Lungs

Nicholas Culpeper said "Some of the root in powder … helpeth the pleurisy, as also all other diseases of the lungs and breast, as coughs, phthysic (wasting diseases of the lungs) and shortness of breath; and a syrup of the stalks do the like".

Angelica is traditionally used in bronchitis and for chronic lung diseases. It is a useful antispasmodic expectorant, which relaxes and dilates the bronchioles, helping to clear phlegm and reduce coughing.

Heart/Circulation

Angelica is a circulatory and heart tonic, helpful for congestive heart failure, angina, or a weak circulation. It is beneficial in Reynaud's syndrome and poor circulation to the extremities. It helps with congested blood conditions and is safe to be used regularly in teas and tonics. The infused oil applied over the heart also provides a warming activating stimulant.

Urinary system

Angelica is a warming tonic for the kidneys, it has a gentle diuretic effect, and is an effective urinary and bladder disinfectant.

Rheumatics

A useful herb for gout and chronic rheumatism. It clears swelling from the joints, the oil is particularly helpful for muscular weakness and pain if used as a rub. It can be used as in a footbath to help aching feet and legs especially when accompanied by poor circulation.

Nervous system

When cold conditions affecting the head cause vertigo, migraines, palsy, or faintness, angelica will warm the brain and revitalise the nerves. It reduces cramps, muscular spasm, restless legs, and peripheral neuropathy either used as a massage oil or in hand and foot baths.

Gynaecological

A helpful herb for menopause, menopausal weakness, palpitations, and depression. It is helpful for painful periods, hot flushes, pelvic congestion, and fibroids or weak and irregular menstruation.

Doses

Angelica cordial

Cut 180 grams fresh angelica root into thin slices, pour on 1 litre of boiling water, add 225 g of honey, the juice of two lemons, infuse for 1/2 hour then add 200 ml of brandy. Drink 20 ml neat or diluted with an equal amount of water.

Tincture

10–35 ml 1:3 tincture a week is useful when added to 140 ml of a herbal tonic. (taken in a dose of 10 ml twice daily)

Candied angelica root

Make a syrup, gently simmer the chopped root in it for 20 minutes until the root goes translucent. Strain, roll in brown sugar, and dry in a low oven or a de-hydrator until leathery but not rock hard.

Angelica digestive bitters mix

33% angelica tincture,
33% elecampagne tincture.
16% dill aromatic water.
16% gentian (*Gentiana lutea*) tincture.

Bay

Sweet Bay. Bay laurel. Noble laurel. Daphne
French: Laurier d'Apollon

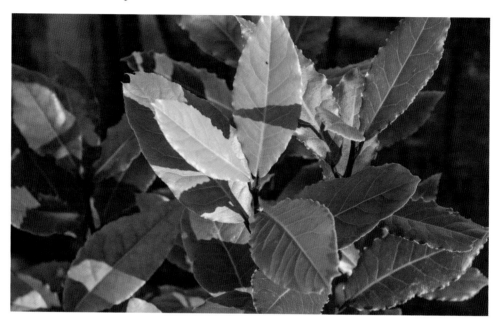

Latin:	*Laurus nobilis*
Family:	Lauraceae

Element	Fire
Planet	Sun
Humour	Choleric
Quality	Hot and dry in the second degree, cleanses phlegm from the head, lungs and stomach, protects the vital spirit

Organs

Stomach
Spleen
Liver
Heart
Brain

Actions

Gastric tonic
Carminative
Cholagogue
Antiseptic
Anti-inflammatory
Antifungal
External healer
Stimulant

Constituents

Volatile oil: cineole, linalool, limonene
Sesquiterpines
Lignan glycosides

Traditional uses and humoral influences

Bay is under the dominion of the sun, being hot and dry in the second degree. It is also under Leo, the astrological sign that rules the heart, pericardium, thoracic vertebrae, stomach, the sides, and jointly the midriff with the sign Virgo.

The vital spirit, which resides in the heart, carries the essence of life and through generating innate heat both activates the organs, and protects the body through resisting and expelling poisons. When this internal warmth is low and we have become vulnerable to the invasion of external toxins, bay will strengthen the vital spirit and protect the body. Bay was believed to protect against the plague, and wreaths were hung over doorways to keep sickness out. Bay is recommended for treating all diseases coming from a cold cause. Its heating and cleansing action makes it very beneficial for those diseases caused by Saturn, the ruler of the earth element, which has a cold and dry temperament. Diseases of Saturn include melancholy, obstructions of the spleen and liver, bone pains, migraines, palsies, and paralysis. Nicholas Culpeper commented that it will "help all cold and rheumatic distillations from the brain to the eyes, lungs, or other parts, and being made into an electuary with honey do help the consumption, old coughs, shortness of breath and thin rheum's; as also the migraine" The thin rheum's refers to excess catarrh, and as the eyes are associated with the Sun, bay can also be used to help clear eye infections. To help all cold conditions affecting the womb, bladder, and bowels, Culpeper also recommended using a bath made from the decoction.

Mythos

The bay tree was sacred to both the Romans and the Greeks and dedicated to Apollo and his twin sister Artemis/ Diana. Apollo the sun god provided cleansing and purification. Crowning a person with a wreath of laurel was considered both purifying and a recognition of divine authority. Asclepius the god of healing, was also traditionally crowned with bay. In early Christianity the evergreen bay symbolised eternal life and became a symbol of resurrection, accounting for it often being planted in and around graveyards.

Culpeper dramatically expressed this belief in its ability to give protection saying that it "resists witchcraft very potently, neither witch nor devil, thunder nor lightning, will hurt a man in the place where a Bay tree is".

The Greek myth of the water nymph Daphne, who was the daughter of the river god Peneius, explains where this belief arose; Eros had fired an arrow of love that had split apart, with each part flying in opposite directions. Half of it struck Apollo filling him with passion and lust while the other part struck Daphne producing the opposite effect, ensuring she would be forever chaste. As soon as he caught sight of Daphne Apollo fell deeply in love with her and was determined to make her his own. However, her pure chaste character bound her to do everything she could to resist him. She managed to run and hide from him for a long time, but eventually, having the endurance of a god, Apollo finally chased her down and pinned her to the ground. At this point Daphne called out to the earth goddess Hera to save her, who in an instant whisked her away to Crete replacing her with a bay tree. The tree subsequently came to represent purity and chastity, and became dedicated to the oracles of Delphi. The oracles remained chaste and pure so that their sacred visions would be free of any contamination, leading them to be named the "Daphnemancies" after the water nymph. The leaves have a slight narcotic effect, and by chewing them the oracles would enter a sacred trance enabling them to communicate better with the divine realms.

The leaves were presented to Roman generals returning from battle to cleanse them of the blood of war before they re-entered the city, and in this way such "laurels" became a symbol of victory. A period of peace would often follow the victory and the laurel wreath therefore also became a symbol of peace. The word "baccalaureate" combines the words laurel and bachelor, a bachelor is unmarried and therefore chaste, and the title was awarded for completing three years devoted to remaining pure while on the search for truth and wisdom.

Emotional

Bay helps to clear feelings of negativity, bringing back a more joyful view of the world. It refreshes the spirits, helping us to feel cleansed of all that has been overwhelming us. When we are feeling exhausted, tired of life, and find it difficult to see any brightness in the world around us, a bay bath has a wonderfully uplifting effect. I recommend using it when we have been through a time of sickness, trauma, or feel overwhelmed by the negativity of others. As the ancients

proclaimed, it is a powerful plant of the sun, and of the essence of life itself, enabling it to give us encouragement even in the darkest moments of our lives. When we use bay in this way we are also acknowledging our own divine nature and sacred vision.

Stomach, spleen, liver

The Stomach is under the rulership of the moon and the phlegmatic humour, it is particularly susceptible to an excess of cold and damp, reducing its ability to break down food. The heating effect of bay warms the stomach, helping it to "apprehend" the nutritious elements in food, it eases cramps and colic, which are caused by excess cold, and expels wind. The warming effects help to clear congestion of the liver and spleen, the spleen is the seat of the retentive faculty in the body and if it gets blocked by excess cold we find that stasis, constipation, bloating, and wind may follow. We are still familiar with bay being added as an aromatic digestive herb to meals, especially to fatty stews, and to help in the digestion of meats.

Brain

The brain has a cold damp phlegmatic temperament, and is easily affected by an excess of cold damp congestion. When this happens we suffer from lethargy, dullness, dumbness and faintness, convulsions, palsies, and migraines. The ears are effected by cold conditions and dropping in some bay oil, or using a steam with bay can help all cold conditions of the head, sinuses, and any respiratory congestion.

Skin

The skin can be washed with bay water for itches and scabs. It is particularly useful for acne, eczema, and rosacea. A cleansing wash can be made by combining the distilled waters of bay, witch hazel, and rose geranium. It can be used to cleanse the skin two or three times a day applied on a damp pad.

Joints

When the joints are painful and stiff massaging with bay infused oil is very helpful. Having a bay bath, or using a footbath or hand bath also helps with pain, exhaustion, and tiredness.

Doses

Acne rosacea skin wash

Aromatic waters of
Bay: 60%
Witch hazel: 30%
Pelargonium: 10%

Bath or steam

Fresh or dried leaves made as a decoction with 100 g of leaves to one litre of water gently simmered for 5 minutes in a covered pan then added to the bath.

Infusion

Is made by infusing a fresh or dry bay leaf in a cup of hot water for 10 minutes, may be drunk three times daily.

Birch

White birch. Silver birch

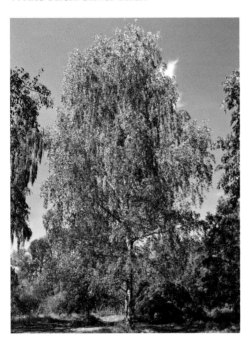

Latin:	*Betula alba / pubescens / pendula.*
Family:	Betulaceae

Element	Water
Planet	Venus
Humour	Phlegmatic
Quality	Warm and dry in the first degree. Clears and dries excess phlegm, dries swellings especially from the kidneys and joints, pain relieving.

Organs

Kidneys
Joints
Heart
Skin

Actions

Astringent
Bitter
Anti-inflammatory
Anticancer
Diuretic
Antipyretic

Constituents

Betulinic acid
Flavonoids
Saponins, glucosides, glycosides
Volatile oils: methyl salicylate, butenols, anthocyanins

Traditional uses and humoral influences

Birch is ruled by Venus, who governs the sexual organs, kidneys, throat, and breasts. It is warm and dry in the first degree, and is used for fevers, rheumatism, gout, and for strengthening the reproductive and urinary system.

Venus rules the cool "venous" circulation, and birch will help clear any excess fluid from the circulatory system, making it useful in the oedema that occurs due to a weak and failing heart, a condition originally called "dropsy".

Birch resists putrefaction and is protective against infection, both externally as a poultice of the bark, leaves, and shoots, and internally as an infusion or expressed juice of the leaves and shoots. It is particularly useful to protect the kidneys and urinary passages from inflammation and infection. In Russia the cinder birch conk mushroom, which grows from the side of the trunk, has long been used traditionally for treating cancers and chronic disease. The mushroom itself has high concentrations of betulinic acid, which is in high concentrations in the bark. The acid shows activity against carcinoma cell lines for skin cancer, including melanoma, and is also active against brain tumours and is a specific inhibitor of HIV.

By heating the bark, a thick tar-like gum called birch tar is produced. This has been used since Neolithic times, both as an adhesive for tool making and as a healing agent. One of its uses was as a chewing gum, which reduces oral inflammation and infection and also helps with sore throats and upper respiratory infections. The tar has also commonly been prescribed for treating skin inflammations, eczema, boils, and abscesses.

Mythos

Its name is thought to derive from the Sanskrit word "bhurga"—to write upon. It may also be a derivation of the Anglo Saxon word for shelter, "beorgan", the strips of bark being used as protection. The druidic name was "Beth", which was the first letter in the ancient Ogham tree alphabet. It was considered the tree of beginnings and the birth of the year, protecting the young sun as it begins its growth into the new year. In the ancient Druidic "song of Amergin", the line for birch is "I am a stag of seven tines", referring to the age of a stag when it emerges as a mature or royal stag. In ancient Welsh poetic myth, a sea stag was also the name given to an ocean wave, connecting birch to the water element, which is also ruled by Venus—commonly the great mother of all life in ancient myth.

Birch is the first forest tree to come into leaf and was considered the tree of inception and new beginnings, able to cleanse the past and any negativity that may remain. In fact, it was said that delinquents and lunatics were struck with the birch rod, as it was a certain way to cleanse all the evil that resided within them. The druids consecrated their places of learning and new students with a birch twig and dew, the twigs being thought to pass the vital spirit of enlightenment into the person, awakening new wisdom within them. A birch rod of life was used for bestowing blessing and protection. In the spring cattle in Bavaria and Slovakia are beaten as a way of keeping the cattle healthy all year round and to promote fertility.

The birch tree is the symbolic tree of Imbolc, the ancient Celtic festival of spring and new light, which later became Candlemas. Birch was considered protective against witches and evil, being hung over doorways, stables, and cradles to offer protection. In the Hebrides it was believed that birch branches hung over a cradle would protect the child from being taken by fairies.

For Siberian peoples the birch represented the world tree, and during the initiation rites of Shamans birches would be felled from the place of burial so that the ancestors could be present. Nine trees would be cut and ribbons attached, representing the link between the initiate and the world of spirit.

Emotional

Birch cleanses the spirit and gives a feeling of renewal and the return of light and hope. It can be used to cleanse after periods of depression, and following times when we have felt stuck and unable to move on. It protects us from the negativity of others and helps us to move beyond self-judgement and the scorn of others, allowing liberation from restrictive self-beliefs and self-condemnation. It is herb of new beginnings and letting go of old unhelpful negative patterns.

Skin

The distilled oil from the bark is known as birch tar and has been used for skin complaints, such as eczema and psoriasis. The twelfth century mystic healer Hildegard of Bingen prescribed the leaves and flowers for treating open wounds and ulcers.

Urinary and reproductive systems

The leaves are used to treat inflammations and infections of the bladder, kidneys, and urethra. It was a traditional remedy for dissolving and flushing out kidney and bladder stones, with Nicholas Culpeper saying "being drunk for some days together, is available to break the stone in the kidneys and bladder". Usually drank as a tea, I have found that it is an invaluable remedy for urinary, pelvic, and reproductive inflammation and pain. Commonly, I prescribe a fresh juice made from the leaves and twigs or alternatively an infusion of the tops three times a day.

Heart

There is a tradition of using birch for the heart, particularly for fluid retention and a weak heart. I once had a Romanian woman come to my shop asking for birch leaves to use as a poultice to treat her heart, she told me that her Grandmother used to place a poultice over her heart when it felt weak.

Joints

The salicylates in birch help with the pain of rheumatism and gout. Birch is also a gentle enough remedy to be used for age related osteoarthritis and also for hip and back pain. Its anti-inflammatory action and cleansing action also make it useful in rheumatoid arthritis. It can be taken as a tea or as a juice, the tea made with leaves, tops, or the bark.

Doses

Infusion

One teaspoon of leaves infused in a cup of hot water, drink up to 3 cups a day.

Juice

10–30 ml three times a day.

Bath

A double chopped handful of tops and leaves simmered in 2 litres of water for 20 minutes, added to the bath.

Borage

Borage. Bugloss. Burrage. Bee plant. Starflower

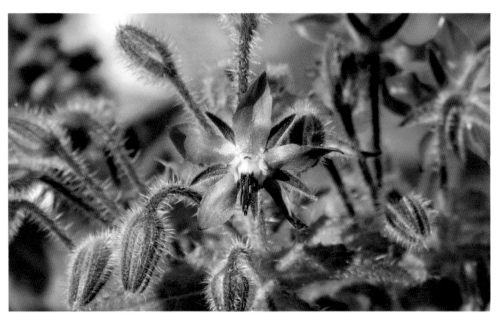

Latin: *Borago officinalis*
Family: Boraginaceae

Element   Air
Planet   Jupiter
Humour   Sanguine
Quality   Warm and moist in the
          first degree, It clarifies the
          blood, cheers the heart,
          purges melancholy.

Organs

Heart
Head
Lungs
Kidneys
Liver

Actions

Tonic
Diuretic
Soothing
Demulcent
Temperate (balances heat and cold)
Anti-melancholic
Antipyretic
Adrenal restorative
Galactagogue

Constituents

Saponins
Mucilage
Tannins
Alkaloids: very low levels of
pyrrolizidine alkaloids
Lipids: essential fatty acids—
stearidonic and linolenic acid.

Traditional uses and humoral influences

Borage is under Jupiter, the ruler of the liver, and also the sign of Leo, the ruler of the heart. It is warm and moist in the first degree. The liver is a warm and moist organ responsible for producing the blood and replenishing the radical moisture. This moist substance in the blood enables the transportation of innate heat around the body keeping its heat in balance while delivering energy to the organs.

Borage shares the warm and moist temperament of the liver and blood, and through its association with Leo, it also lends this moistness and warmth to the heart. This highlights the fact that borage was considered a cordial herb; a prime herb for warming, moistening, and nourishing the heart.

Jupiter is the ruler of the planets and represents strength and protection. Borage shares this quality making it especially helpful in protecting the heart from being scorched by extreme or hot emotions. Being warm it will also maintain the hearts natural heat when it becomes overwhelmed by cold melancholic vapours. The herbalist John Gerard said, "Those of our time do use the flowere in salads to exhilarate and make the mind glad. There be also many things made of them, used for the comfort of the heart, to drive away sorrow, and increase the joy of the minde" (Gerard, 1636).[1]

The heart is particularly prone to being overwhelmed by the cold and dry vapours of the melancholic humour emanating from the spleen, as it lies immediately below the heart. Borage with its gentle warmth and moisture is considered particularly helpful as an antidote to these melancholic vapours. Externally the leaves can be used as cooling poultices for skin inflammations and are also traditionally used for inflammations of the eyes.

Culpeper comments, "It helps the itch, ringworms and tetters, or other spreading scabs or sores."

Both borage seeds and leaves have traditionally been recommended to mothers to increase the flow and production of breast milk. The seeds are very rich in essential fatty acids containing up to 25% omega 3 and omega 6 fatty acids. The leaves have a gentle diuretic action, and through combining soothing, moistening, and tissue restorative actions it is very beneficial in inflammatory conditions of the urinary and reproductive tracts.

Mythos

It is said that the name "Borago" comes from a corruption of the Latin "Corago" derived from the word for the heart "Cor" and "ago"–I bring, in essence meaning; I bring "heart" or courage.

There is a well-known Roman saying quoted by John Gerard in his herbal, "Ego Borago, gaudia semper ago". Gerard translates this as, "I, Borage, bring always courage" (Gerard, 1636).[2] However, the Latin word "gaudia" actually translates as "joys", which corresponds closely to the Roman name for the herb; Euphrosynon, derived from the word for Euphoria, showing the value that they gave borage as a bringer of joyfulness. In Fernie's Herbal (1897) he tells us; "According to Diocorides and Pliny, the Borage was that famous nepenthe of Homer which Polydamus sent to Helen for a token "of such rare virtue that when taken steep'd in wine, if wife and children, father and mother, brother or sister and all thy dearest friends should die before thy face, thou could'st not grieve, or shed a tear for them" (Fernie, 1897).[3]

In the Greek myths the herb was sent to Helen of Troy by her lover Polydamus as a token of his unending love. Another suggestion is that the name derives from the Celtic word "barrach" meaning a man of nobility.

Emotional

Borage is above all a calming herb. It soothes a wounded heart and helps those suffering from both grief and anguish. It doesn't cloud the mind or have a sedative effect, but gives a soothing feeling of relaxation, protection, and ease.

Heart

Borage is included in Nicholas Culpeper's five cordial herbs; rose, violets, balm, borage, and bugloss. He considers it to protect the heart from poisons and to "clarify the blood, and mitigate heat in fevers"

Gerard says, "Syrup made of the floures of Borage comforteth the heart, purgeth melancholy and quiteth the Phrenticke and lunatic person." (Gerard, 1636).[4] Traditionally the heart is considered especially vulnerable to heat, either from external causes, such as fever, or from internal causes, such as extreme emotions or worry and fear. Protecting and defending the heart from such challenges was considered a major duty of the physician. It has been shown that

high levels of stress hormones, such as adrenaline and cortisol will increase inflammation of blood vessels. In extreme cases, adrenaline has been shown to bring on "broken heart syndrome", which is now recognised as a medical syndrome called Takotsubo cardiomyopathy. This happens when excessive emotion or stress induce a heart paralysis resulting in a heart attack even though there is no physical blockage to the coronary arteries or any other physical heart problem.

Borage is likely to be a very wise choice of herb for anyone who is at risk of such events.

Lungs

With its mucilaginous qualities, borage has often been used to help soothe bronchitis and other pulmonary complaints. Maude Grieve in A Modern Herbal (1931) notes, "Borage is much used in France for fevers and pulmonary complaints". This is confirmed by the French folk herbalist Maurice Messegue commenting,

> "My father used to call it a 'soothe-all' and indeed it does bring a most soothing and comforting sensation to those suffering from bronchitis, catarrh, and congested membranes; in pleurisy and rheumatism. I have successfully treated colds with foot baths or hand baths of Borage" (Messegue, 1981).[5]

Liver

Borage has always been considered an effective blood tonic, with Culpeper praising its ability to "clarify the blood". He also says of it, "The juice made into a syrup ... is put, with other cooling, opening and cleansing herbs to open obstructions, and to help the yellow jaundice, and mixed with fumitory, to cool, cleanse, and temper the blood thereby;"

Borage is warm and moist in character, which is the same temperament as the liver. It therefore helps to bring balance back to the liver, whether it is suffering from either heat and dryness, or coldness and blockage. Gerard stated, "The leaves eaten raw ingender good bloud, especially in those that have been lately sicke" (Gerard, 1636).

There has been concern expressed that any plants containing pyrrolizidine alkaloids may cause liver damage. However, in borage these alkaloids occur in very low concentrations, estimated to be less than ten parts per million, a level that is unlikely to pose a significant risk.

Doses

Tea

One teaspoon (2–4 g) to a cup. Two cups daily.

Tincture

1:3 5 ml 1–3 times daily.

Broom

Scotch broom. Irish tops. Bizzom. Genesta

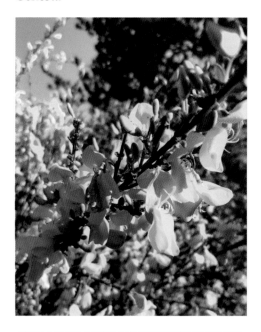

Latin:	*Cystisus scoparius,*
	Sarothamnus scoparius
Family:	Fabaceae

Element	Fire
Planet	Mars
Humour	Choleric
Quality	Hot and dry in the second degree. Dries and purges phlegm.

Organs

Heart
Kidneys
Joints

Actions

Cardiac tonic
Antiarrhythmic
Diuretic
Antihaemorrhagic

Constituents

Alkaloids: sparteine, lupanine
Flavonoids: genistein, scoparin
Phenethylamines
Volatile oils: eugenol, isovaleric acid, benzoic acid

Traditional uses and humoral influences

Broom is ruled by Mars and is hot and dry in the second degree. According to Culpeper, along with elder and hyssop, it will purge and clear phlegm downwards. In very strong doses it acts as an emetic and purgative, and in lower doses is an effective diuretic. It was recommended by Culpeper for treating dropsy, or the accumulation of fluid as a consequence of a failing heart. This excess of cold dampness was seen to inhibit the flow of the animal spirit to the heart, leading to it losing rhythm and activity, a condition to which one becomes more susceptible to with age.

Nicholas Culpeper also recommends it for gout, pains in the hips and the joints, and sciatica. Maurice Messegue, the French folk herbalist recommends using it for low blood pressure, lung infections, uterine haemorrhage, and deficiencies of the endocrine glands, particularly the thyroid.

Mythos

The broom is the badge of English Plantagenet kings who took their name from the medieval Latin name for the plant, *Planta genista*. Although a broom covered in blooms was an omen of fertility, it was considered very bad luck to make a broom out of it when in flower. With the old saying proclaiming, "If you sweep the house with blossomed broom in May, you are sure to sweep the head of the house away".

It was said that the five angled stem correlated to the doctrine of signatures, as the internal angle of a pentagon is seventy-two degrees, which is the perfect rate at which the heart should beat. It was a favourite herb of King Henry VIII who was said, by the herbalist Gerard in 1597, to have taken the distilled water of the flowers to help recovery from overindulgence or what was called "surfeits".

Emotional

Broom helps when emotional endurance is required. It keeps the heart strong when we are under pressure and need reassurance.

Heart

The alkaloid sparteine contained in broom is known to be gently cardioactive. Unlike digitalis, it doesn't act on the heart muscle and it doesn't accumulate in the body. Its action is to slow down pathologically accelerated stimuli in the conductive system of the heart, and to reduce the increased irritability of the conduction system. This regulates the action of the heart reducing fibrillation and arrhythmias. The other alkaloids, sarothamnin and genistein, help with the inhibition of extrasystoles. Whilst the flavonoids it contains have been shown to have a beneficial effect on heart muscle function and the initiation of cardiac impulses. These combined actions all make broom an effective treatment for arrhythmia and ectopic beats. Broom also increases return of blood to the heart via a vasoconstrictive effect, which makes it a helpful herb in low blood pressure.

Kidneys

Nicholas Culpeper said of broom that it "cleanses also the reins or kidneys and bladder of the stone, provokes urine abundantly, and hinders the growing of the stone in the body". It has often been recommended as a helpful diuretic, especially when weakness of the heart is a contributory factor.

In A Modern Herbal, Maude Grieve gives the following recipe, "A compound decoction of Broom is recommended in herbal medicine as of much benefit in bladder and kidney affections as well as in chronic dropsy. To make this, 1 oz Broom tops and ½ oz. of Dandelion roots are boiled in one pint of water down to half a pint, adding towards the last, ½ oz. of bruised Juniper berries. When cold, the decoction is strained and a small quantity of cayenne added. A wineglassful is taken three or four times a day".

Doses

Infusion

Of dried herb and flowers; 1–2 g three times a day.

Tincture

1:5, 0.5–2 ml three times a day.

The infusion and the tincture must be prepared from recently harvested material, as its quality deteriorates with keeping.

Do not use in high blood pressure and in pregnancy.

Burdock

Burdock. Lappa. Fox's clote. Herrif

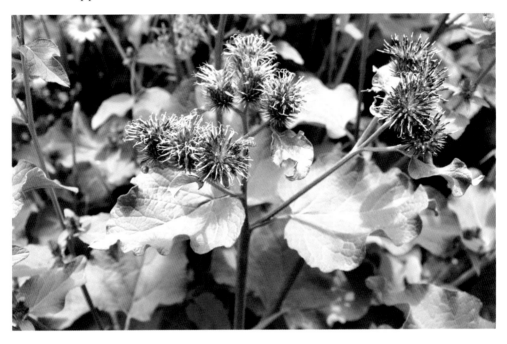

Latin:	*Arctium lappa*
Family:	Asteraceae/compositae

Element	Water
Planet	Venus
Humour	Phlegm
Quality	Leaves: cold and dry in the first degree, a cooling and cleansing diuretic that strengthens the womb. Root: temperately warm and dry, nourishes the liver and cleanses the blood.

Organs

Liver
Skin
Kidneys
Lungs
Womb

Actions

Tonic
Cleansing
Cooling diuretic
Diaphoretic
Antibacterial
Antioxidant
Drawing and healing

Constituents

Polysaccharides: inulin
Volatile oil
Phenolic acids: caffeic acid,
cholorogenic acid
Flavonoids: luteolin, quercertin, rutin
Lignans: arctin, arctigenin
Vitamins: A, B, C, P
Iron, calcium, copper, iodine, silicon,
sulphur, zinc

Traditional uses and humoral influences

Burdock is ruled by Venus, the planet that holds sway over the reproductive organs, especially the womb. It has a connection with the phlegmatic organs, such as the lungs, kidneys, and bowels. The leaves are cold and dry, which is not surprising as they are very bitter in taste, and are considered to be very effective as a blood cleanser and a cooling diuretic. The root is warm and dry in the first degree and has a sweet nourishing taste. This makes it a valuable remedy in cases of excess heat or choler, helping to ripen and soften any blocks that have arisen and open the passages of the liver and kidneys to ease their elimination. Its cleansing action has been considered valuable in gout and rheumatic conditions and in hot inflamed skin disorders. As a cleanser and purifier burdock has long been used in folk and country medicine. The French herbalist Maurice Messegue says, "My Father was once visited by a farmer who was covered in boils and was in very great pain and distress. The treatment prescribed was entirely that of Burdock; infusions to be taken internally, and baths and tinctures externally. In eight days all the boils had disappeared. Burdock is a most wonderful purifying agent.- put a handful of sliced fresh roots and freshly picked leaves into a litre of water. (2 or 3 cups a day) Note: The treatment should be supported with baths [hand and foot-baths] – one and a half handfuls of roots and leaves into a litre of hot water, 2–3 baths a day.)"[1]

In all of these cases, the leaves are included in the prescriptions, like Dandelion, the leaves seem to be most often preferred for treating the kidneys and as a diuretic, and for their strong cleansing quality. However the roots have also been considered as an effective blood cleanser, they have a slower more gentle action, warming the kidneys and liver, clearing excessive heat through gently softening hard cold congestion in the liver and other organs, and ripening and softening cold raw undigested humours that are causing stasis and congestion. It clears excess heat in inflammatory conditions, such as eczema and other skin conditions and has been used for cooling fevers. These uses correspond to its modern reputation as an immune strengthener, and a remedy for viral illnesses such as colds and flu. It has been shown through scientific research to be a powerful antioxidant herb with antibacterial activity.

Mythos

The common name comes from "dock" meaning large leaves and the Latin "burra" meaning a lock of wool, it being common for sheep's wool to become entangled in the seed heads.

The old English name for burdock was "herrif", "aireve" or "airup" from the Anglo Saxon *Hoeg* hedge, and *Reafian*, meaning to seize. A probable reference to its burr's getting hold of any passerby. Culpeper gives its popular names of the time as personata, happy major, and clot burr. The Latin word for face is "persona", and it is thought that the leaves were used by Italian actors to hide their faces when the drama required it.

The name arctium comes from the Greek for bear, "arctos", and is said to derive from the similarity of the seed head to the shaggy fur on the head of a bear.

Emotional

Burdock is a grounding nourishing herb, giving us a sense of stability in an impermanent world, allowing a sense of rootedness and foundation to arise within us. It helps us to cast off old debilitating emotions, enabling us to connect with the spiritual nourishment held in our quiet inner depths.

Liver

Burdock root helps to clear congestion from the liver, gently increasing secretions and the movement of bile. It is a powerful detoxifier and liver restorative, its gentle temperate warmth enables it to bring the liver back to its natural warm moist temperament. I once had a naval officer who was needing treatment for "Gulf War Syndrome", a condition believed to have been caused by the over use of vaccination, anti-malarials, and organophosphates as prophylactic treatments before going into a tropical warzone. I prescribed a daily decoction of burdock root, dandelion root, and angelica root; 15 g of the mixed roots to be decocted in 1 pint and left to steep overnight, it was then drunk in divided doses over the next day. After three months of treatment the patient was able to return to full duties once again, much to her relief.

Skin

In "A Modern Herbal" (Grieve, 1931) states that burdock is "alterative, diuretic and diaphoretic. One of the best blood purifiers. In all skin diseases, it is a certain remedy and has effected a cure in many cases of eczema, either taken alone or combined with other remedies, such as yellow dock and Sarsaparilla". Culpeper also recommends using the leaves externally for skin conditions: "The Burdock leaves are cooling, moderately drying, and discussing withal, whereby it is good for old ulcers and sores"

Kidneys

Culpeper considered burdock to be a cooling diuretic, which is used to help open and cool the urinary passages when they are excessively hot, dry, and inflamed. The kidneys have a cool moist temperament, and when there is a hot distemper causing inflammation it must be corrected to enable the cleansing of excess heat or excessive amounts of watery humours. Burdock and dandelion are considered two of the most cooling in these circumstances. Nicholas Culpeper recommends the leaves as diuretic and of benefit in bladder pain; "The juice of the leaves being drunk with honey provokes urine and remedies the pain of the bladder"

Lungs

The root is demulcent and mucilaginous, making it a soothing remedy for the respiratory system. It was recommended for treating consumption (TB) and the continual cough that accompanied it. The root was used for coughing blood and as a warming strengthening remedy for the lungs, a recommendation first made by the ancient Greek herbalist Dioscorides. Modern research shows that the lignans, which are most concentrated in the seeds, but also occur in the roots have an antiallergenic action.

Womb

Burdock has always been considered able to strengthen the womb, with the leaves being applied abdominally to stop miscarriage. Burdock is considered useful in all conditions of heat and congestion in the reproductive organs.

Doses

Root

3–5 g decocted in a cupful of water, up to twice daily.

Leaf

One teaspoonful to a cup three times a day.

Tincture

Root and/or leaf 1:3 strength, 10 ml twice daily.

Chamomile

Roman chamomile. English Chamomile. True Chamomile. Sweet scented Chamomile. Maythen. Manzanilla

Latin: *Anthemis/Chamaemelum nobile*

German Chamomile. Scented mayweed. Wild Chamomile.

Latin: *Matricaria recutita/ chamomilla*

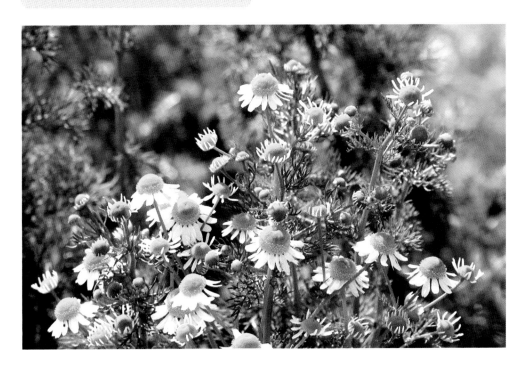

Family: Asteraceae

Element   Fire
Planet   Sun
Humour   Choleric
Quality   Warm and dry in the first
           degree, Heats the head,
           liver and joints, clears
           fever and pain, especially
           from a cold cause.

Organs

Stomach
Head
Liver
Joints
Kidneys, Womb
Skin

Actions

Relaxant
Sedative
Nervine
Antispasmodic
Bitter
Stomachic
Carminative
Vermifuge
Antimicrobial
Imunostimulant
Anti-allergic
Anti-inflammatory
Analgesic

Constituents

Anthemis nobile: Volatile oils: angelic
acids – chamazulene, pinocarvone
Lactones
Flavonoids: anthemoside, luteolin,
apigenin
Coumarins, phenolic acids
Matricaria recutita: Volatile oils:
alpha-bisabolol, chamazulene,
matricine
Flavonoids: apigenin, luteolin
Coumarins

Traditional uses and humoral influences

Chamomiles are ruled by the sun and
are warm and dry in the first degree.
Both Roman and German Chamomile
have been used interchangeably over
time and location. Nowadays the German chamomile is the one that we are
most familiar with, however it is likely
that Culpeper and the earlier herbalists were more often referring to the
Roman Chamomile. It was reputed as
a prime fever medicine, a tradition said

to go back to the time of the Egyptians:
Nicholas Culpeper says;

> "This is Nechesor, an Egyptians
> medicine, it is profitable for all
> sorts of agues that come from
> either phlegm, or melancholy
> or from an inflammation of the
> bowels, being applied when the
> humours causing them shall be
> concocted: there is nothing more
> profitable to the sides and the
> region of the liver and spleen
> than it."

It is a gentle bitter, which helps to open
the liver and release heat, thus helping to
clear a fever, while its sedative and pain
relieving effects help aches and pains. It
has always been held in such high regard
by country people that there are many
traditional sayings, a typical example
from Germany proclaims:

> "A good cup of Chamomile tea
> does more good than three Doc-
> tors!" (De Cleene & Lejeune, 1999).[1]

It is a traditional eye remedy, useful in
conjunctivitis, blepharitis and styes, best
prepared as a hot poultice or compress
over the eyes.

The polysaccharrides in chamomile are
immunostimvulant, and German chamomile has been shown to be antimicrobial
against staphylococcus, streptococcus,
leptospira, and candida, as well as acting
against certain tick-borne viruses.

Mythos

The name chamomile comes from the
Greek *kamai*—ground, and *melon*—
apple, which alludes to the strong and

distinctive apple-like perfume of the "true" or Roman Chamomile.

An old English saying goes:

"Like a camomile bed-
The more it is trodden
The more it will spread."[2]

Chamomile was considered to be one of the St John's worts, which are flowering herbs with health giving and protective qualities collected at the midsummer solstice to be hung in the rafters of the house to protect from misfortune, evil, and spells. The herb was sacred to the Norse god Balder, and in Greek legend was said to grow in the garden of Hecate, the Goddess of magic. The bright yellow flowers of chamomile are a reminder of the two flaming torches that Hecate used to guide Persephone through the darkness of the underworld.

Emotional

There are few better herbs to bring balance to the emotions, and to bring a lighter vision in times of darkness. Roman Chamomile has a more euphoric and uplifting action on the spirit, while German Chamomile is calming and soothing. Chamomile is a herb which helps us to reconnect to the heart, bringing our vital spirit into alignment and balance. It helps us to regain composure when in a state of panic, and to be able to release ourselves from the grip of negative thinking. It calms the mind, bringing back focus when we are feeling scattered and dispersed.

Skin

Washes can be used for treating burns, a use backed up by research into the oil,

alpha-bisobolol, that it contains. Eczema, acne, and psoriasis are all helped by both external application, as well as internal use.

Boils, abscesses, and areas of inflammation on the skin all benefit from a wash, poultice, or compress. Adding 15 drops of the essential oil of German chamomile to 50 ml of ointment or cream will clear patches of psoriasis when applied twice daily.

Head

There is a Scottish saying; "To comfort the braine, smell to camomile".

To aid sleep chamomile tea is a tried and trusted remedy, and although today we most often use German Chamomile it is likely that in former times the Roman or True Chamomile was most valued for this purpose. As a treatment for anxiety associated with an overactive mind, a strong German Chamomile infusion steeped overnight, taken daily on waking is very effective. I have found the aromatic water of Roman Chamomile an effective insomnia remedy; 10 ml before bed, or in the middle of the night when sleep has deserted us. Using a ten-minute steam inhalation of German chamomile flowers before bed is an effective way of breaking a cycle of chronic insomnia, it calms the brain and is especially good for those in states of high anxiety. I once had a young patient with chronic insomnia who came in a very distressed state, having not slept at all for the three previous nights. She was sceptical that I could help and was only there to placate her mother, when I told her that I intended to use chamomile she got up and shouted "Don't you think I've already tried that!" and promptly went to leave the room. I stopped her in her tracks by asking if she had tried it as an inhalation, and by suggesting that she had nothing to lose and everything to gain by giving it a go. She agreed to try it, albeit with great scepticism, only to find that unlike everything else she had tried it immediately helped her from the very first night. After using it for two weeks her sleep had completely returned to normal. Alongside the inhalations we used a herbal pill containing rose, hawthorn flowers and lemon balm herb, and some St John's wort pills.

Stomach and Liver

For indigestion, diarrhoea, and stomach pain in general, it should always be the first response. It may be combined with mint, fennel, or aniseed to increase its carminative effects, and can be drunk freely or sipped as an infusion throughout the day. A hot poultice applied to the abdomen is very helpful for relieving stomach and bowel pain. It is always helpful for children's complaints, especially colic, when it can be given in teaspoonful doses throughout the day— either using the infusion or the aromatic water. I once treated a three-month old baby who was in continual distress due to suffering from constant reflux and colic. As he was bottle fed I prescribed an infusion of German Chamomile flowers and aniseed, two teaspoons of each to a pint and made as an infusion. This tea was then used to make up the baby's milk, with such beneficial effects that the mother continued to use it throughout his infancy whenever a problem arose.

Joints

"The bathing with a decoction of Chamomile takes away weariness, eases pains, to what part of the body soever they are applied." (Culpeper,).

The anti inflammatory chamazulene compounds found in the essential oil of German chamomile are some of the most potent of the plant world. Adding 10–15 drops of the essential oil of German Chamomile to a 50 g jar of cream or ointment makes a very effective rub for painful, arthritic, or inflamed joints.

Womb

The name *Matricaria* derives from matix, meaning womb or mother. It is variously referred to as the "caring mother" or "the herb that cares for the mother". Strong infusions, baths, and compresses are helpful for period pains, and also for assisting in the birth process. It is a very useful herb to help counter menopausal symptoms, such as insomnia, anxiety, night sweats, and hot flushes. It combines especially well in this case with angelica, lovage root, and sage. It has been shown to be safe throughout pregnancy.

Doses

German Chamomile flowers

Tea

One heaped teaspoon to a cup.

Tincture

1:3; 5 ml as needed up to three times a day in a little water.

Roman Chamomile aromatic water

10 ml before bed for insomnia, 10 ml twice daily for anxiety.

For any kind of pain, neuralgia, toothache, muscle spasm

Apply as a hot poultice and place a hot water bottle on top.

Chamomile bath

Use 20 g in 1 litre of hot water, leave to steep for 30 minutes, then add to a full bath.

Cleavers

Goosegrass. Hedge rife. Burweed. Clitheren. Sticky willy

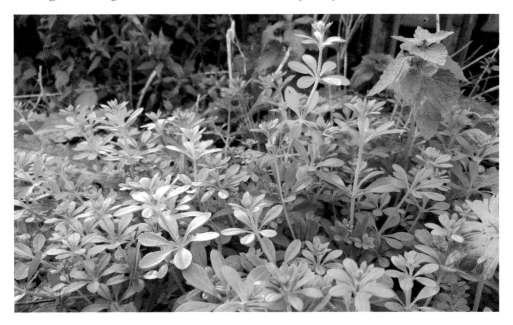

Latin: *Galium aparine*
Family: Rubiaceae

Element   Water
Planet   Moon
Humour   Phlegm
Quality   Warm and dry in the first
           degree, cleanses the blood
           and strengthens the liver.

Tonic
Astringent
Antiseptic
Anti-inflammatory
Febrifuge
Haemostatic
Anticancer

Organs

Kidneys
Liver and blood
Skin

Actions

Alterative
Diuretic

Constituents

Chlorophyll,
Iridoids: asperuloside, asperulosidic
acid.
Polyphenolic acids: p-coumaric,
caffeic acid, gallic acid.
Flavonoids: luteolin
Fatty acids
Sterols, linolenic, lauric acid,
stigmasterol, campesterol,
Anthraquinones

Traditional uses and humoral influences

Cleavers is ruled by the moon and is warming and drying in the first degree. It is cleansing and opening, traditionally being used in the spring to clear the system of crude or undigested humours that may have accrued in the body and blood over the winter months. Nicholas Culpeper comments;

"It is a good remedy in the spring, eaten in water gruel to cleanse the blood and strengthen the liver, thereby to keep the body in health, and fitting it for that change of season that is coming"

The moon rules the phlegmatic season, the last part of the winter preceding the spring. It is a time of dampness, with water building up, lying on the ground causing flooding and stagnation. Cleavers, with its warm and dry quality and association with water and the moon, is seen as being especially powerful in shifting this seasonal dampness from the body. By taking spring tonic herbs at this point in the year, we greatly benefit from the rising vitality contained in the green shoots of the emerging plants, similarly allowing them to transform the wet cold dampness in the body into vital new growth. They not only act as spring cleansers but are full of vitamins, minerals, and micronutrients, providing a natural supplement to our diets after the winter. The thirteenth century herbalists from Myddfai in Wales suggested that taking the infused water of the whole plant in the spring as the only thing you drink each day for nine weeks would "completely destroy and expel eruptive poisons in the blood and humours" (Pughe, 1861).[1] They recommended pounding the fresh plant, leaving it to steep for six hours overnight in spring water, drinking the water in the day, then drinking a decoction of the remaining herbal mash before bed.

In Grieve's A Modern Herbal (1931), she reports its traditional use as a calming herb for the mind and as a cure for insomnia. She also notes its use in folk medicine as a tea for treating head colds.

Mythos

The name *Galium* comes from the Greek "gala", meaning milk, which the herb was used to curdle, and *aparine* comes from the Greek verb "apairo" meaning to take hold of, due to the propensity the herb and especially the burrs to stick to clothing. The Galium family include the bedstraws, which were considered to be sacred to the Norse goddess Freya, and are associated with fertility, spring, and birth.

The bedstraws and woodruffs, of which there are about 300 hundred species, are the European representatives of the Rubiaceae family. This large plant family provides the quinine tree from South America and the original native coffee plant that grows in Ethiopia. If the seeds of cleavers are dried and gently roasted over a fire, they can then be infused to make a coffee substitute. The roots of cleavers produce a red dye, whilst the madder plant, another member of the Rubiaceae family, provides the red stain used for colouring the wood of musical instruments.

Emotional

Cleavers clears emotional baggage and and gives us the courage to follow new directions and explore new horizons. It brightens our outlook on the world, enabling us to shrug off current concerns as well as past worries and regrets. If you need to clear out some stagnant emotions and negative thought patterns, a fresh cleavers bath and period of cleansing with the tea is very helpful.

Skin

The juice of the herb can be used externally for all kinds of wounds, sores, eczema, and skin eruptions. It is very effective as a poultice for treating non-healing leg ulcers, the fresh herb being crushed and applied twice or three times daily in muslin. The traditional treatment also recommends that the wound be left open to the air, covered but not occluded. The ulcer is only treated with the herb and not washed out between applications. This treatment was used successfully by Dr Quinlan, a surgeon from Dublin in the early 1900s and an account of the results was published in the medical journals of the time. I have used it successfully on a number of patients who had not been helped with conventional care, having been given the directions for its use from Mrs Mary Barnes from Suffolk, the daughter of a district nurse who used the remedy in the 1930s. The decoction is a traditional folk remedy for treating sunburn and freckles. The oil made from the fresh herb is useful to massage onto sore breasts, and enlarged glands.

Liver

The liver is the organ associated with blood, and cleavers is a powerful blood purifier cleansing excess phlegm, damp, and cold congestion from the liver. By clearing damp congestion it improves the expulsive faculty of the body, and therefore accelerates the elimination of waste products.

Cancer

There is a history of use for treating hard swellings and malignancies with cleavers. In his "Botanic Guide to Health"[2] published in 1855, Dr Coffin recommended treating cancers by taking two fluid ounces of the juice (60 ml) three times daily, whilst a contemporary, Dr Boyce, suggested five fluid ounces (150 ml) twice daily. If the tumour was externally accessible the fresh herb would also be used as a poultice. It was recommended for hard scrofulous swellings of the neck, and the "king's evil", both referring to glandular swellings associated with tuberculosis.

Kidneys

For urinary system pain, inflammation, and infections, drinking an infusion throughout the day is very helpful when made to a medicinal strength of 30 g to one pint of water. The old herbalists recommended it for stranguary (the difficulty in passing urine) and for urinary stones. In my experience, it combines well with shepherd's purse and horsetail in equal parts for treating urinary infections, bleeding, and chronic cystitis. I usually prescribe this strength of infusion (30 g to a pint) to be left overnight and then strained in the morning, and the resulting liquid to be drunk over two days. It should be taken at the first sign of infection and then continued for eight days, or until the infection has cleared. It can be safely drunk over an extended period of time to return a chronically inflamed bladder back to health, as is the case with interstitial cystitis.

Doses

Infusion

3–5 g dried herb infused in hot water and drunk 3 times a day.

Juice

15 ml–60 ml up to three times a day.

Clover

Meadow trefoil. Honeysuckles. Suckles. Cocksheads.
Bee-bread. Smere. Shamrock

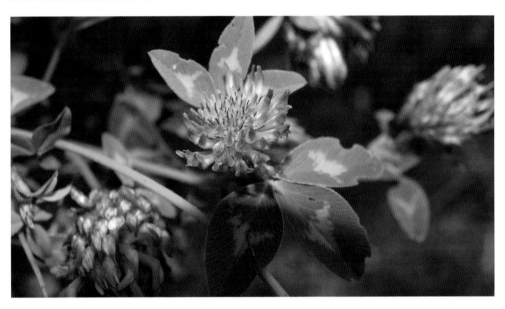

Latin:	*Trifolium pratense*
Family:	Fabiaceae (formerly Leguminoseae)

Element	Ether
Planet	Mercury
Humour	Etheric humour
Quality	Cold and dry in the first degree

Organs

Lungs
Skin
Liver and blood
Reproductive organs

Actions

Antispasmodic
Expectorant
Sedative
Anti-inflammatory
Blood cleanser
Hormonal balancer
Anti-tumour

Constituents

Flavonoids:
flavones, isoflavonesL genistein,
daidzein, pratensin
Phenolic acids: salicylic, coumaric,
caffeic acids
Procyanidins: epicatechin, catechin
Volatile oils, sterols, fatty acids.
Vitamins: A, B complex, C, F, P
Magnesium, calcium, potassium,
copper, selenium, zinc

Traditional uses and humoral influences

Clover is under the rulership of Mercury, aligning it with the etheric element. Like many other members of the bean or legume family, such as lentils, it has a cold and dry temperament. Mercury and the etheric element are closely associated with the nervous system. Stress and emotional upset often manifest in an exacerbation of eczema and other skin conditions, the cooling and calming effect of clover will reduce these symptoms and help to temper the heat that is being felt in the skin. The flowers have been widely used for skin conditions, both used externally and taken internally. In recent times clover flowers have been considered an alterative agent, helping the body to change its function when out of balance and to help clear toxins via the lymphatic system. Clover has high levels of nutrients alongside its wide range of anti-inflammatory plant sterols and antioxidants, which may well account for these actions. It became a traditional treatment for whooping cough, its antispasmodic actions being beneficial in calming the paroxysmal cough.

It may also be used as an external and internal treatment for gout and is helpful for any condition indicating excess heat in the blood. The phenolic acids, such as salicylic acid and caffeic acid, are anti-inflammatory and are likely to help reduce the swelling and pain of inflammation.

It was common to use both the white and red clovers. Other closely related members of the family were also used in a similar fashion, including the lesser yellow trefoil and the bird's foot trefoil. Culpeper also gives bird's foot trefoil a cold and dry quality, but puts it under the dominion of Saturn not Mercury. He also specifically recommends it for kidney problems and kidney stones, as well as for use as a powerful wound healing herb.

Mythos

"With a four-leafed clover, a double-leafed ash and a green tipped seave, You may go before the queens daughter without asking leave" (De Cleene & Lejeune, 1999)[1]—old English proverb.

(The traditional name for a rush is seave)

The word clover is a corruption of the Latin word for a club, alluding to the shape of the leaves. According to William Fernie in 1897, "Its charm has been ever supposed there is an unfailing protection against evil influences, as is attested by the spray in the workman's cap, and in the bosom of the cotters wife".[2] The ancient phrase "to be living in clover" is an allusion to it being a plant that grows in rich and fertile pastures. It is believed that the ancient Celtic druids greatly revered the clover, the number three being an important sacred number. The interconnected triple spiral design resembling a clover leaf, called the triskele, is an ancient druidic emblem that is found carved into many ancient monuments and standing stones. The number three signified the spirits of air, earth, and water and was connected to the triple aspect of the ancient Indo-European white goddess. In European folk stories, the number arises as the three tasks, the three wishes, the three children, and the three challenges of a task. The shamrock of Ireland is a clover, most probably the lesser yellow trefoil, and it was said that St Patrick the patron saint of Ireland explained the Christian trinity to the Celts by using the three leaves of clover. In heraldry a clover leaf represents the possession of meadowland, ears of corn represent farmland, whilst acorns represent the possession of woodland. It was also believed that dreaming of lying in a field of clover would mean that one was about to receive a financial reward. There are many stories about the beneficial powers of four leaf clovers, they are said to bring good fortune, protect from spells and evil, work as a love charm and confer on the carrier the ability to see through all trickery and witchcraft.

It was an ancient belief that the clover's protective abilities extended to it working as an antidote to the bites of venomous creatures, such as snakes and scorpions. Pliny the elder recommended taking twenty seeds in wine or a decoction of the flowers as an antidote, and he claimed that one would never find a snake in a field of clover.

Emotional

It makes a gentle calming tea, helping those who feel weighed down by responsibility. It helps with sleep and relaxation, reduces stress, tension, and anxiety. It can help us feel more nourished and supported when we are feeling vulnerable, enabling us to find the strength to face difficult times.

Lungs

Clover has a long tradition for treating coughs, bronchitis, and whooping cough. William Fernie said in his 1897 Herbal Simples; "A syrup is made from the flowers of the red clover, which has a trustworthy reputation for curing Whooping cough, and of which a teaspoonful may be taken three or four times in the day".[3]

Skin

Red clover has been thought to be a beneficial herb in chronic skin diseases, such as eczema and psoriasis, and in the British Herbal Pharmacopeia is recommended as a specific treatment for these conditions. In Thomas Bartram's Encyclopaedia of Herbal Medicine[4] he recommends using clover with yellow dock. Yellow dock is considered an effective purgative of excess heat in the blood so this would be traditionally considered a useful adjunct in chronic conditions alongside a cooling herb such as clover. The etheric element is considered to be an integral aspect of the nervous system, itching and irritation is seen as excess heat or agitation of the etheric humour, so the coldness of clover is therefore likely to be a beneficial antidote.

Hormonal

There have been a number of studies that have shown clover to benefit menopausal symptoms, improve vaginal tissue structure, and to improve blood pressure and bone density, it is believed that this may be due to the isoflavone content. I have had a number of patients who have benefitted from drinking red clover tea throughout menopause and found it very helpful. I often prescribe a menopausal tea which combines red clover flowers, chamomile flowers, lovage root, and rose petals.

Anticancer

There is evidence that diets rich in the isoflavones, such as genistein contained in clover, are protective against certain forms of cancer, with research confirming it to be particularly helpful in prostate cancer. There was a lot of interest in red clover as a treatment for cancer in the nineteenth century. It was reported in the New York tribune in September 1884 that a case of breast cancer of six years standing had been cured with a prolonged internal use of an extract of red clover. In the Botanic Guide to Health,[5] written in 1848 by Dr Coffin, he suggested using a red clover salve for treating cancer. It was made by simmering red clover flowers in water for an hour, with the strained liquid being simmered repeatedly with a second or third batch of flowers until the liquid resembled the consistency of tar, it was then applied externally twice daily to growths and swellings.

Doses

Tea

A heaped teaspoon to a cup, infuse for 5–7 minutes, drink two or three cups daily.

Medicinal infusion

30 g to 500 ml, infuse for 15 minutes, one cup twice daily.

Tincture

1:3 tincture, 5mls three times daily—the isoflavones are not effectively dissolved in alcohol; a tea may be preferable for treating hormonal issues.

Comfrey

Knitbone. Bruisewort. Consolida. Ass ear. Yalluc (Saxon)

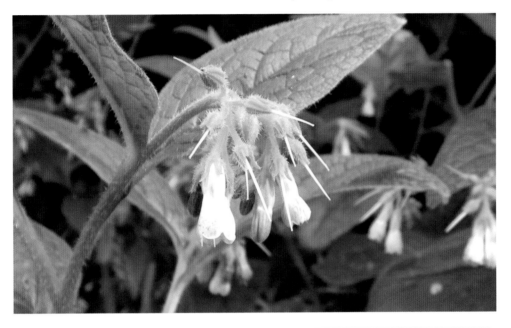

Latin:	*Symphytum officinale*
Family:	Boraginaceae

Element	Earth
Planet	Saturn
Humour	Melancholic
Quality	Cold and dry in the first degree, strengthens tissues, cools heat in lungs, stomach and bowels.

Organs

Joints, skin, bones
Stomach, bowels
Lungs
Kidneys

Actions

Demulcent
Soothing
Antihaemorrhagic
Anti-inflammatory
Healing
Expectorant

Constituents

Allantoin
Mucillage
Tannins
Phytosterols
Polyphenols: rosmarinic, caffeic, chlorogenic acid
Vitamins: A, B12, C
Calcium, potassium, phosphorous, selenium, sulphur, copper, zinc, magnesium

Pyrrolizidine alkaloids (0.02–0.18% in leaf, 0.25–0.29% in roots)

Traditional uses and humoral influences

"This is a herb of Saturn … cold, dry, and earthy in quality" (Culpeper).

Saturn rules the melancholic earth humour and is associated with the spleen, the bones, the teeth, the ears, and the sediment of the blood. Comfrey strengthens, consolidates, dries blood, and heals internal and external wounds. It is undeniably one of the most valued wound herbs, being used for everything from bruises to broken bones. Traditionally both the root and the leaf have been used internally and externally.

Culpeper considered it to help with "all those inward grief's and hurts … and for outward wounds and sores in the fleshy or sinewy part of the body whatsoever".

Comfrey's cold and dry quality not only consolidates, but also cools fevers and will "allay the sharpness of humours", an allusion to its ability to soften and soothe any hot or irritated tissue or organ. Its healing and soothing effect extends to the lungs, stomach, intestines, bowels, and kidneys.

Its dryness refers to its ability to arrest haemorrhage and bleeding, and historically it has been prescribed for bleeding from the lungs, stomach, bowels, or bleeding piles. According to Maude Grieve (1931), 15 g (1/2 oz) of the crushed root is combined to 2 pints of water (1.1 litres) and is boiled to make a decoction, which is drunk in wineglassful doses (200 ml) hourly until the bleeding stops.

Teas or decoctions are also recommended for treating bleeding and painful gums, as well as a gargle for sore throats and pharyngitis.

Mythos

The name is said to come from the Latin "con firma", meaning to bring together, and the family name is derived from the Greek word "sympho", meaning to unite. As a country medicine, it was widely grown in gardens. Country people in earlier times ate the herb as a green vegetable, and it is said that in some parts of Ireland it was also taken as a cure for defective circulation and "poverty of blood" (Grieve, 1931). Traditionally the root is combined and roasted with dandelion and chicory roots to make a popular coffee substitute.

Skin/Joints

Allantoin has been recognised as a potent agent able to stimulate tissue formation and hasten wound healing. A synthetic version is produced for use topically in skin and wound care preparations.

Grieve (1931) says, "Comfrey leaves are of much value as an external remedy, both in the form of fomentations, for sprains, swellings and bruises, and as a poultice, to severe cuts, to improve suppuration of boils and abscesses, and gangrenous and ill conditioned ulcers. The whole plant beaten into a cataplasm and applied hot as a poultice has always been deemed excellent for soothing pain in any tender, inflamed or suppurating part. It is useful in any kind of inflammatory swelling".

Nicholas Culpeper also extolled its viruses saying, "The roots being outwardly applied, help fresh wounds or cuts immediately, being bruised and being laid thereto; it is especial good for ruptures and broken bones: yea, it is said to be so powerful to consolidate and knit together, that if they be boiled with dissevered pieces of flesh in a pot it will join them together again". Although all of the plant can be used, along with Culpeper, most records in folk tradition show a preference for using the roots; they are usually peeled, pounded, or grated and applied as a thick paste, sometimes with the addition of hot water.

After a sprain or an injury, the roots can be chopped and steeped in hot water and the injured part immersed. This can be repeated three times daily for 20 minutes reusing and heating the same liquid.

It may also help to drink the herb as a tea to aid the healing of broken bones. I have had two separate patients with ruptured Achilles tendons who had quick and complete healing having used comfrey leaf tea twice daily; in one case the surgeon couldn't believe that the patient returned without even the slightest limp.

An oil or ointment made from the leaves or the roots can be a very effective way of applying the herb externally for painful joints, arthritis, and joint pain, including spinal pain.

Lungs

Nicholas Culpeper, speaking of its action on the lungs says: "Comfrey helps those that spit blood … the root boiled in water or wine and dunk … It helps the defluction of rheum from the head upon the lungs … and causes the phlegm that oppresses them to be easily spit forth" This is further attested to by Maude Grieve (1931) who says:

"For its demulcent action it has long been employed domestically in lung troubles and also for quinsy and whooping cough. The root is more effectual than the leaf and is the part usually used in cases of coughs".

As well as its soothing demulcent activity, it works as a gentle expectorant.

Stomach

There has been a long term use of comfrey as a soothing mucilaginous remedy, often in the same way as marshmallow root and slippery elm powder. All have been used for heartburn, stomach pain, diarrhoea, bleeding, and piles. It was considered one of the best remedies for ulcers of the stomach and the liver, this recipe was recorded by Maude Grieve in her modern herbal (1931) where she quotes from a contemporary publication—the "Chemist and Druggist" (August 13th 1921.)[1]

"For ulcers of the stomach and liver especially, the root (the part used) was regarded as sovereign … The old Edinburgh formula is the simplest and probably the best: Fresh comfrey and fresh plantain leaves, of each 1lb (450g), bruise them and squeeze out the juice; add to the dregs spring water 1lb (400ml) boil to a half, and mix the strained liquor with the expressed juice; add an equal quantity of white sugar and boil to a syrup".

I have found that the powdered root can be used as a capsule to treat inflammatory bowel disease, diverticulitis, and anal fissures, given in a dose of up to four capsules three times daily after food. In line with the current guidance I would suggest only using it in this way under the supervision of a qualified herbalist.

Safety

Since it has been discovered that animals which ingest pyrrolizidine alkaloids (PAs) have shown to develop liver damage, it has been presumed that plants containing PAs are a danger to health. Comfrey was particularly targeted as a potential risk because it also has a history of use as a food. The evidence against comfrey has been based on animal studies that involved ingestion of large quantities of the plant, much larger than any dose that might be recommended therapeutically. Liver function tests on long-term human comfrey users were normal, even though some of them had consumed up to 25 g of the herb daily for up to 30 years.

In 1989, the World Health Organisation recommended the dose of the leaf should not exceed 5 g daily, or 25 ml of a 1:5 extract. Currently the National Institute of Medical Herbalists recommends using the infusion of the leaf for no more than six weeks under the supervision of a qualified herbalist.

Doses

Tea

1 teaspoon of leaf (1.5 g) up to three times daily, discontinue after six weeks use.

Tincture

1:5 up to 20 ml daily.

Externally the pulverised root or leaf can be applied as a fresh poultice, left in place or repeated throughout the day.

Cowslip

Our Lady's keys. Mayflower. Palseywort. Fairy Cups.
Plumrocks. Paigle. Peter's flower. Arthritica. Keyflower. Key of Heaven
Anglo-Saxon: Cuy lippe
Greek: Paralysio

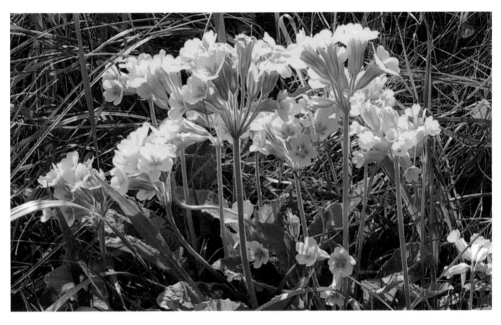

| Latin: | *Primula veris* |
| Family: | Primulaceae |

Element	Water
Planet	Venus
Humour	Phlegmatic
Quality	Warm and dry in the first degree, clears heat and wind from the head, strengthens the nerves

Organs

Head
Nerves
Heart
Lungs
Joints

Actions

Anti-inflammatory
Analgesic
Sedative
Antispasmodic
Vasodilator
Anti-rheumatic

Constituents

Saponins
Glycosides
Flavonoids
Tannins

Traditional uses and humoral influences

Cowslips are both warm and dry in the first degree, are ruled by Venus, and are in the zodiacal sign of Aries—the sign that governs the head and all the structures above the first vertebrae, highlighting their particular relationship with the head, brain, and nerves. We read in John Pechey's herbal of 1706;

> "The leaves and flowers are used in apoplexies (stroke), palsies, and pains in the joints".[1]

He also valued its pain relieving and restorative powers, adding;

> "The water of the flowers, the conserve, and the syrup are anodyne, and gently provoke sleep; and are very proper medicines for weakly people". (Pechey, 1706)

Venus has command over the phlegmatic or watery humour in the body and also rules the radical moisture, which cools and mollifies the innate heat contained in the vital spirit, lubricating its flow and movement around the organs, balancing the body's natural heat. It provides the colder, slower, moist, and blue looking part of the circulation that is contained in the veins, which is still called the 'venous circulation' after her. Cowslips strengthen this cooling moisture enabling them to reduce excess heat in the head and nerves and to also gently warm and strengthen the nerves and brain when they have become too cold and congested by phlegm.

Mythos

In Shakespeare's The Tempest, the spirit Ariel sings the following poem when he hears that he is about to receive his freedom from the service of his master, Prospero;

> "Where a bee sucks, there suck I,
> In a Cowslips bell I lie
> There I couch when Owls do cry.
> On the bats back I do fly,
> After summer merrily,
> Merrily, merrily, shall I live now,
> Under the blossom that hangs on the bough".

The name "cowslip" is thought to come from when the flowers grew abundantly in pastures, the belief being that the flowers grew from what the cows had slupped! Another theory is that the name derives from the Anglo Saxon "cow's leak", meaning cow's plant.

Cowslip is also a flower of the spring goddess, who was variously known as Olwen, Freyer, Ceres, Helle, and Demeter. The return of the yellow flowers to the land in spring was likened to the return of the blond flowing tresses of the spring goddesses reappearing. Spring is associated with fertility and new life, and in Norse legend the flower is associated with the goddess Freyer. She was also the overseer of the entrance to the underworld or Valhalla, the realm where one enjoyed eternal feasting and infinite pleasures after death.

The flowers resemble a bunch of keys, their shape being similar to the keys used in medieval locks. The flowers were therefore considered to resemble the keys to paradise and the afterlife. When such paganistic beliefs were later Christianised, the flowers became known as the keys of the "Virgin Mary", or "Our Lady", and Valhalla became heaven so we also find the names "Our Lady's keys", "Peter's keys" or "Herb Peter" being given to the plant.

This association of cowslips with love and fertility still existed until recently in country tradition. Young girls would tie the flower heads together to make round balls or "Tisty tosty's" and would sing; "Tisty Tosty, tell me true, who shall I be married to?" (Hatfield, 2007).[2] While singing this ditty they tossed the balls of flowers from hand to hand reciting the names of possible suitors, when the ball dropped it would indicate which one was the lucky boy.

Emotional

Cowslips help to restore us to a happy smiling countenance, like spring itself returning. They have a gentle calming effect on the heart and emotions, allowing us to let troubles slip quietly away, enabling us to maintain a meditative, peaceful and liberated mind, free from the troubling thoughts that so frequently cloud our vision. They protect us from extreme and troubling emotional states and help us to better go with the flow.

Head

The flowers have a reputation as one of the best gentle sedatives and relaxants, especially valued for their effect in strengthening the nerves and the brain. Nicholas Culpeper said, "The Flowers … remedy all infirmities of the head coming

of heat and wind, as vertigo, ephialtes (nightmares), false apparitions, phrensies, falling sickness, palsies, convulsions, cramps, pains in the nerves". The brain has a cool, moist, and watery temperament and can be prone to cold congestion. This coldness was thought to be a potential cause of palsy, lethargy, and convulsions due to phlegm obstructing and excessively cooling the animal spirit that activates the nervous system.

In Estonia the flowers are still collected in the forests by country people, and dried and stored for use throughout the year. The flowers or "Umbels" are strung together and then pulled tight into a ball, then hung in a warm place until dry and stored in an airtight container. If any moisture gets to the flowers they quickly spoil, and the yellow flowers turn green.

The Austrian folk herbalist Maria Treben recommended a tea for insomnia made with cowslip flowers, lavender flowers, St John's wort herb, hop strobiles, and valerian root. She also suggested taking it for migraines and nervous headaches.[3]

Lungs

Cowslip's anti-inflammatory and sedative properties make it a useful and calming drink for irritant coughs. The roots have been made into a cough syrup, and the tea drunk as an infusion.

Joints

The analgesic and anti-inflammatory properties of the flavonoids aid joint pains, with Nicholas Culpeper recommending the flowers for pains in the back, as well as the bladder. Sebastian Kneipp, the founder of naturopathy in the 19th century said;

> "He who has a tendency to rheumatism and gout, should drink 1 to 2 cups of Cowslip tea daily over a long period. The intense pain will slacken and with time disappear". (Kneipp, 1896)[4]

Heart

Venus has a relationship with the cool venous side of the circulation and heart, and cowslip has a history of being used in country remedies for a weak heart and dropsy (oedema). Maria Treben writes in Healing Through God's Pharmacy (1980) that both the tea and the wine may be taken to strengthen the heart.

Doses

Tea

3–5 g (a large pinch) infused before bed, up to 3 times a day for chronic rheumatic complaints, or as a refreshing spring tea.

Maria Treben's insomnia tea

50 g cowslip flowers,
25 g lavender flowers,
10 g St John's wort herb,
15 g hops strobiles,
5g valerian root.

Maria Treben's blood purifying spring tea

50 g cowslip
50 g elder flower shoots,
15 g stinging Nettle,
15 g dandelion roots.

Take one teaspoon of this mixture to ¼ litre of boiling water, infuse for 3 minutes. It may be sweetened with a little honey.

Dandelion

Piss en lit. Priest's crown. Swine's snout

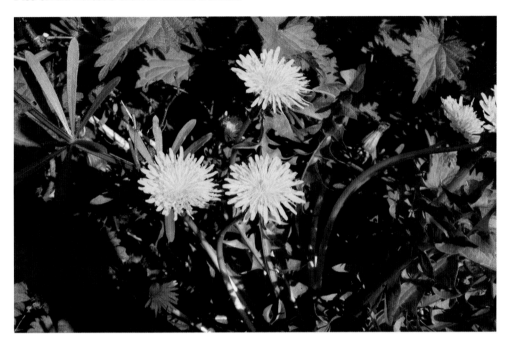

Latin:	*Taraxacum officinale*
Family:	Compositae/Asteraceae
Element	Air
Planet	Jupiter
Humour	Sanguine
Quality	Cold and dry in the second degree, opening and cleansing, cools the stomach, liver and kidneys

Organs

Liver
Gall bladder
Kidneys
Stomach
Joints
Skin

Actions

Liver stimulant
Diuretic
Bitter tonic

Constituents

Sesquiterpine lactones
Polyphenols
Coumarins
Triterpenes
Vitamins: A, B, C, D
Potassium, zinc, iron
Inulin

Traditional uses and humoral influences

Dandelion is ruled by Jupiter, having a cold and dry quality, both in the second degree. It is opening, cleansing, healing, and is considered specifically cooling for the stomach and liver. It is often said that the leaf is one of the strongest of the herbal diuretics.

Culpeper comments that "It is of an opening and cleansing quality, and very effectual for the obstructions of the liver, gall and spleen, and the diseases that arise from them, as the Jaundice and hypochondria".

Anatomically the "hypochondrium" is the uppermost part of the abdomen, from the Greek "hypo", under and "khondros", cartilage, in this case of the sternum. Unlike today's understanding of the word hypochondria, meaning an imagined set of symptoms, it referred to the physical symptoms and diseases that arose from an excess of cold and dry humours blocking the spleen and the liver producing melancholic vapours. These melancholic vapours cause morbid feelings and a wide range of symptoms associated with congestion and depletion of innate heat.

Dandelion is one of the main spring tonic herbs, the leaves and flowers being gathered fresh in the spring when it first appears. During the winter when the digestive heat is at its lowest, food is less likely to get broken down into to its constituent parts, with the food and humours it contains remaining "crude" and unrefined. These crudities may cause blockage and stasis in the blood and organs, so in the spring blood cleansing tonics, such as dandelion, nettle, and cleavers, may all be used to help detoxify the system.

Country uses

It was very common for dandelion to be gathered by country people to eat fresh in salads in the early spring. The roasted roots have long been used as a coffee substitute.

In the book Country Remedies by Gabrielle Hatfield (1994), the following country uses are recorded;

> "Infusion for indigestion, Tea for 'spring humours', infusion of flowers for cough, Juice to remove cancer on lip, Juice used for warts, leaves chewed for arthritis, infusion of leaves applied for eczema, roots used to purify blood and restore appetite". (Hatfield, 1994)[1]

Mythos

The name is from the Greek, taraxos (disorder) and akos (remedy). Hecate is said to have entertained Theseus on his journey to defeat the minotaur, during which time she fed him for thirty days on dandelion roots. This gave him the strength to complete his mission. November is the month associated with Hecate, and this is also an indication of when the root should be gathered, as at this time it was considered most nutritious, and was when it was traditionally harvested. In fact, the levels of the powerful gut probiotic inulin, a polysaccharide that improves gut microbiology, as well as other nutrients now have been clearly shown to be at their highest concentration in the root during the autumn.

Emotional

Dandelion is above all a nourishing herb, both the leaves and roots give one a feeling of being strengthened, restored, and nourished. It brings a sense of grounding, allowing ones energy to settle, making it feel like everything is falling into its correct place. It helps promote a positive outlook enabling one to maintain a good emotional and mental balance.

Liver

The liver is the seat of the blood humour and the organ that controls the digestive faculty of the body. The temperament of the liver is hot and moist. However it can be blocked by cold melancholic vapours arising from the spleen, or from the residue left behind after a period of excessive heat as will occur during acute illness, repeated fevers, excess alcohol, and overwhelming emotional states. This cold residue left after such a period of excessive heat was called burnt choler, black bile, or atribilis. The blockages caused by this residue can have far reaching consequences, often being the cause of poor liver function, reduction of detoxification, and reduction of blood flow to the organs. Dandelion has bitter digestive tonic effects, it opens the passages of the liver increasing the flow of bile, flushing the gall bladder, and helping to clear out any blockage. By increasing the flow of bile through the liver, the organ that is responsible for breeding blood and producing balanced humours, dandelion directly cleanses and nourishes the blood at its source. Its bitterness improves digestion by stimulating the release of digestive juices in the stomach, and activates the liver, gall bladder, and pancreas. Traditionally the root has been considered the most appropriate part to use to help the liver, and the leaves most useful for the kidneys. However, all parts of the plant share the beneficial properties regarding the liver, so it would make sense to use the most active and available parts of the plant according to the season; the leaves and flowers in the spring and summer, and the roots in the autumn and winter.

Kidneys

The leaves are often considered to be the most powerful of all the herbal diuretics and are also high in potassium, which often becomes depleted when a conventional chemical diuretic is used. It provides 397 mg of potassium per 100 g of leaf, making it one of the most concentrated natural sources—juicing the leaves makes a very effective natural potassium supplement. Traditionally dandelion was used for dissolving kidney stones, and according to Culpeper "it opens the passages of urine in young and old; powerfully cleanses imposthumes- (a swelling containing puss, such as an abscess) ... and inward ulcers in the urinary passages, and by its drying and temperate quality doth afterwards heal them; for which purpose the decoction of the roots or leaves in wine, or the leaves chopped as pot herbs, with a few Alisanders, and boiled in their broth are very effectual".

Joints

Dandelion has been considered helpful in rheumatic conditions, especially gout, and for hot inflammations of the skin and the joints. It has confirmed anti-inflammatory activity in animals, as well as antioxidant, and anti-tumour activities.

Doses

Infusion

The traditional amount for the infusion is 1 oz to a pint, or 30 g to half a litre, take 3 wine glass (125 ml) doses each day.

Juice

30 ml of the fresh juice taken in the morning, the fresh leaves used in salad.

Tincture

30 ml of 1:3 tincture of root or leaves per day.

Dock

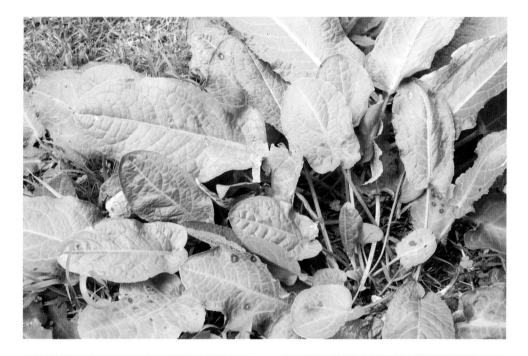

Yellow dock. Curled dock
Latin: *Rumex crispus*
Red dock. Blood wort. Water dock
Latin: *Rumex aquaticus*
Patience dock. Monk's dock
Latin: *Rumex alpines*
Common dock. Round leaved dock.
                Butter dock

Latin: *Rumex obtusifolius*
Family: Polygonaceae

Element   Air
Planet   Jupiter
Humour   Sanguine

Quality   Cold and dry in the
            first degree, cleanses
            the blood, purges hot
            humours from the liver,
            blood and bowels

Organs

Bowels
Stomach
Skin
Liver
Spleen
Joints

Actions

Laxative
Alterative

Lymphatic
Cleansing
Externally healing
Drawing
Cancer remedy

Constituents

Hydroxyanthracenes:
Anthroquinones, chrysaphanol,
    emodin
Anthrone—rumexone
Tannins
Oxalates (leaves)
Volatile oils
Vitamin: A, C
Iron, manganese, calcium,
    phosphorous, potassium, sulphur

Traditional uses and humoral influences

Nicholas Culpeper said that "All Docks are under Jupiter ... All of them have a kind of cooling, drying quality: the sorrels being the most cooling and the bloodworts being the most drying ... the red dock, which is commonly called Blood wort, cleanseth the blood and strengthens the liver, but the yellow dock is best to be taken when either the blood or the liver is effected by Choler".

The root was often boiled and the liquid drank to "purify the blood" and specifically to cure boils. This is a folk recipe collected by Gabrielle Hatfield in Bedfordshire in 1985 (Hatfield, 2007).

"This is a cure for boils, which has been proved in my own family. Dig up five dock roots, wash them so that they are very clean, put two cupfuls of clean water in a saucepan, also the five dock roots, and let them boil for thirty minutes. Strain with a fine muslin, and put into a bottle. Drink one teaspoonful night and morning".[1]

Dock is considered helpful for glandular swellings and has come to be regarded as a powerful lymphatic tonic by present day herbalists. The cooling properties of dock were also considered to help with headaches if it was thought that heat was the cause, a country remedy was to place fresh dock leaves on the temples to ease pains in the head. Traditionally dock root is harvested in the winter or early spring, when the roots have the richest nutrient levels.

Mythos

The name 'dock' refers to large leaved wayside weeds, with the name possibly also being connected to the name of the hard part of an animal's tail, similar to the hard and brittle roots of the plant. When the root is dug it frequently breaks leaving a blunt end, rather like a tail that has been cut short or "docked". The docks used to be in the plant genus *Lapathum*, which comes from the Greek word for cleanse.

In Orkney it is said that on docken stems the trows (trolls) will ride.

Liver and spleen

The liver is ruled by Jupiter and is the seat of the digestive faculty, where the chyle is broken down into its constituent humours and is then passed in the blood to the organs. Diseases of heat, such as inflammatory skin conditions, inflammatory joint conditions, itching, irritability, PMT, and constipation, can all be signs of excess choler in the blood, liver, and spleen.

Nicholas Culpeper says, "Bloodwort is exceedingly strengthening to the liver and procures good blood, being as wholesome a pot—herb as any growing in a garden". The roots have high levels of nutrients and trace elements, they deeply penetrate the ground, enabling them to draw out iron, potassium, phosphorus, sulphur, manganese, and calcium from the soil. The bitter principles also stimulate liver function and bile flow, aiding digestion and intestinal absorption.

Cancer

Yellow dock is closely related to rhubarb root, which is used as part of the Essiac cancer remedy. Scientific research into the anthroquinones contained in both rhubarb and dock has shown that they have antitumour properties for a number of cancer cell lines, including liver, gastric, lung, prostrate, ovarian, leukaemia, breast, epidermal cancers, and myelomas. There are also records for its use as a cancer remedy in country medicine; a remedy from Norfolk in the 1920s recommends that the dock was to be boiled and the growth steeped in the resulting liquid. The growth was then poulticed with the boiled dock itself. In Grieve's herbal (1931), she says "The Yellow dock has also been considered to have a positive effect in restraining the inroads made by cancer in the human system, being used as an alterative and a tonic to an enfeebled condition caused by necrosis, cancer, etc".[2]

Bowels

The anthraquinone constituents are laxative and purgative, and the tannins help to give the herb an astringency, which balances its laxative effects making it much milder than senna. Anthroquinones also have antiviral, antifungal, and antibacterial activity. The seeds are astringent and were commonly used for dysentery. Culpeper suggested that the seeds were helpful for diarrhoea and looseness of the bowels, saying

> "The seed of most kinds, whether garden or field doth stay laxes and fluxes of all sorts and is helpful for those that spit blood".

Skin

"Nettle out, Dock in-
Dock remove the nettle sting"—traditional English saying.
Dock is traditionally used to treat all kinds of skin problems, Culpeper says:

> "The roots boiled in vinegar helpeth the itch, scabs and breaking out of the skin if it be bathed therewith."

From Gabrielle Hatfield's research into English country uses we have the following in her book "country remedies": "An interesting remedy for dermatitis, which became locally famous, was recommended by a man then living in Ingham, Norfolk. Again the patient had had unsuccessful treatment from the hospital. She was advised to gather the roots of the marsh dock (take the plants that grow with their feet in the water) and boil them and use the resulting liquid to bathe the rash. She used it with such success that in subsequent years she always made up a bottle for this, which was used for treating any rash, sunburn, etc., and was lent to neighbours with great success" (Hatfield, 1994).[3] Dock leaves applied to chapped skin, and dock leaves steeped in brandy applied to the skin are all country variants of the use of dock for skin inflammations. The decoction or extract of the roots has also been used as an internal remedy for skin conditions, Maude Grieve (1931) says, "It is excellent for dispelling any obstinate itching of the skin".[4] Combined with other herbs the roots can be decocted and drank over a period of time, especially when there are long term hot and itchy skin conditions.

Joints

Poultices of the leaves can be applied to help hot and swollen joints, as well as the decoction of the root being used internally.

Doses

Decoction

15 g of root simmered in 500 ml of water for ten minutes, ½ a cup once or twice daily.

Tincture

1:3, 5 ml twice daily.

Capsules

400 mg; one or two daily after food.

Elder

Black Elder. Elderflower. Bore tree.
Anglo Saxon: Eldrun. Ellhorn. Burtre. Hylder.
Ogham: Ruis
Gallic: Scovies
Ancient British: Iscaw

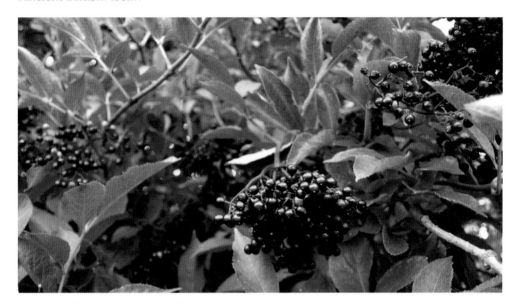

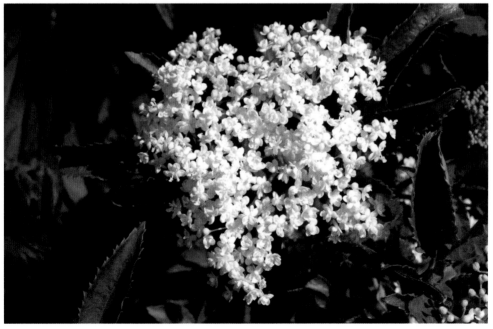

Latin:	*Sambucus nigra*
Family:	Caprifoliaceae

Element	Water
Planet	Venus
Humour	Phlegmatic
Quality	Warm and dry in the first degree, cleanses phlegm and choler, strengthens the expulsive virtue

Organs

Heart
Head
Stomach
Lungs
Kidneys
Joints
Womb
Eyes
Skin

Actions

Anti-inflammatory
Antiallergenic
Sedative
Diuretic
Diaphoretic
Externally healing
Antipyretic

Constituents

Triterpines: ursolic acid
Sterols
Vitamins: A, C, B1, B2, B6
Fatty acids: linoleic, linolenic
Flavonoids: rutin, quercertin, kaempferol

Cyanogenic glycosides: prunasin, sambunigrin
Anthocyanadins
Resins

Traditional uses and humoral influences

> "If the medicinal properties of its leaves, bark and berries were fully known, I cannot tell what our countryman could ail for which he might not fetch a remedy from every hedge, either for sickness, or wounds". (Evelyn, 1664)[1]

Elder is ruled by Venus and is hot and dry in the first degree. The flowers have always been valued for their cooling effects and are often included in traditional recipes for fevers and colds. According to traditional therapeutics, the gentle warmth of the flowers helps to move excess phlegm and loosen congestion and to thin and expel excess heat or choler. Venus governs the expulsive virtue in the body, and therefore herbs that work in sympathy with Venus, such as elder, will strengthen the cleansing and purging activities of the body. Its drying action is particularly helpful for excess catarrh, helping to reduce inflammation of the sinuses, sneezing, and the symptoms of hay fever. Its diaphoretic action promotes sweating, which helps to bring the body's temperature down when feverish. A herbalist colleague told me that one evening when she was a student of herbal medicine, her young baby came down with a raging fever. The shops were shut and she had no paracetamol. However, she had recently learned about elderflower in her plant studies and so decided to make up a tea of the flowers to give to her baby. As soon as he was given the bottle he drank it until it was empty, within an hour the fever had passed and he was soon enjoying a peaceful sleep. When he woke in the morning he was completely recovered. From then onwards she gave it every time her child became unwell and always found it effective. Due to the wide range of medicinal properties it has, elder has often been considered a cure-all; there is an old English country saying that when you get sick you should take elderflowers for three days—if then you don't get better, it may be time to call the doctor!

The berries have a warming, nourishing, and strengthening action, and are particularly helpful to resist the cold damp effects of winter on the phlegmatic organs, such as the lungs and the joints. The flower water, distilled or infused, is traditional as a remedy for the inflammation of the eyes, used as a compress or as a wash.

Mythos

Throughout Europe elder has a sacred history. It was said to be the wand of Medea the Greek goddess of magic and sorcery, the tree of Freyer, the Norse goddess of fertility and also the tree of Thor, the god of Thunder. The name may well come from the name of the queen of the elves "Eldrun", whilst other European names, such as Elhorn and Frau Holle, derive directly from the association with Freyer the spring goddess. The Russian deity Pushkaitis who ruled over gnomes and goblins was said to live under the roots of elder trees, which in many other countries was also believed to be the abode of fairies, tree deities, and supernatural beings. In Romany plant lore it was advised never to sleep under an elder or the fairie folk would spirit you away. A high level of respect for the elder was widespread; country people would not only leave offerings at the base of elder trees, but would only cut the tree after performing prayers and rituals to the elder mother. As late as 1983, one such country custom was still recorded in this rhyme from Leicestershire;

> "Old Woman, Old Woman,
> Give me some of your wood,
> And when I am dead
> I'll give you some of mine".
> (De Cleene & Lejeune, 1999)[2]

The elder also has an association with death. In the Ogham tree alphabet it is the thirteenth tree, corresponding to the last lunar month of the year, the month of the death of the year.

Emotional

Elder is the herb of release. It helps us to release and shed limiting thoughts, feelings, and behaviours. It also helps us to release ourselves from the negativity of others. If we have felt that we have been set upon, denigrated, attacked, or criticised, elder will provide a feeling of protection and impermeability. It helps us to shapeshift into new ways of being in the world, reinventing ourselves as magical beings with cunning and artistry. You are never alone with elder, she is our mother, protector, and companion and is always waiting to support us in our time of need.

Heart

Elder has a calming and soothing action, which makes it a gentle calming remedy for those who feel emotionally stressed and overheated. The roots were formerly prescribed to treat the excess fluid associated with dropsy, or the oedema caused by heart failure.

Head

Elderflower clears the head, refreshing the nervous system, and has a tonifying and reviving effect on the brain. In 1677 Dr Martin Blochwich wrote 'The Anatomy of Elder', a book solely dedicated to the medicines that can be made from elder. Pertaining to the head he says, "To mitigate headache and to remove the distress it causes, use the cake of the flowers of the Elder that is left in the vesica after distillation of the water. It must not be burned. Sprinkle it with vinegar of the flowers, apply it to the head, and use additional vinegar to renew the treatment as necessary. It opens the pores of the skin, and dispels the headache when inhaled".[3] In humoral medicine the natural temperament of the brain is cold and moist, and the etheric element that activates the nervous system and the brain is also considered to be cold. Therefore the head is particularly susceptible to problems associated with coldness, congestion, and chills. Elderflower has a gentle warming action, as well as the ability to expel excess moisture and dampness, enabling it to help clear the head, and bring it back into a balanced temperament, neither too hot nor too cold.

Lungs

Elder is one of my favourite gentle lung remedies. The berries are gentle expectorants and the flowers soothe inflamed and irritated mucous membranes. Combined with lime flowers, thyme and chamomile, it can be drunk freely as a tea throughout the day to help with coughs, asthma, and respiratory irritation associated with allergies.

Blochwich (1677) has the following recipe for

> "cases of extreme coughing with expectoration of phlegm and risk of further infections: take a handful of fresh or shadow dried Elder leaves, boil them in a quart of fountain- or clear river-water down to a third of the original volume. The strained drink should be sweetened with sugar or scummed honey, drink a warm draught of it in the morning and evening every day. The same is recommended in cases of hoarseness resulting from catarrh impairing the windpipe".[4]

The Rob, made by gently simmering the juice of the berries with sugar until it has the consistency of a syrup, was a traditional home remedy for colds and coughs. Fernie in his herbal of 1897 recommends "one or two tablespoons mixed with a tumbler of very hot water. It promotes perspiration, is demulcent to the chest. Five pounds of the fresh berries are to be used with one pound of Loaf sugar, and the juice should be evaporated to the thickness of honey".[5]

Elderberry is antiviral and protective, and combined with elecampagne root and hyssop makes a very beneficial winter tonic, both to protect against winter viruses and also to help clear them when they arise.

Stomach

The roots and bark have been considered an effective purgative since the time of Hippocrates. A fresh infusion made from the bark of the young branches is very helpful for nausea and a bloated stomach. It can be prepared at any time from the young branches; scrape a large handful of the thin bark from young branches, it will come away easily. Add 250 ml of boiling water and leave to stand for 15 minutes, drink in small doses (75–100 ml) throughout the day.

Skin and wound healing

A simple ointment of the leaves made by infusing them in oil and thickening with beeswax (1 oz to ½ a pint) is effective for treating all skin afflictions, including wounds, burns, and ulcers. I have found that it is very effective in healing long-standing leg ulcers. It can be combined with other wound herbs, such as marigold, woundwort, and mallow, and then applied as a fresh poultice for an hour twice daily.

Joints

Elderberry juice was often used as an adulterant of port and claret and therefore was banned in Portugal from being grown at all. In Mrs Grieve's A Modern Herbal (1931), she tells this elderberry story; In 1899 a physician in Prague was told by a sailor that whenever he drank port on a long journey his rheumatic pains cleared. The physician tried to replicate the effect by prescribing port to his other rheumatic patients, but met with little success. When he realised that the sailor had actually been drinking cheap port adulterated with elderberry, he pre-scribed that instead, and finally had very good results. The dose suggested at the time was 30 g of elderberry juice mixed with 10 g of port wine. Elderberry consequently gained a renewed reputation for helping with rheumatic pains, joint pain, and sciatica in European medicine generally. We now know that the Anthocyanadins, which constitute the red pigment in the berries, are both anti-inflammatory and reduce the degeneration of cartilage and connective tissue.

Doses

Tincture

The tincture may be taken 10–30 ml a day.

Tea

The tea made from the flowers can be drunk freely.

Juice

10 ml, three times a day.

Elderflower champagne

In the spring a traditional drink known as elderflower champagne is made.

Place six large heads of elderflowers in one Gallon of water (4 ½ litres), add 1 ½ pounds of sugar (700g), gently dissolve the sugar in the water, when cool add one squeezed and chopped lemon including the peel, 2 tablespoons of cider vinegar with the mother. Leave to stand for 24–48 hrs in a lightly covered vessel. Strain into bottles, seal and drink 4–6 weeks later. It is best to use plastic bottles as they will expand if the pressure gets too great rather than explode like glass ones!

Elecampagne

Scabwort, Elfwort. Horseheal. Elf dock. Velvet dock. Starwort
Welsh: Machalan y llwyglas

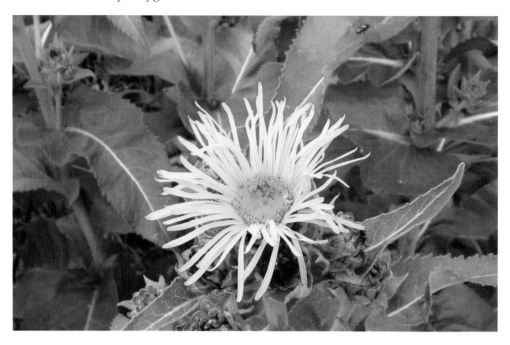

Latin:	*Inula helenium*
Family:	Asteraceae/compositae

Element	Ether
Planet	Mercury
Quality	Hot and dry in the third degree, cleanses damp from the lungs, stomach and bladder, invigorates the nerves and heart

Organs

Lungs
kidneys
Stomach
Womb

Actions

Expectorant
Diuretic
Diaphoretic
Stomachic
Immune stimulant
Antibiotic
Antiviral
Anti-inflammatory

Constituents

Essential oils: incl. camphor, alantol,
    thymol
Sesquiterpene lactones:
    alantolactone, inulin
Triterpenes: stigmasterol, sitosterol
Polyacetylenes

Traditional uses and humoral influences

Elecampagne is ruled by the planet Mercury, it is warm and dry in the third degree and is softening and loosening.

Culpeper calls it "A warm, invigorating, animating medicine". It was well known by the ancients, and there was a Latin saying "Enula campana reddit praecordia sana" meaning "elecampagne will the spirits sustain".[1]

It was a traditional restorative after periods of ill health, and it protects against the recurrence of infections.

Herbs ruled by Mercury are associated with the etheric element and the animal spirit, which resides in the head and nerves. The etheric element and the animal spirit are cold and dry, they activate the brain, connect the organs, and stimulate the movement of the vital spirit around the body. During the eleventh century in Salerno, Italian translators of the Arabic writer Serapio suggested elecampagne would help when the nerves are afflicted by cold- this being a cause of diseases such as sciatica and migraine.

Elecampagne will clear cold stagnation and stimulate movement when cold is a cause of congestion. It helps to strengthen the heart, is useful in dropsy (heart failure), and conditions where the heart seems to have been affected by stasis, coldness or excess damp. The spleen is a cold and dry organ, which is the seat of the retentive faculty and is easily blocked by excess melancholy; cold vapours that rise up from it will block the vital spirit in the heart causing depression and melancholy. Elecampagne is a loosening medicine, which has a warming and softening effect helping to ripen and clear blocked humours and is especially helpful to clear excess cold hard melancholy from the spleen.

In Roman times eating elecampagne daily was recommended not just for the digestion but also to bring mirth and joyfulness, a belief shared by Hippocrates who thought it would take away both anger and sadness. Culpeper also suggests that the fresh roots and leaves if beaten into beer and drunk daily "cleareth, strengtheneth and quickeneth the sight of the eyes".

Culpeper praised it for treating infections saying, "It cures putrid and pestilential fevers". It is also a diaphoretic, inducing sweating, thus helping to break a fever. More recently it has been found that the sesquiterpene alantolactone, found in the volatile oil and giving the plant its distinctive smell, is both anti-inflammatory and immunostimulatory and has been demonstrated to have natural antibiotic properties against both TB and diptheria.

I often use it for treating a weakened immune system and have found that it is particularly helpful for treating herpes virus infections, such as chickenpox, shingles, and outbreaks of genital herpes.

William Fernie (1897) tells us; "Prior to the Norman conquest, and during the Middle Ages, the root of Elecampagne was musch employed in great Britain as a medicine; and likewise it was candied and eaten as a sweetmeat. Some fifty years ago the candy was sold commonly in London, as flat, round cakes, being composed largely of sugar, and coloured with cochineal. A poece was eaten each night and morning for asthmatical complaints".[2]

Mythos

The Latin name *Inula* is thought to be a derivative of the Greek name Helenion, said to come from the belief that when Helen of Troy was kidnapped from Sparta she took elecampagne flowers with her and wherever her tears fell elecampagne sprung up.

The plant was traditionally used for treating those who had been "elf shot", a condition caused by mischievous elves in which one's vital energy becomes drained. It was also said to be helpful in divination rituals, being used as an incense to assist in scrying—gaining divinatory visions from watching the smoke of the burning herb over the surface of a bowl of water. It was recommended by Dioscorides for the bites of wild animals, and it had a reputation as an "alexipharmic" or resister of poisons, with William Fernie in his 1897 herbal saying; "it was customary when travelling by a river to suck a bit of the root against poisonous exhalations and bad air".[3]

Emotional

The seventeenth century herbalist John Parkinson was correct when he said that elecampagne will "expel melancholy and sorrow" (1640).[4] It gives us a boost when the spirits are low, and when we have lost hope and feel emotionally and spiritually exhausted. It brings a sense of lightness when we have become overwhelmed, liberating us from darkness. Like the planet Mercury, it offers magical transformation and divine inspiration.

Lungs

The lungs have a moist and wet, temperament and are prone to conditions of coldness and damp. The warming action of elecampagne clears damp from the lungs and restores the natural level of warmth and dryness in the respiratory system.

It is expectorant, cleansing, and warming for the lungs, helping to expel catarrh and excess mucous. It is particularly helpful to protect against infections of the respiratory system, especially those occurring in the autumn and winter. Culpeper considered it a warming pectoral for coldness in the lungs along with balm, betony, hyssop and liquorice. He recommended it for the consumptive, for whooping cough, and for wheezing. As early as 1885, it was discovered to have highly effective antibacterial properties, particularly against the *Mycobacterium tuberculosis* a disease for which it had always been used from ancient times. It has since been found to also have good antimycobacterial activity against *M. diptheriae* (Diptheria) (Fisher, 2018).[5] The fresh candied roots, or lozenges made from the dried powdered root, were used for asthma and weak lungs, especially when it was associated with coldness. A recipe from the Herbalists of Myddfai for cough and Dyspnoea;

> "Take the root of Elecampagne, two pennyworth of black pepper, and the same of the roots of mallows, let them be powdered and made into a confection with clarified honey. Take as much as a pigeons egg the first thing in the morning and the last at night. It is proven". (Hoffman, 1978)[6]

Womb and kidneys

It has a gentle warming action on the womb, kidneys, and bladder, increasing urination and menstruation. It helps with stagnation, congestion, and with blood stasis in the reproductive organs, which is commonly a cause of endometriosis, fibroids, and period pains.

Stomach

A warming aromatic bitter, the Roman writer Pliny said, "Let no day pass without eating some of the roots of Enula condited to help digestion and cause mirth" (Fernie, 1897).[7]

Culpeper recommends it as "very effective to warm a cold, windy stomach, or the pricking therein or the stitches caused by the spleen". It is anthelmintic, meaning that it kills parasites and worms, and is useful in treating worms in children; it can be given in regular small doses in capsules, being both safe and well tolerated.

I have often found it helpful in treating intestinal infections, such as norovirus, and especially for protecting ME patients who are vulnerable to intestinal infection.

Skin

Culpeper recommends the ointment for scabs and itch and the decoction for washing old sores and cankers. There is some evidence that in some people the external application of elecampagne may cause a sensitivity reaction, so it should be used with care and possibly used only as a wash, and not through application of the essential oil.

Doses

Tincture

Up to 5 ml three times a day.

Decoction

A heaped teaspoonful to a mug as a decoction, it is bitter but it if you add a squeeze of lemon juice it transforms the taste and makes it quite palatable. The presence of vitamin C also increases its bioavailability.

My "Three root decoction" for bronchial coughs and lung infections, and for treating viral illness:

Combine one heaped teaspoonful of elecampagne and valerian root, and three slices of fresh root ginger, decoct gently for ten minutes, add two teaspoons of elderberry juice (if available), and honey and lemon to taste. Drink three times a day for chest infections.

Fennel

Sweet fennel. Common Fennel. Fenkel. Spingel

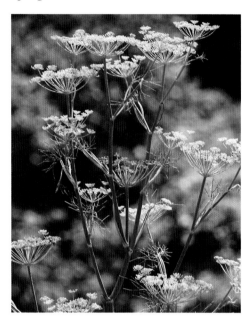

Latin:	*Foeniculum vulgare*
Family:	Apiaceae

Element	Ether
Planet	Mercury
Humour	Etheric
Quality	Hot in the second degree, dry in the first, expels phlegm from the stomach and brain

Organs

Stomach
Bowels
Head
Kidneys
Liver
Spleen
Womb
Breasts
Ovaries

Actions

Digestive
Carminative
Diuretic
Expectorant
Decongestant
Relaxant
Hormonal balancer
Antiseptic
Anti-inflammatory
Anti-parasitic
Antimicrobial
Galactalogue

Constituents

Volatile oils: fenchone, anethole, limonene, pinene, thymol
Flavonoids: rutin, quercitin, kaempferol
Coumarins: bergapten
Phenols: chlorogenic acid
Sterols

Traditional uses and humoral influences

Fennel is under the rulership of Mercury, is hot in the second degree, and dry in the first degree.

Mercury and the etheric element are connected to the animal spirit, which is cold and dry in temperament and resides in the head. The warming quality of fennel helps assist in keeping the nervous system active and warm. It is this warmth that also makes fennel beneficial for any organs that have a damp, phlegmatic character, such as the lungs, stomach, bowels, kidneys, bladder, and brain. Hildegard Von Bingen, the twelfth century mystic said; "Even eaten raw fennel does not harm the body in any way. In whatever form one eats fennel, it makes us happy, gives us a good skin colour and body odour and promotes good digestion".[1]

John Milton—Paradise Lost

> "A savoury odour blown,
> Grateful to appetite, more pleased my sense
> Than smell of sweetest Fennel".

As a warming herb for the stomach, Nicholas Culpeper considered fennel an essential addition to meals with fish; "it consumes the phlegmatic humour, which fish most plentifully afford and annoy the body with" Fennel oil has been shown to be antibacterial and antifungal, with activity against *E.coli*, *Salmonella* and *Helicobacter pylori*, both of which can infect the digestive system (Fisher, 2018).[2]

Fennel was considered to strengthen the mind and the sight, for which it was recommended to use the juice from the leaves and stem. Hildegard (1998) also values fennel for its ability to calm the mind and the emotions, and considers it especially helpful for insomnia; "One who is unable to sleep for being occupied by some difficulty should, if it is summer, cook fennel and twice as much yarrow. When the water has been squeezed out, he should place the warm herbs around his temples, forehead, with a cloth over them. He should also take fresh sage and sprinkle it with a bit of wine, and place this over his heart and around his neck, and he will be soothed for sleeping".[3]

Mythos

The name fennel derives from the Latin word for hay, "foenum". The Greeks gave it the name marathron, deriving from "maraino", meaning to grow thin, alluding to its fine feathery leaves or possibly the belief that eating fennel would help one lose weight: "Both seeds, leaves and roots thereof are much used in drink or broth, to make people more lean that are too fat" (Culpeper).

Fennel is associated with the Titan Prometheus, his name meaning "forethought". By hiding an ember of the sun in a fennel stalk, he is credited with smuggling fire out of Olympus and bringing it back to the mortals after the Gods confiscated it from them. This is a mythological allegory of the benefits of fennel, which like Prometheus helps to bring the messages of divine light through the ether, thus activating the mind and nourishing the animal spirit.

Fennel was also believed to be used by serpents to help them grow a new skin each time one was shed, and it was said that they also rubbed their eyes on the stalks to give them clearer vision.

Along with other umbelliferous plants, such as dill, celery, parsley and caraway, fennel has always been considered an antidemonic remedy. It was an old English custom to attach fennel and St John's wort over doors and windows on Midsummer's Eve (St. John's Eve) to protect the household from evil powers. The stalks were also considered efficacious in removing curses.

Emotional

Fennel calms, warms, and settles. It gives us clarity and clear vision in times of confusion, helping us to let go of fears and worries about the unknown. It balances emotions, with the medieval mystic Hildegard recommending that taking the seeds will force the emotions of the heart back into the correct balance.

Stomach and bowels

In the Compleat Herbal of Physical Plants (1706), by John Pechey he says; "The seed strengthens the stomach and takes off nauseousness … This has done much good for those that have been troubled with wind in their stomachs".[4] Fennel warms the stomach, clears biliousness and wind, reduces nausea, and settles indigestion. Fennel along with dill, caraway, and sweet cicely was traditionally used in "gripe" water, a traditional remedy for colic in babies. As well as helping to clear wind, it has a gentle laxative effect.

Liver

Fennel warms and activates the digestive function in the liver, improving production of digestive juices and the secretion of bile. Nicholas Culpeper said that "The roots are of most use in physic, drinks and broths, that are taken to cleanse the blood, to open obstructions of the liver".

It is commonly taken after food in the form of a tea, as a digestive alcoholic spirit, or the seeds themselves can simply be chewed. It is interesting that in the myth of Prometheus, who is so strongly associated with fennel, it is said that his liver would regenerate every night after it had been consumed by eagles as a punishment for helping the mortals, once again serving as an allegorical reminder of another medicinal benefit of the herb.

Lungs

"There is nothing like fennel for the lungs and the bronchial tubes; it brings ease in bad attacks of coughing, whooping cough, and asthma, and clears the worst blockages" (Messegue, 1981).[5] Fennel is traditionally used in asthma, Culpeper attests; "The seed is of good use in medicines to help shortness of breath and wheezing by the stopping of the lungs" . In country medicine it was given as a syrup prepared from the juice. It has warming and clearing properties, gently assisting expectoration and relaxing the bronchioles, helping to reduce wheezing.

Hormonal remedy

The sterols in fennel have gentle hormonal effects, it has been used to help with lactation and to encourage a regular hormonal cycle. It has a gentle relaxing oxytocic action that helps to encourage a good flow of breast milk. A traditional recipe for a nursing tea is equal parts of fennel, aniseed, and nettle.

Kidneys

Culpeper mentions its ability to "provoke urine" and with its ability to disinfect and reduce inflammation it can be used alone or added to other urinary herbs for conditions such as cystitis. It is often considered to be a good detoxifying herb, both helping to cleanse the liver and to enable the kidneys to flush out waste products.

Doses

Fennel tea

One teaspoon of seeds infused in ½ a pint of boiling water.

Tincture

1:3 tincture; 5 ml 1–3 times daily.

Nursing tea

Equal parts fennel seed, aniseed, nettle herb.

One teaspoonful to a cup, three cups daily.

Fenugreek

Bird's foot. Greek hay. Greek fennel
Sanskrit: Methi

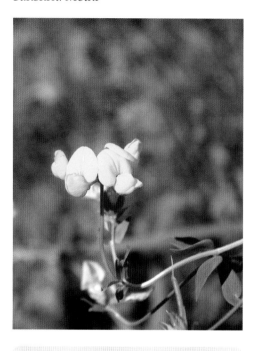

Latin:	*Trigonella foenum–graecum*
Family:	Fabaceae

Element	Ether
Planet	Mercury
Humour	Etheric
Quality	Hot in the first degree, dry in the second degree, softening and dissolving, cleanses and purges the bowels, chest and lungs of congealed phlegm

Organs

Bowels
Stomach
Liver
Lungs
Womb

Actions

Laxative
Demulcent
Emollient
Drawing agent
Expectorant
Galactagogue
Anti-inflammatory

Constituents

Steroidal saponins: diosgenin, yamogenin
Alkaloids: trigonelline
Mucilage (up to 30%)
Flavonoids
Vitamins: A, C, D, B1, B2, Niacin
Calcium, phosphorous, iron

Traditional uses and humoral influences

Fenugreek is under the rulership of Mercury, the planet of connection, communication, and movement. When the etheric humour becomes excessively cold it leads to blockage and sluggishness. Unlike its close relative clover, which is cold and dry, fenugreek is both gently warming and drying. It clears excess dampness, and is a stimulating tonic herb that enlivens the liver, stomach, and lungs, purging excess thickened or congealed phlegm from these organs. It is soothing and mucilaginous, and is very helpful for irritation and inflammation throughout the digestive system. It improves the appetite and is considered nutritive and restorative. Fenugreek is particularly helpful after periods of debilitating illness, having a reputation of helping to aid recovery and to put weight back on. It was used for gout, fevers, aiding childbirth, and healing both external and internal ulcers. It has a gentle warming and nourishing effect on the female reproductive organs, helping to increase lactation, strengthen the womb, and clear damp congestion. It has been shown to be antioxidant, anti-inflammatory, and antibacterial, specifically against *E.coli*, *Staphylococcus aureus* and *Yersinia enterocolitica* (Fisher, 2018).[1]

Mythos

Fenugreek was used by the ancient Egyptian, early Greek, and Roman civilisations as both a medicinal and culinary herb. Its name, *feonum-greacum*, means "Greek hay". It was often used as a nutritious additive to conditioning mixes for horses and cattle and also to improve their taste and digestibility.

Maurice Messegue (1981), the French folk herbalist, says "It always gives me pleasure to see the pale yellow flowers of this modest cousin of clover and lucerne … because it is a herb of joy, and I put it in my love potions along with savory, hogweed and celandine".[2]

Bowels and stomach

Fenugreek is a gentle but effective colonic lubricant that soothes the passage of stool and enables the passing of complete evacuations. Nicholas Culpeper said "The decoction or broth of the seed, drank with a little vinegar, expels and purges all superfluous humours which cleave to the bowel".

The seeds reduce inflammation and discomfort associated with inflammatory bowel disease and diverticulitis, thus helping with both diarrhoea and loose stools as well as with constipation. Fenugreek helps to normalise gut flora, thus reducing bloating and distension. The seeds may be eaten after soaking, or the powder can be made into a drink or can be taken in capsules. It is one of my favourite gentle laxative herbs, which isn't habit forming and can safely be used over extended periods of time, I have found that taking two capsules before bed is quite adequate to keep the bowels moving effectively in most cases, and can be increased if necessary.

For gastritis and heartburn, the powder taken as a drink is equally effective, it provides a protective, healing and anti-inflammatory coating, and is an alternative to marshmallow root powder and slippery elm.

Liver

Fenugreek is a gentle bitter remedy, the seeds can be eaten after soaking or a decoction of them may be drunk. The seeds have also been shown to be liver protective, having a similar effect to the protective silymarin compounds found in milk thistle. The liver is the seat of the blood humour and fenugreek is known to have a beneficial effect on blood sugar levels, benefiting patients with both type 1 and type 2 diabetes, improving glucose tolerance, and reducing insulin resistance. In clinical trials, fenugreek has also been observed to reduce levels of LDL cholesterol by up to 30%.

Lungs

Nicholas Culpeper suggests that the "decoction, first made with dates, and afterwards made into a syrup with honey, cleanses the breast, chest and lungs, and may be taken for any complaint thereof".

Womb

In Egyptian times it was considered helpful to aid childbirth, and it is an effective herb to increase the flow of breast milk. Diosgenin, one of the steroidal saponins that it contains is gently oestrogenic, making it a helpful remedy during menopause and when the female reproductive system is weak or depleted.

External use

The seeds boiled and crushed are used like linseed as hot poultices to draw the poison out of boils and abscesses.

Doses

Dried herb or seed up to 2g three times daily.

The seeds may be taken as a decoction, a powder or a paste.

400 mg capsules: two capsules up to three times daily.

Feverfew

Featherfew, Bachelors buttons. Midsummer daisy. Flirtwort.
Pyrethrum parthenium, Chrysanthemum parthenium

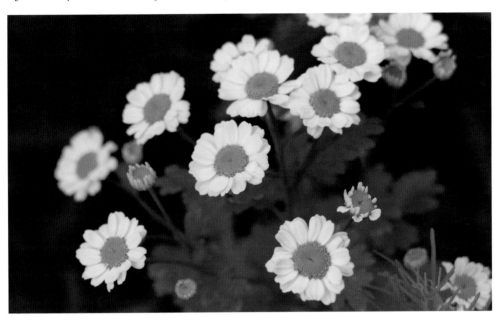

Latin:	*Tanacetum parthenium*
Family:	Asteraceae/Compositae
Element	Water
Planet	Venus
Humour	Phlegm
Quality	Hot in the third degree, dry in the second, heats the head and womb, purges choler and phlegm, clears melancholy and raises the spirits

Organs

Stomach
Womb
Head
Joints
Lungs

Actions

Febrifuge
Anti-inflammatory
Antispasmodic
Analgesic
Anti-rheumatic
Stomachic
Anthelmintic
Antimicrobial

Constituents

Volatile oil: α and β pinene, camphor
Lactones: parthenolide, chrysantholide
Monoterpenes
Resins
Tannins

Traditional uses and humoral influences

Feverfew is ruled by Venus and is considered hot in the third degree and dry in the second degree.

Nicholas Culpeper tells us, "Venus commands this herb, and has commended it to succour her sisters, to be a general strengthener of their wombs, and to remedy such infirmities as a careless midwife has there caused; it cleanses the womb, expels the afterbirth, and does a woman all the good she can desire of a herb". He also considers that it will "purgeth both Choler and Phlegm", making it a powerful cleansing herb that activates the expulsive faculty of the body, a faculty that is also under the rulership of Venus and associated with the phlegmatic humour. An excess of the phlegmatic humour brings on all cold and rheumatic diseases, such as fluid retention, dropsies, oedema, discharges and abscesses. It also causes coughs, excess mucous from the lungs, head pain, lethargy, palsy, convulsions, and epilepsy, due to phlegm obstructing the animal spirit. Cold also causes cramps and colic, and so may be a cause of digestive pain.

Culpeper also advises its use for those "troubled with melancholy and heaviness, or sadness of spirits", a use confirmed by Mrs Grieve (1931) in the early 20th Century recommending its use in "hysterical complaints, nervousness and low spirits, and as a general tonic. The cold infusion is made from 1 oz of the herb to a pint of boiling water, allowed to cool, and taken freely in doses of half a teacupful". Fernie in his 1897 Herbal Simples says "It is a positive tonic to the digestive and nervous systems … [and] is best calculated to pacify those who are liable to sudden, spiteful rude irascibility, of which they are conscious but say they cannot help it, and to soothe fretful children".[1] He advises taking 10–20 drops of the tincture with a spoonful of water three times daily.

Externally the flowers can be used as a pain relieving poultice, especially thought to be helpful for facial pain and neuralgia. The ancient welsh herbalists of Myddfai recommended an ointment made by pounding together in butter equal parts of fresh feverfew, plantain, sage, and bugle to be used as a treatment for bruises.

Mythos

The heat of the herb is reflected in the old name *Pyrethrum*, coming from the Greek "pur" for fire, and the common name feverfew is a corruption of the medical term febrifuge, meaning to break a fever. The flowers are long-lasting and the generic name *Tanacetum* derives from the Greek word "athanato", meaning long-lasting or immortal. The herb was often used to strew around coffins, as a sign of immortality and perhaps also as it is a powerful repellent of flies and to allay odours. The tincture or a wash may also be applied to exposed parts of the skin for protection from biting insects.

Emotional

Feverfew helps to move stuck, heavy feelings, it stimulates renewal and helps us to feel cleansed of old redundant ways of thinking. It clears anger and resentment while calming and clearing the mind, helping new visions to arise and fresh perspectives to open up. It helps to motivate us to move on from habitual patterns of negative thought, whilst removing emotional stagnation.

Fevers

Fevers may be due to cold and moist conditions, such as external cold, low vitality, physical stagnation, and exhaustion, which can all diminish innate heat and vital spirit and allow external poisons to enter the body. The ability of feverfew to purge both the excess heat of the fever and also purge and dry the excess moisture that has caused the fever makes it an excellent herb for breaking the fever. Its large range of antimicrobial compounds provided by volatile oils, monoterpenes, and lactones, combined with its anti-inflammatory and relaxant properties make it an ideal treatment for all the stages of fever—it is especially helpful in relieving the aches and pains that accompany viral infections. It can be taken as a strong infusion (30 g to 500 ml, three doses of 100 ml daily) or combined with other fever reducing herbs, such as lime flower, elderflower, yarrow, eyebright, and catmint.

Stomach

John Pechey in his 1706 Compleat Herbal of Physical Plants praises its ability to stimulate the appetite and activate the stomach saying it, "does all that a bitter herb can do".[2] The stomach is considered to be a phlegmatic organ, under the rulership of the moon, so often problems such as colic and indigestion may be caused by excess cold and dampness, reducing stomach heat. Its antispasmodic effects compliment the gentle bitter action,

helping to both activate digestion and enable good effective peristalsis.

Head

Culpeper says "It is very effectual for all pains in the head coming from a cold cause" He also suggests its use for vertigo. John Pechy in his herbal of 1706 also recommends it for headaches; "Take of feverfew one handful, warm it in a frying pan, apply it twice or thrice hot: this cures an Hemicrania".[3] This word means "half head", and is the word from which the term migraine is derived. In recent times, clinical trials have shown the herb to be an effective prophylactic for migraine, with the fresh herb being recommended—one or two leaves eaten daily. The lactones are believed to inhibit prostaglandin and arachidonic acid release, both of which have been implicated in the genesis of migraines.

It is also interesting to note that migraines are often associated with weak digestion, nausea, bloating, and are often triggered by intolerance to certain foods. The bitter tonic action of feverfew helps to strengthen the digestion and enable better digestive activity, as well as strengthening the expulsive virtue and improve elimination of waste products.

Joints

Rheum comes from the Greek word "to flow", and when excess cold and damp phlegm congest flow in the body, it frequently impacts on the joints, with rheumatic pain ensuing. The hot cleansing action of feverfew helps to clear such dampness, reducing stiffness, pain, and swelling. In Thomas Bartram's

Encyclopeadia of Herbal Medicine (1995) he states the following case, "After 12 years with osteo-arthritis of the hands a patient ate three leaves a day and was soon able to turn most taps".[4] The sesquiterpene lactone parthenolide from feverfew is now known to inhibit the action of the inflammatory compound interleukin-12 produced by the immune system, giving modern confirmation for this traditional use.

Womb

Feverfew's warming, antispasmodic action makes it very useful for period pain, the tincture can be taken in small doses of twenty drops hourly throughout the day. It has an activating effect on the reproductive system and can be used to help regulate periods when they are absent and bleeding is minimal. More than 30 ml of the tincture weekly may increase bleeding and shorten the cycle, so in such cases caution should be taken. However, it will improve fertility when pelvic congestion is present.

Lungs

The lungs have a cold and moist temperament, making them susceptible to the effects of excess phlegm, when the warming properties of feverfew are particularly helpful. Traditionally, a decoction of the herb would be taken with sugar or honey to help with difficulty in breathing, wheezing, and coughs.

Doses

Infusion

A simple infusion can be made with one ounce to a pint and drunk in divided doses over two days.

Tincture

The tincture can be taken 20 drops hourly for period pain.

Fever tea

Equal parts of:
Feverfew
Elderflower
Lime flower
Mint
Chamomile
Yarrow
  Prepare with one heaped teaspoon to a cup, drink freely throughout the day.

Guelder rose

Cramp bark, Guelder rose. Water elder. Red elder. Rose elder. Gaitre berries. May rose. Sambucus aquatis

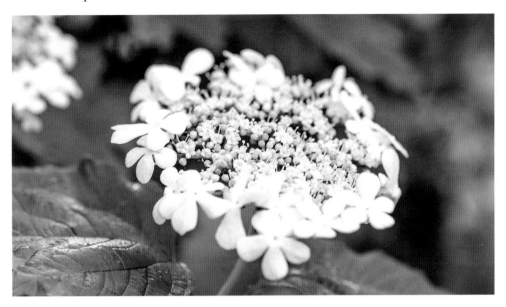

Latin:	*Viburnum opulus/viburnum prunifolium*
Family:	Caprifoliaceae
Element	Water
Planet	Venus
Humour	Phlegmatic
Quality	Warm and dry in the first degree, clears cold damp congestion from the lungs, heart and womb

Organs

Lungs
Heart
Womb
Stomach and digestion
Bladder

Actions

Antispasmodic
Relaxant
Sedative
Astringent
Antidiarrhoeal

Constituents

Bitter: viburnin
Valeric acid
Salicosides
Tannins
Hydroquinones: arbutin
Coumarins: scopoletin, scopoline
Calcium, potassium, magnesium, phosphorous, and iron

Traditional uses and humoral influences

Like the common elder, guelder rose is ruled by Venus and is considered warm and dry in the first degree. It relieves any congestion or obstruction associated with coldness and it warms the blood and circulation, enabling the blood to flow freely and easily. Its warmth relaxes blood vessels improving blood flow to the extremities and improving the flow of oxygenation to the heart. The respiratory passages are particularly prone to cold and damp, they have both a wet phlegmatic temperament and being open to the air they are prone to being affected by cold. Guelder is considerably warming and activating, helping to clear phlegm and catarrh through warmth. Its relaxant effects extend to the nervous system, reducing nervous tension due to the gentle warmth that it imparts to the nerves and brain. It contains similar compounds to valerian, which may account for it also being considered a useful sedative.

The name cramp bark has come from America, where European settlers found the similar tree *Viburnum prunifolium* being used by the First Nations people. They used a decoction of the bark to treat gynaecological conditions, aiding recovery after childbirth and the effects of menopause. In particular, it was very effectual in relieving menstrual cramps and other spasmodic conditions. Consequently, herbalists also used the plant for treating spasm of the digestive tract or the bile ducts.

Mythos

The guelder rose grows throughout Europe, North Africa, Asia, and North America. In America it is called cramp bark or black haw and has its own subspecies, *Viburnum prunifolium*. Although it has a different leaf shape it shares similar five-petalled flowers and an almost identical chemical composition. The geulder rose is related to the common elderflower and is placed under the same plant family, although the botanist Carl Linnaeus correctly recognised the bush was distinctly different from the common elder (*Sambucus nigra*) and included it in a different genus that he called *Viburnum*.

Guelder rose is not a herb that appears in any of the older herbals, it is however referred to in the writings of Geoffrey Chaucer who names it "gaitre berries". He suggests that it is among the plants that "Shal be for your hele" and to "Picke hem right as they grow and ete hem in" (Grieve, 1931).[1] The name geulder rose could be a degradation of "water elder" to "guelder" or it may be in reference to the Dutch region Gueldersland where the cultivated non-fruit-bearing *Viburnum opulus* "roseum" or the "snowball" tree comes from.

Emotional

Geulder rose is a very helpful herb for nervous agitation and tension, especially when it is caused by emotional overload. It calms the heart, strengthens the spirit, and reduces panic attacks and fearfulness.

Lungs

Like elder flower, guelder rose is particularly helpful for lung conditions associated with catarrh, bronchial spasm, and irritation. Its sedative and relaxant properties make it particularly helpful for asthma, and persistent, irritating coughs. It makes a good addition to cough syrups combining particularly well with rosehip syrup.

Heart

Cramp bark is particularly helpful for cold congestion of the circulatory system due to aging, exhaustion, or heart problems. Traditionally it was used to treat palpitations and a weak heart, and in more recent times herbalists have found it valuable for treating high blood pressure. The salicylate compounds that it contains are known to be anti-inflammatory and they have been shown to reduce the stickiness of the blood whilst having the added advantage of increasing peripheral blood flow.

Womb

Both cramp bark and guelder rose can be helpful for dysmenorrhea (painful periods), threatened miscarriage, pelvic pain, and for labour and postpartum pains. Both varieties can be useful for congestive and inflammatory pelvic pain, such as endometriosis.

Stomach and digestion

The gentle bitter properties activate the digestive organs and release spasm. This makes it a useful remedy for colic, indigestion, and irritable bowel syndrome. It is specifically recommended for spasm of the bile ducts and gall bladder pain.

Bladder

Its anti-inflammatory effects and relaxant properties account for it also being recommended for urinary stones and bladder pain.

Doses

Decoction

2–4 g one to three times daily.

Tincture

1:3 5–10 ml up to three times daily.

Capsule

400 mg three times daily.

Hawthorn

May, Maybush. Haw. Quickset. White thorn. Gazels. Bread and Cheese tree

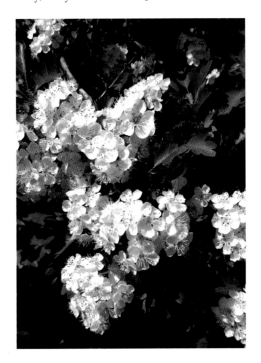 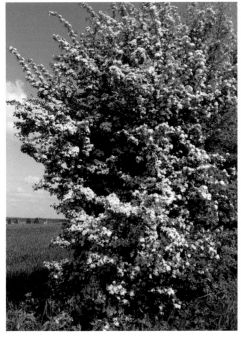

Latin: *Crateagus oxycanthoides*
Family: Rosaceae

Element   Fire
Planet   Mars
Humour   Choleric
Quality   Cold and dry in the first
          degree, astringent and
          diuretic, clears excess
          moisture

Organs

Heart and circulation
Kidneys
Head

Actions

Hypotensive
Cardiac tonic
Antiarrhythmic
Vasodilator
Astringent
Antispasmodic
Diuretic

Constituents

Flavonoids: viexin, quercetin, rutin
Procyanidins
Amines: dopamine, acetylcholine
Triterpines: ursolic acid, oleanic acid

Traditional uses and humoral influences

Hawthorn is a tree of Mars, but unlike the hot choleric humour that Mars rules, it is cooling and drying in its action. Hawthorn is a member of the rose family, the family that also contains brambles and apples and is notable for its cooling and drying properties. Mars has a relationship with the choleric humour and the hot aspects of the blood, and hawthorn is especially useful in cooling and calming hot distempers affecting the heart, reducing arrhythmias, and normalising blood pressure. Its antispasmodic effects help to improve blood flow to the heart and also improve the circulation generally. It is considered protective for the heart and circulation with Culpeper recommending the seeds as being "good for the Dropsy". Maurice Messegue (1981) says; "My father used to prescribe the bark of the plant for fever, the fruit for diarrhoea, and the flowers to regulate the heartbeat and the blood pressure. I myself make use of Hawthorn for nervous spasms, arteriosclerosis, angina and obesity, and it is one of my best 'tranquiliser' herbs".[1]

Its antispasmodic actions are very helpful for pain associated with tension or constriction of organs due to spasm. Once when treating a patient for the extreme pain caused by an ovarian cyst, I remembered Messegue's advice for using the herb in cases of spasmodic pain. I combined hawthorn flowers with rosemary and suggested using a hand and foot bath. Within two minutes of using the hand bath the patient described the most profound tranquilising and painkilling effects travelling throughout her body—she said that it was similar to taking the strongest conventional painkiller but without the side effects. She continued the treatment and after three days the three weeks of ever increasing pain she had been having had completely subsided.

Culpeper was also greatly impressed by the hawthorn's ability to draw things out;

> "If cloths or sponges be wet in the distilled water; and applied to any place wherein thorns and splinters, or the like, do abide in the flesh, it will notably draw them forth, and thus you see the thorn gives a medicine for its own pricking, and so doth almost everything else".

Mythos

The scientific name *Crateagus oxycanthoides* comes from the Greek "kratos", meaning hardness, "oxus", meaning sharp, and "akantha", meaning a thorn. The Greeks dedicated the hawthorn to Maia, the goddess of spring and midwifery. She was the mother of Hermes and also connected to the death aspect of the triple goddess of ancient Europe who conducts the souls to Hell. Hawthorn both combines the energy of the divine maiden and her renewal of life and the aspect of the death goddess and her powers of decay. The blossoms exude a foul smell, which attracts the carrion insects that are the tree's main pollinators. May, the month of Maia and the time of the blossoming of hawthorn, was also the traditional month of cleansing the temples in Greek and Roman custom. They would wash and cleanse the sacred statues and throw out the old gifts and offerings from the previous year, it was a time when old clothes would be cast off, and the new robes worn during the midsummer festivities would be prepared. This may well be connected to the old saying; "Ne'er cast a clout before May is out".

Hawthorn has been regarded as a tree with special powers throughout its history. Ruled by Mars and said in Teutonic legend to have sprung from a bolt of lightning, hawthorn thus has the power to also protect from lightning strikes. An old English saying goes;

> "Beware of an Oak, it draws the stroke,
> Avoid an Ash, it courts a flash,
> Creep under a thorn,
> It will protect you from harm".

As well as lightning, hawthorn was believed to protect against witches, evil spirits, vampires, and was said by the Romans to prevent hauntings by the spirits of the deceased. As well as Maia, the Romans also dedicated the tree to Flora, the goddess of spring, and also to Cardea. Cardea is the goddess associated with the hinge, and therefore the threshold. Her wand of hawthorn was especially protective against witchcraft and spells crossing the threshold and was particularly effective against those cast on children. Ovid said; "Her power is to open what is shut, and to shut what is open" (Tarrant, 2004).[2] She was associated with the north/south axis around which Roman towns were planned, and it is from her that we get the name for the "cardinal" points of the compass.

In ancient British mythology, the hawthorn is named "Hauth" and is the sixth tree of the ancient Ogham tree alphabet. In the ancient song of Amergen, said to have been sung as the first druid stepped onto the shore of Ireland, the corresponding line for hawthorn is: "I am fair amongst the flowers" (Graves, 1948).[3]

In the ancient Welsh book, the Mabinogi, the tree is said to belong to the great hawthorn giant Yspaddaden, whose beautiful daughter Olwen was the princess of spring and fertility and was known as "She of the White track". Olwen is the guardian of sacred wells and springs, and it is traditional in May, the month belonging to her, to dress and cleanse springs and wells with flowers welcoming her fertility back to the land. The hero Culwych had to defeat the giant Yspaddaden to gain the hand of Olwen in marriage and release the lands from his dark spells and terrible rule. Culwych succeeded with the help of the knights of King Arthur to complete the thirty-nine impossible tasks that Yspaddeden had set him to gain the hand of Olwen. Finally Culwych slayed the tyrannical giant and brought peace and prosperity back to the land.

Large and ancient hawthorn trees often marked the locations of the ancient administrative Moot and Manorial courts, and in Ireland hawthorns are still considered to be the meeting places of the little people or fairies and should not be cut down lest you want to suffer terrible ill fortune.

Emotional

Mars and the giant Yspaddadan represent the anger that often resides in our hearts, feeding feelings of hurt, resentment, and revenge. If like Culwych we are to find fulfilment then we must release love (Olwen) into the world by overcoming the burning hatred (Yspadaden) that arises when we feel wronged. Hawthorn softens and draws out poisonous and deep set toxic emotions allowing us to regenerate the joy in our lives. Like the rose, hawthorn helps to open our hearts allowing us to develop kindness and compassion towards others. It is only by having an open and loving heart that we can protect ourselves from the damage caused by negative emotions, ironically it is only by letting go of our own anger that we can protect ourselves from the effects of the anger of others.

Like the physical ability of hawthorn to draw out and cleanse the things that pierce the skin, it also has the ability to help draw out the feelings and hurtful actions of others that have got under our skin. Like the Greeks and Romans seeing the month of May as a time of cleansing and casting off the old, hawthorn helps us to finally let go of all that poisons our heart and spirit.

Heart

The heart is especially susceptible to being scorched by too much heat, this may be caused by extreme emotions, especially anger, as well as mental agitation, fevers, overwork, or a stressful life. Trauma and crises, such as the death of a loved one, can also leave us broken-hearted. Hawthorn calms, cools, protects and also "heals" a broken heart. It relaxes the coronary arteries, increasing blood flow, oxygenation, and nourishment

of the heart muscle. We now recognise that stress hormones and high levels of adrenaline increase oxidative damage to the tissues, corresponding to the historic idea of excessive heat scorching organs. The flavonoids in hawthorn help to strengthen and regenerate inflamed and damaged tissues, and rutin helps to stabilise and regenerate blood vessel walls and reduce oxidative damage. In this way, hawthorn combines powerful emotional benefits with physical benefits to the heart and circulatory system.

A combination which I have found most useful is to use equal parts of hawthorn, rose flowers, and melissa, made as a tea or administered as a pill, powders, or tincture. It releases feelings of tension, helps grief and the broken-hearted and also benefits those who suffer with deep set feelings of anguish and despair.

When treating high blood pressure, it is helpful to combine the cooling effects of hawthorn with the warming and releasing effects of herbs such as guelder rose, lime blossom, and yarrow.

Doses

Tincture

1:3, 5 ml 1–3 times daily.

Infusion

3–5 g once or twice daily.
Because of its potential blood pressure lowering effects, care should be taken by those who have low blood pressure. Start with a low dose, and then slowly increase.

Hops

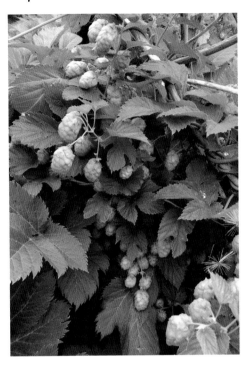

Latin: *Humulus lupulus*
Family: Cannabaceae

Element   Fire
Planet   Mars
Humour   Choleric
Quality   Hot and dry in the second
           degree, cleanses and
           purges phlegm, warms
           and opens the passages of
           the liver clearing excess
           choler, warms the spleen
           and bowels.

Organs

Stomach
Head and nerves
Liver
Spleen
Kidneys

Actions

Sedative
Nervine
Digestive
Antispasmodic
Antimicrobial
Diuretic
Aromatic bitter

Constituents

Bitter principles
Volatile oils, mainly humulene
Flavonoids
Resins
Tannins
Phenolic acids

Traditional uses and humoral influences

Hops are ruled by Mars, and have an opening and clearing action. Mars is associated with the gall bladder and the hot choleric humour in the body. In people with choleric temperaments there is a danger that heat may build up, causing choleric afflictions, or diseases of heat. Signs of this imbalance include; feelings of heat, sweating, thirst, acidity, nausea, constipation, fury, irritability, skin problems, acne, carbuncles, fevers, shingles, frenzy, poor sleep, cystitis, bladder and kidney blockage and stones, menstrual irregularity, light and scant periods. Heat can also build up in the liver and organs due to stagnation, so the opening, clearing effect of hops helps to flush out any congestion, or stagnation.

Nicholas Culpeper says; "A syrup made of the juice and sugar, cures the yellow jaundice, eases the head-ache that comes of heat, and tempers the heat of the liver and stomach, and is profitably given in long and hot agues that arise from choler and blood". He continues; "In cleansing the blood they help … all manner of scabs, itch, and other breakings out of the body" One of the main symptoms of liver disease and congestion is itching and the development of boils and scabs. The powerful bitter digestive tonic effect of hops helps to activate the liver clear the congestion, warming the spleen, and activating the bowels.

Externally hops work well as a poultice for inflammations, neuralgic, and rheumatic pains. A warm pillow of hops is very helpful for toothache, ear ache, and according to Mrs Grieve in A Modern Herbal (1931) will also "allay nervous irritation". She goes on to say, "An infusion of ½ oz to a pint … has proved of great service also in heart disease, fits, neuralgia, and nervous disorders, besides being a useful tonic in indigestion, jaundice, and stomach and liver afflictions generally … it gives prompt ease to an irritable bladder".

In her Physica (1998), Hildegard Von Bingen writes the following. "Hops is a hot and dry herb, with a bit of moisture. It is not much use for a human being, since it causes his melancholy to increase, gives him a sad mind, and makes his intestines heavy. Nevertheless, its bitterness inhibits some spoilage in beverages to which it is added, making them last longer."[1] This depressing effect is associated with the cooling action of the herb, which in some cases may exacerbate internal states of coldness, especially in those who have a cold stagnant temperament such as melancholics. For those with depression caused by anxiety and agitation, as is often seen in those with a hot firey choleric disposition, hops are entirely appropriate.

Recent research has focused on a number of anticancer activities of hops, including the inhibition of cell growth in breast, colon, prostate cancers, and leukaemia (Fisher, 2018).[2]

Mythos

Wild hops are native to Britain, but probably not Scotland. Beer or ale has been brewed since ancient times, but it wasn't until some point in the 14th century that hops were added to preserve it for longer—the powerful antimicrobial and antifungal properties of the resins stop the brew from going mouldy.

According to a Flemish myth, a lowly apprentice glassmaker named Gambrinus was given hops and taught how to make beer by the devil to enable him to forget his broken heart. In return he had to give the devil his soul after thirty years, but when the devil returned Gambrinus used magic chimes that the devil had also given him to trick him into dancing until he was so exhausted that he gave up on demanding his soul.

Head and nerves

Hops will cool and calm the head and the heart clearing excess heat and agitation, helping to release tension and relieve stress. Hops have a gentle euphoric action on the nervous system and can help to relieve depression when its cause is overworrying, anguish, and anxiety. They are also very helpful for menopausal hot flushes, night sweats, and anxiety.

Stomach and digestion

The bitter acids are antimicrobial and antifungal, which helps to reduce dysbiosis of the gut flora and increase the secretion of stomach juices. Hops also have an antispasmodic effect on smooth muscle easing digestive spasm. Hops were considered helpful to "loosen the belly", clearing constipation, especially that which would be considered to be coming from hot and dry conditions.

Bladder and kidneys

Hops are a gentle diuretic and reduce spasm and cramping associated with the bladder and urinary passages. Its antimicrobial properties are also beneficial in clearing cystitis.

Doses

Tincture

As a tincture 5–10 ml can be taken up to three times a day, and can be combined with valerian and passionflower as an aid to sleep, 5–10 ml before bed.

Hops infused in Sherry is a traditional bitter stomach tonic.

Tea

Traditionally hop tea was made from the dried leaves combined with Ceylon tea.

For a medicinal strength infusion

½ oz (15 g) of the strobiles are infused in 1 pint (450 ml) of water, and drank over 24 hours.

Hyssop

Hyssop, Azob (Dioscorides)

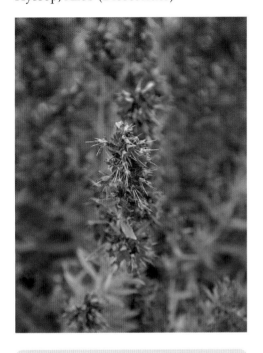

Latin: *Hyssopus officinalis*
Family: Lamiaceae/labiateae

Element   Air
Planet   Jupiter
Humour   Sanguine
Quality   Hot and dry in the
           second degree, warms
           the stomach, liver, lungs,
           clears and cleanses
           dampness.

Organs

Lungs
Stomach
Liver
Heart

Actions

Antispasmodic
Expectorant
Antimicrobial
Vermifuge
Carminative
Diaphoretic
Stimulant
Sedative

Constituents

Volatile oils: camphor, thujone,
    linalool
Polyphenols: caffeic acid, rosmarinic
    acid
Flavonoids: diosmin, hesperidin
Diterpenes: marrubiin
Triterpenes: oleanoic acid, ursolic
    acid
Polysaccharides

Traditional uses and humoral influences

Hyssop is ruled by Jupiter and associated with the astrological sign Cancer. It is both hot and dry in the second degree. Jupiter rules the Liver, the lungs and inhalation, the ribs, and the veins. Cancer is associated with the water element, which has a correspondence to the stomach, bowels, the bladder, and the skin.

The hot and dry temperament of hyssop makes it particularly helpful for all conditions affecting those organs in which there is excess cold and damp phlegm. Conditions caused by excess phlegm are: all cold and rheumatic diseases, fluid retention, dropsies, oedema, discharges and abscesses, coughs, and excess mucous in the lungs. Cramps and digestive colic are also caused by excess cold and damp. The warmth of hyssop also helps to reduce fever through promoting perspiration and is a traditional remedy for children's fevers.

Hyssop is mentioned by Hippocrates and the Roman writer Pliny, they list a wide range of uses including: snake bites, as an emetic, toothache, laryngitis, asthma, cough, for stimulating bile, epilepsy, jaundice, abscesses and inflammations, sores, hysteria, and for eye conditions. The antimicrobial properties of the essential oils and the anti-inflammatory properties of polyphenols, such as rosmarinic acid, give hyssop a powerful role in helping with scabs, itches, and external sores and ulcers, as well as internal infections.

Jupiter has rulership over the mid brain, the area where judgement is considered to take place. The warmth of hyssop activates this part of the brain, clearing any cold obstructions which may be diminishing the function of this discerning part of the brain. The brain is the seat of the cold Mercurial etheric humour, which is antipathetical to the warm temperament of Jupiter and may itself be the cause of an excessively cold brain. The other cold humours, the melancholic and phlegmatic humours, may also lead to the brain losing its activating innate heat and therefore be a cause of the animal spirit becoming too cold and stagnant—potentially bringing on lethargy, palsy, convulsions, and epilepsy.

In Maude Grieve's A Modern Herbal (1931), she draws our attention to hyssop's traditional use in joint problems; "A tea made with fresh green tops, and drunk several times daily is one of the old fashioned country remedies for rheumatism that is still employed".

Mythos

> "Purge me with Hyssop, and I shall be clean: wash me, and I will be as white as snow"
>
> Psalm 51:7

Hyssop has a long tradition as a herb of purification and cleansing. The Greeks used hyssop to cleanse their temples and it was a sacred Jewish herb symbolising forgiveness. In the gospel of John the sour wine given to Jesus on the cross was passed to him on a stem of hyssop. The use of the herb as a purgative remedy for the body and the mind made it a symbol of purity and regained innocence, and consequently a herb of baptism representing the renewal of life as a Christian.

Emotional

Fear and worry are emotions that are traditionally associated with the water element, the moon, and the zodiacal sign of Cancer. Hyssop clears the mind, helping us to let go of dark and long-term fears and anxieties. It is often the fear of being wrong or of losing face that stops us from allowing forgiveness into our hearts. A hyssop bath can cleanse us after trauma, sickness, or periods of worry and fearfulness. Jupiter represents strength and protection, he gives back courage, pride and improved self-esteem. When we feel overwhelmed, weakened, or diminished, hyssop is one of the greatest allies we can call upon.

Liver

Nicholas Culpeper says of Hyssop "It amends and cherishes the native colour of the body, spoiled by yellow jaundice." The liver has a warm and moist temperament, its role is to digest the raw crude humours in food and to distribute them to nourish the organs. When there is poor digestive heat, or the flow of bile through the liver is obstructed due to cold constrictions a warming digestive herb such as hyssop is considered very beneficial.

Lungs

The lungs are ruled by Jupiter, but have a cold and moist temperament, making them particularly prone to conditions of excess phlegm. The volatile oils in hyssop are stimulating and promote expectoration, volatile oils are excreted through the Lungs and as they have a slightly irritant action on mucous membranes they clear and move phlegm. However the expectoration is only very gentle, enabling thick congestion to be gently loosened and moved. The tea is particularly helpful for long term chronic lung conditions, protecting them from infection and clearing excess mucous, it can be drunk over long periods without causing any problems.

Stomach

The astrological sign Cancer associated with hyssop corresponds to the stomach. In William Fernie's 1897 Herbal Simples, he says "Hyssop tea is a grateful drink, well adapted to improve the tone of a feeble stomach, being brewed with the green tops of the herb".[1] In more recent times the use of hyssop as a digestive has not been so common. However, it is one of the most pleasant and effective digestive teas, particularly helpful for those of a cold constitution or with a weak phlegmatic digestion. The tea speeds recovery from food poisoning and is helpful for reducing nausea. Drinking the tea consistently will cleanse the gut of pathogenic microflora, being a useful treatment to keep *H. pylori* and small intestinal bacterial overgrowth at bay (Fisher, 2018).[2]

Doses

Tea

One heaped teaspoonful to a cup, three cups daily.

Tincture

5 ml up to four times daily.

Juniper

Common Juniper. Fairy circle. Gorst. Melmont berries. Genevrier.

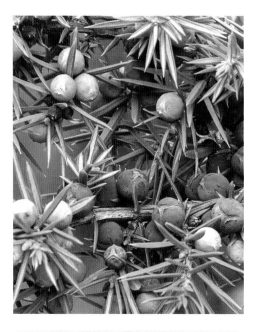

Latin:	*Juniperis communis*
Family:	Cupressaceae

Element	Fire
Planet	Sun
Humour	Choleric
Quality	Hot in the third degree, dry in the first. Resists poisons, strengthens the brain, heart, stomach and liver, clears phlegm from the lungs, bladder and kidneys.

Organs

Head
Heart
Lungs
Stomach
Kidneys
Joints

Actions

Diuretic
Expectorant
Antiseptic
Stomachic
Carminative
Anti-rheumatic

Constituents

Volatile oils: α and β pinene, sabinene, limonene
Sesquiterpenes: caryphyllene, cadinene,
Flavonoids
Phenols: resveratol
Resins
Bitter glycoside: juniperin
Tanins: condensed types including oligomeric procyanidins

Traditional uses and humoral influences

Juniper is a herb of the Sun, hot in the third degree and dry in the first degree. Its heat and dryness chases away excess moisture or phlegm. The head, heart, stomach, lungs, kidneys, bladder, and joints all benefit greatly from its activating and warming actions. Culpeper says:

"This admirable Solar shrub is scarce to be paralleled for its virtues. The berries are hot in the third degree, and dry but in the first, being a most admirable counter poison, and as great a resister of the pestilence as any growing … they are admirably good for a cough, shortness of breath and consumption … pains in the belly, ruptures, cramps, and convulsions … they strengthen the brain exceedingly, help the memory, and fortify the sight by strengthening the optic nerves: are excellently good in all sorts of agues; help the gout and sciatica, and strengthen the limbs of the body".

Juniper is governed by the sun, which rules the heart, the seat of the vital spirit. It is the innate heat, the warm aspect of the vital spirit, that primarily protects the body from infection, and "resists poisons". In folk traditions throughout Europe the berries were chewed as protection against infections and flu, as well as a cure for wind, bloating, and colic. It is the activity of the innate heat in the stomach that enables food to be broken down into chyle, and the innate heat that allows the liver to extract the constituent humours from the chyle in what is called the "first concoction". When innate heat is lacking in the stomach and liver, herbs like Juniper may be used to warm and activate the digestion. Modern research has shown that the berries are active against a range of bacteria including *Staphyloccocus aureaus, Enterococcus faecalis, Salmonella enteriditis,* and even have mild activity against *Helicobacter pylori* (Fisher, 2018)[1]—the bacteria believed to trigger stomach ulcers. They are also antifungal and are active against

candida organisms, which often colonise the gut causing dysbiosis, bloating, and inflammation.

The condensed tannins in juniper, known as oligomeric procyanidins (OPCs), are responsible for many of its beneficial effects and are also found in red wine and green tea. The OPCs are up to 20 times more antioxidant than vitamin C, making them effective at reducing antioxidative damage to tissues, as well as protecting the circulation by reducing the build up of atherosclerotic plaques in the vascular system and elsewhere (Pengelley, 2004).[2] These procyanidins are also recognised as being beneficial in eye health, giving modern confirmation of Culpeper's seventeenth century belief that juniper may strengthen the optic nerve and the sight. Tannins and phenols are found in the berries, and one well researched phenol, resveratol, has been shown to be antioxidant, anti-inflammatory, antiplatelet, and antiallergenic with demonstrated anticancer activity.

Mythos

Junipers are either male or female and are found throughout the northern hemisphere, including the Americas and the whole of Eurasia. In ancient times, Juniper was dedicated to the Furies, the three goddesses of the underworld who were sent out to bring justice to wrongdoers. The branches would be burned as offerings to Hecate, the goddess of magic and the underworld, and would be used to fumigate houses after a death. In all the areas that it is found, Juniper has been regarded as a protective plant, strong enough to ward off demons and disease alike. In Tuscany there is a belief that if Juniper is hung on the door it will keep witches away, as before entering the house they will have to count all the needles, and as this takes them all night they will finally have to leave in a great hurry before the sun rises at dawn. There is also an Italian saying "If you eat juniper berries every day you will acquire eternal life" (De Cleene & Lejeune, 1999).[3] It was an Italian custom to travel with a stick made from juniper. which would offer the traveller protection. While in Wales it was believed that anyone who chopped down a juniper tree would die within a year. The plant was considered so powerful that beakers manufactured from its wood would offer magical protection from spells and pestilence, and in some areas of Europe the tree was completely wiped out as the demand for these cups was so high. It was also thought that a drink made from the berries would help one see into the future, and anyone sitting on a juniper stool would be able to see witches entering the room.

Emotional

Juniper is a remedy that encourages and strengthens us when we are feeling weakened and emotionally vulnerable. It drives away fear and sadness, replacing it with a sense of resilience and hope.

It will protect us from negative influences and puts up a shield around us when we have to deal with difficult or obnoxious people. I often give patients a small dropper bottle of the tincture made from the fresh berries and leaves to take when they are facing difficult situations or feel under emotional attack.

Head

Culpeper believed that the berries "strengthen the brain exceedingly, help the memory … convulsions … and are excellently good for all palsies, and falling sickness"

Juniper counters excess coldness of the brain and restores the activity of the animal spirit. It is excess coldness of the brain that leads to convulsions, headaches, migraines, palsies, poor memory, and reduced mental function.

As we age, or when we get tired, the brain is seen to lose its heat and activity, the warmth of juniper enlivens the brain and the animal spirit. It is interesting to note that degenerative diseases, such as dementia, are associated with the depletion of blood flow to the brain and that Alzheimer's is associated with the development of amyloid plaques, both of which are potentially helped by juniper berries.

Heart

Culpeper says; "It is so powerful a remedy against the dropsy that a very Lye made of the ashes of the herb being drank, cures the disease".

Dropsy is the name that was given when fluid builds up in heart failure, a lye is made by mixing the ashes with cold soft water, such as rain water, and once they have separated, drawing off the water.

The antioxidant effects of the berries make juniper a valuable heart tonic, they improve circulation and reduce the inflammation within the vascular system that it is now recognised to lead to the formation of cholesterol plaques and the eventual blockage of the arteries seen in circulatory and heart disease.

Lungs

Culpeper states of the berries that "they are admirably good for a cough, shortness of breath, and consumption". One of the symptoms of TB is a chronic cough, and recent research has confirmed that the oils from the berries are active against the TB bacillus (Fisher, 2018).[4] These warming oils also make it a gentle expectorant, having an attenuating (thinning) action and moving and clearing thick phlegm from the lungs. When giving an inhalation for bronchitis, respiratory infection, and chronic coughs, I find it helpful to add juniper berries to a mix of thyme and chamomile flowers.

Stomach

Culpeper said that taking the berries "strengthens the stomach exceedingly, and expels the wind, indeed there is scarce a better remedy for wind in any part of the body, or the cholic".

The stomach and bowels are considered to be governed by the phlegmatic humour, its cold moistness being liable to weaken digestion, resulting in flatulence and colic. The berries work as a warming digestive tonic, which also neutralise pathogenic bacteria and yeasts that may threaten the digestive system. The berries were recommended to be eaten in the morning, with Culpeper saying that one should eat ten or a dozen of the berries each morning fasting.

Kidneys

Nicholas Culpeper says of the berries; "They provoke urine exceedingly, and are very available to dysuries and stranguraries". As well as having diuretic effects, it is known that the oils are highly antiseptic, making juniper a valuable addition to remedies for cystitis and any other infective condition of the urinary tract.

Doses

10–12 berries before food, three times daily.

Tea

Tops and/or berries 5 g infused in a cup of hot water, up to three times a day.

Tincture

1:3, 2–3 ml three times daily.

Not to be used in pregnancy, and usually advised to be used for no more than six weeks continuously, especially if being used in higher doses.

Lavender

Spikenard

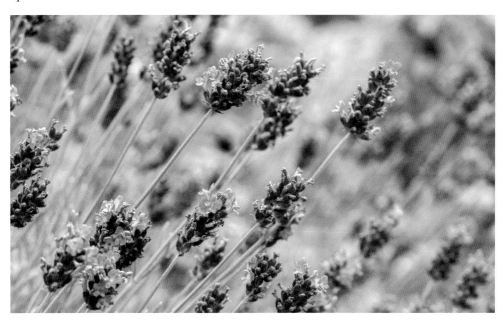

Latin: *Lavandula vera*
Family: Lamiaceae

Element   Ether
Planet   Mercury
Humour   Etheric
Quality   Hot and dry in the third
          degree, heats the head,
          is opening, cleansing,
          diaphoretic, and diuretic.

Organs

Head
Stomach
Liver
Spleen
Skin

Actions

Stimulant
Carminative
Antispasmodic
Euphoric
Sedative
Antiseptic
Restorative tonic

Constituents

Volatile oils: linalyl acetate, camphor,
     linalool, limonene
Coumarins
Triterpines
Flavonoids
Caffeic acid, rosmarinic acid

Traditional uses and humoral influences

Lavender is ruled by Mercury and is hot and dry in the third degree. Mercury rules the brain and the animal spirit. As well as the apprehending activity of the brain, it also rules the tongue, hands, and the feet. Mercury is considered to have a cold and dry quality, as does the etheric element to which Mercury is related. When there is an excess of coldness in the brain or nerves lavender is helpful with its hot, clearing, cutting, and warming aromatic action. As Nicholas Culpeper says, "lavender is of special good use for all griefs and pains of the head and brain that proceed from a cold cause. This can include, migraine, vertigo, fainting, pain, apoplexy (stroke), cramps, convulsions and palsies". Cold blockages of the animal spirit were considered to be the cause of stroke, and lavender with its warmth opens and cleanses such obstructions. There is now pharmacological confirmation for this ancient indication, as the coumarins contained in lavender are known to have an anticoagulant action conferring protection against blood clots (Pengelley, 2004).[1]

Lavender comes into the category of "discutient" or "diaphoretic" medicines—these have the property of aiding elimination through sweating. Often like lavender, herbs in this class have a gentle warming action, activating and moving the blood. This movement distributes and dispels heat, meaning that they balance heat in the body, which sometimes leads to an overall cooling effect. This explains why herbs like lavender and mint, which are paradoxically classed as warming herbs, can actually tend to cool the body when it is over heated.

Lavender strengthens the stomach, and according to Culpeper "frees the liver and spleen from obstructions". The liver is the organ that breeds blood, and the spleen retains and stores it; if either are blocked by excess cold, the free flow of vitality and nourishment carried in the blood will not reach the organs and tissues.

The London Pharmacopeia suggested the compound tincture of lavender for "falling sickness, and all cold distempers of the head, womb, stomach and nerves" (Grieve, 1931).[2] It was made of the oils of lavender and rosemary, which were steeped in a spirit of wine with cinnamon bark, nutmeg, and red sandalwood for seven days. This was to be taken in a teaspoon dose in a little water, considered especially helpful after an indigestible meal.

Mythos

"As Rosemary is to the spirit, so Lavender is to the soul" – English saying.

The spirit resides in the heart, and in the form of the vital spirit activates the organs and tissues giving them life. The soul corresponds to the divine element within us, passed on from generation to generation through procreation and able to receive inspiration from the divine realm. The soul corresponds to the highest realm in Hermetic cosmology, the realm of intellect, mind, and the angels, it is illuminated from above by the realm of light and divine creation where God resides. Mercury is the winged messenger of this divine illumination, bringing its wisdom and enlightenment to the mind, it is the planet of connection and communication carrying divine light through the ether, nourishing the soul, which resides in each physical body. When the body dies the vital spirit ceases to exist, but the divine soul that the body contains continues.

Lavender is native to the Mediterranean, and the cultivated varieties still grown today came from the Middle East to England in the seventeenth century. In Egypt, Phoenicia, and Arabia, lavender was used as a perfume and for mummification. It spread across Europe around 600 BC, with the Romans making use of it in their elaborate bathing rituals. By the early Middle Ages, washerwomen were known as lavenders, as they spread the clothes to dry upon the bushes and for scenting clean clothes with it while in storage. It was during the same era that monasteries began cultivating lavender in their physic gardens.

The medieval mystic Hildegard von Bingen (1998) recommended lavender water, a mixture of lavender and gin or brandy, as a remedy for migraine. She said "lavender is hot and dry, and its heat is healthy, whoever cooks this lavender in wine and if he has no wine in honey and water, and frequently drinks it when it is warm, will lessen the pain in his liver and lungs, and stuffiness in his chest, it also makes his thinking and disposition pure".[3]

Cleopatra is said to have worn its scent (her secret weapon!) to seduce Julius Caesar and Marc Antony, and some claim that the asp that delivered the fatal bite was hidden among her lavender bushes. Adam and Eve are credited with bringing the plant with them when expelled from the Garden of Eden. In the Gospel of Luke, Mary washed the feet of Jesus and anoints them with ointment containing spikenard, one of lavender's other names.

Head

Lavender is considered a "cephalic", which is a herb for the brain. Mercury is the planet that rules the head, which is cold in temperament. Cold organs such as the brain are often also prone to cold conditions, these may include vertigo, fainting, confusion, migraine, and depression. The vinegar, distilled water, or oil of lavender is a specific remedy when rubbed on the temples for headaches, or any "cold" conditions of the head.

An elderly patient I treated who had been suffering from a burning tongue for some years and had explored every avenue from conventional drugs to acupuncture came for help. Her tongue would start to burn, would curl and shed its coating, leaving sore red patches. It could happen daily, usually when she was tired or if her nerves or emotions had been stirred up, and especially following a poor night's sleep. We found an effective treatment was to use drops of distilled lavender water directly on the tongue at the first sign of a problem. As she had got older her nervous system had become depleted, and the tongue being ruled by mercury and therefore connected to the animal spirit was a prime place for this deficiency to show. The lavender helped by strengthening the animal spirit, clearing any cold blockages, and by countering the nervous depletion.

Lungs

To clear congestion, use as an inhalation, 30g in a litre of boiling water. If you are using the essential oil, use no more than 4 drops in a bowl. It clears the head, the sinuses, and helps with all upper respiratory tract infections. A compress of the flowers applied to the chest as hot as possible can be used with a hot water bottle placed on top. An infusion made with 2 teaspoons of lavender to a cup can be used as a mouth wash for inflammations of the mouth, throat, and tongue.

Stomach

The stomach is considered to have a cold damp temperament. When it is too cold it causes flatulence, distension, or bloating. Lavender used as a tea with chamomile can be particularly helpful. Sipping the distilled water of lavender will also help.

Gynaecological

A hot compress of lavender is very helpful for period pains.

Skin

With its anti-inflammatory and antiseptic properties, it's a very useful skin herb. Baths and washes can be used for eczema and inflamed skin conditions. For burns make a wash from the flowers or use 10 drops of the essential oil in a bucket or large bowl of cold water and immerse the burnt area until the feeling of burning stops.

Doses

Traditional tea recipe

One part lavender flowers to three parts lime flower.

Bath

50 g of lavender flowers steeped in a litre of hot water until cool can then be added to the bath. This helps with fatigue, infections, pain, and also relieves all tension in body, mind, and emotions.

A hot footbath of lavender made either by adding 6 drops of essential oil, or by using 30 g fresh flowers is a powerful tonic and restorative for any case of exhaustion.

Lemon Balm

Melissa. Balm. Sweet balm. Cure all

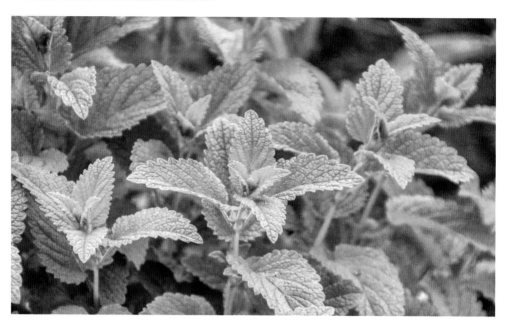

Latin: *Melissa officinalis*
Family: Lamiaceae

Element   Air
Planet   Jupiter
Humour   Sanguine
Quality   Hot and dry in the second
          degree, heats and dries
          heart, lungs and stomach.
          Cheers the heart and
          mind, purges melancholy.

Organs

Heart
Lungs
Brain, nerves
Stomach

Actions

Carminative
Sedative
Diaphoretic
Febrifuge
Anti-Viral

Constituents

Volatile oils; citral, limonene
Flavonoids
Polyphenols; incl rosmarinic acid

Parts used

Flowers and leaves. Gathered;
    July/August.
Loses potency if not stored in airtight
    container.

Traditional uses and humoral influences

Lemon balm is ruled by Jupiter and is under the sign of Cancer. The organs associated with Cancer are the breast, lungs, liver, and stomach, and the sign is aligned with the water element and the moon. This gives lemon balm the combined qualities of Jupiter, the protective and most regal of signs with the cleansing, softening, and nurturing aspects of water and the moon. This results in lemon balm having expansive, warming, cleansing, clearing, and balancing properties. Perhaps the most celebrated quality of lemon balm is its role as a protective herb for the heart. Acknowledged by Culpeper as one of the main cordial herbs, all of which have a cooling and softening effect on the heart, lemon balm provides an antidote to hot and extreme emotions, such as anger, grief, and sorrow.

The liver is also ruled by Jupiter and is the seat of the natural spirit and the organ that facilitates digestion, turning the food in the form of chyle into blood and extracting any harmful substances and clearing them from the system. The liver also governs the discerning or judging part of the mind, helping us to retain beneficial thoughts and ideas and discard the rest. Because of this connection with Jupiter, lemon balm has a clarifying and focusing effect on the brain, whilst calming mental over activity. Its warming effect is strengthening for the memory, as when the brain gets excessively cold and slow the retentive part of the brain stops the free flow of memories and thoughts moving to the active part of the brain, dulling our ability to take on or apprehend new ideas or to recall memories.

"… It causes the mind and heart to become merry, and reviveth the heart … and driveth away all troublesome thoughts and cares out of the mind, arising from black choler and melancholy" (Culpeper)

Excess melancholy arises from congestion in the system from exhaustion, retention of waste products, and poor digestion in the stomach and liver. The effect of melancholy on the brain is to cause an excessive focus on dark thoughts, worries, and pessimism. This is always more of a problem during the cold dark winter months, or the melancholic season. The blockage caused by excess melancholy can be exacerbated by a build up of obstructive "burnt choler" caused by excessive heat, as follows emotional, spiritual, or physical trauma or crisis. Lemon balm's purging action clears the system of such obstructions and will allow the release of excess heat and emotions from the heart, thus cooling and calming the vital spirit.

Mythos

The herb is also called Melissa because of its sacred association with bees, it flowers at a time when the bees are at their most active, and it is said that rubbing beehives with Melissa will ensure that you will never lose the swarm.

The Druids believed that bees came from the paradise like world of the Sun and the Spirit, and in Celtic myth bees were said to possess a secret wisdom garnered from the otherworld, whilst in Norse legend, the tears of Freya were said to be made of bees of gold. Divination by pouring beeswax into water is still a custom practiced by Lithuanian women.

The Kalahari Desert's San people tell of a bee that carried a mantis across a river. The exhausted bee left the mantis on a floating flower but planted a seed in the mantis's body before it died and then the seed grew to become the first human. In the Southern African Sangoma tradition bees are seen as direct messengers from the ancestors, and if a swarm settles in a house a diviner is called to ask what messages the bees bring.

In Greek myth bees were seen as the resurrected form of the sacrificial bull and also as the souls of the dead. The temple priestesses were called Melissae, the Greek word for bee, and the oracular priestess at Delphi was known as the Delphic Bee. Using preparations made with honey these oracular priestesses entered an ecstatic trance or "enthusiasmos", meaning "within is a god", to give divinations, and it was these same Melissae who taught Apollo divination.

The bee was an emblem of Potnia, "The Pure Mother Bee" of the Minoan-Mycenaean culture, with honey playing a central role in the New Year rituals of the Minoans. The Cretan New Year began at the summer solstice, when Melissa is coming into full flower. Then in July, when the great star Sirius rose in conjunction with the sun, a 40-day summer ritual during which honey had been gathered from the hives of wild bees would come to an end. The honey was fermented into a sacred mead, providing a central component of the subsequent ritual celebrations.

Emotions

Lemon balm is helpful for those who feel burnt out, common in those with choleric, firey, personalities, or after long periods of overwork or stress. It warms and moves overwhelming and stagnant emotions, as is often seen in phlegmatic watery and in sanguine airy personalities. It will clear melancholic fearfulness and anxiety arising from dwelling excessively on dark thoughts and worries, as is common with melancholic earthy personalities. Lemon balm raises up the spirits when long-term sadness and despair have taken away all joyfulness and enthusiasm, bringing out the sweet honey of the spirit from the heart, this makes it an especially helpful herb for grief, particularly when combined with rose and hawthorn.

Heart

Lemon balm is a helpful circulatory herb, reducing tension in the heart and circulation, making it useful in high blood pressure and angina. It is difficult to find a better cordial herb or strengthener of the heart, considered a protector against the damage that anxiety, anger, and despair do to the heart. There is now a recognised syndrome called Takotsubo cardiomyopathy, or broken heart syndrome. This occurs when excessive emotion or stress induce a heart paralysis, which can mimic a heart attack, although there is no physical blockage to the coronary arteries or any other physical heart problem. It is now known that this potentially fatal event is caused by an excess release of the stress hormone, adrenalin.

Digestion

Lemon balm makes a soothing tea for indigestion, heartburn, and bloating.

It aids digestion of heavy foods, reducing intestinal spasm, griping, and wind. Jupiter governs the digestive virtue in the body which resides in the liver. Being under the zodiacal sign Cancer, Lemon balm also has an alignment with the stomach, enabling its warmth to strengthen and activate the preparation of foods in the stomach and aid the digestive function of the liver.

Brain and nerves

A spirit of balm, combined with lemon peel, nutmeg, and angelica root, enjoyed a great reputation as "Carmelite water", which was used for nervous headache and numerous other nervous afflictions.

It is a very helpful remedy for tension headaches, stress, and nervous exhaustion. When used as a bath, or footbath, it brings instant relief. Lemon balm works as a gentle sedative on its own, or as an addition to relaxing teas, to both help sleep and in reducing anxiety. It is also traditionally considered helpful for tinnitus and vertigo and any head or nerve pain with a cold cause.

Skin

Rubbing leaves on warts is an old folk remedy, and it can also be used for cold sores and other sores associated with the herpes virus, a traditional use backed up by research into the antiviral effects of rosmarinic acid (Fisher, 2018),[1] which it contains. It is a traditional application for fresh wounds, as a fresh poultice, paste, or as a wash.

Hormones

Lemon balm is a very helpful herb for painful periods, and if drunk daily it can help to regulate the hormonal cycle, as well as aiding depression, palpitations, anxiety, and hot flushes associated with the menopause. It may also be used as a very gentle uterine stimulant during labour. It has been shown to inhibit the effect of thyroid stimulating hormone and therefore reduce the symptoms of hyperthyroidism.

Doses

Tea

A teaspoon to a cup of water as tea.
    10 ml of floral water 3 times daily.

Tincture

5 ml 1:3 tincture 3 times daily.
    For grief, emotional tension and distress, combine it with rose and hawthorn equal parts.
    For digestion, combine with chamomile, mint, and rose petals.

Limeflower

Limeflower tree. Linden. Tilluel. Tila. Common lime

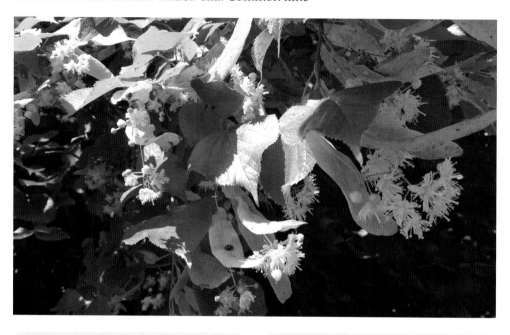

Latin: *Tilia europea/cordata*
Family: Tiliaceae

Element   Air
Planet   Jupiter
Humour   Sanguine
Quality   Warm and dry in the
          first degree. Cleanses the
          blood, strengthens the
          heart, liver, and nerves.

Organs

Liver
Stomach
Brain
Heart

Actions

Sedative
Antispasmodic
Diuretic
Hypotensive
Anticoagulant
Immune enhancer
Antiallergenic
Anti-inflammatory
Soothes epithelium

Constituents

Volatile oils: limonene, anethole
Flavonoids: quercertin, rutin,
    kaempferol
Phenolic acids: caffeic, p-coumeric
Mucilage (up to 10%)
Tannins
Saponins
Mucopolysaccharides

Traditional uses and humoral influences

The lime tree is ruled by the "royal" planet, Jupiter, which also governs the air and blood humour. It is warming and drying in the first degree. It has a strengthening effect on blood vessels and is considered to be a strong blood tonic and cleanser. It also strengthens the liver and digestive faculty and is soothing, moistening, and calming for the nerves and all internal passages, especially the respiratory passages and membranes.

Jupiter is also associated with expansion, and the filling of the chest and inspiration. Limeflower will release tension in the chest and facilitate the smooth flow of respiration, as well as soothing irritation of the respiratory passages, making it very useful in tightness of the chest, coughing and wheezing. Limeflower is a traditional fever remedy, especially for children. It is considered to be warming in the first degree and applicable for use in countering chills. Its diaphoretic action induces sweating, which will bring the temperature down and break a fever. The blossoms of the lime tree have been a favourite ingredient throughout Europe in teas to use during colds, fevers, influenza, and infections.

Both of my herbal mentors had a special place for limeflowers, Christopher Hedley used to say that limeflower takes the fat out of the arteries and puts it on the nerves where it belongs,[1] and my other mentor, the herbalist Julian Barker, used to treat microcirculatory conditions of the arterial system with his triad of herbs combining limeflower, hawthorn, and yarrow.[2]

Mythos

In the Greek myths the oceanid and goddess Philyra gave birth to an illegitimate son after coupling with Kronos. The child was human but with the body of a horse. Philyra was so distraught at being the mother of this strange creature that she begged the gods to transform her out of her pain and was consequently turned into a lime tree. Her son, the centaur Chiron, later taught the healer god Asclepius the sacred knowledge of healing with plants, who then passed it on to the human race.

The Germanic peoples dedicated the lime tree to Freya, the goddess of love, and to Holda, the mother goddess of death and rebirth. Its sacred nature meant the tree became a place to give offerings to the divinities and also a place of Christian pilgrimage. It was believed to have magical healing properties and the wood nymphs and faeries were said to reside between its bark and wood.

Emotional

The lime tree helps us to feel good about ourselves and to overcome mental obstacles. It also helps us to see the best in oneself and others, giving a healthy sense of pride. It helps in mental and emotional agitation, calming an angry mind and resolving depression associated with feelings of failure and desperation.

Heart

Limeflower is a strengthener of the blood vessels and the heart, and an improver of the circulation to the brain. Traditionally thought to prevent atherosclerosis,

In Health Secrets of Plants and Herbs (1981), Messague says, "Thanks to its anti plethoric action it also cleans the blood and makes it more fluid. This makes it is a valuable defence against arteriosclerosis, phlebitis, angina and heart attacks".[3]

Liver

Limeflower is associated with the liver, the blood, and the digestion. It has always been a popular digestive tea taken after meals; it strengthens the digestive faculty that resides in the liver. It is through the digestion of foods into its constituent elements that the blood is made in the liver. The blood carries the vital spirit and the moist fluids around the body. Limeflower improves and lubricates this flow, softening and nourishing the liver, and easing the passage of blood around the body. Through strengthening the liver it has a cleansing action on the blood, clearing putrefaction, poisons, and excess heat from the blood. Research has shown that limeflower contains flavonoids such as quercertin, rutin, and kaempferol and a saponin called scopoletin, all of which are protective of the liver, immunomodulatory, and help to reduce toxic and inflammatory damage to the liver.

Nervous system and brain

The planet Jupiter and the liver are associated with the middle part of the brain. This is the area where judgement and discernment reside. The midbrain digests and judges ideas in the same way that the liver digests foods and discerns nourishment from waste. Limeflower is able to temper and regulate heat in this part of the brain keeping the brain warm enough to freely move ideas around, retrieving memories from the cooler back part of the brain where the retentive faculty resides, while keeping it cool enough not to become overwhelmed by nervous heat from overthinking or anxiety. It was believed that the ventricles in the brain held the nervous "wind", which moved thoughts and ideas around, thus highlighting the connection between the air element, the liver, and the brain. Limeflower is a traditional remedy for epilepsy, fits and anxiety, as well as being a popular aid to a good night's sleep. It has a reputation for calming the nerves and acting as a general tonic for the nervous system. Nicholas Culpeper said;

"The flowers are the only parts used, and are a good cephalic and nervine, excellent for apoplexy, epilepsy, vertigo and palpitation of the heart".

Messegue says, "It is antispasmodic and sedative; there is no better recipe for a good nights sleep than a drink of lime flower tea. I would recommend it to everybody, but in particular to people suffering from nerves, chronic insomnia, anxiety, restless children and old people who find it difficult to sleep".[4] The most recent research has identified that the flavonoids in limeflower have a similar effect on the brain receptors that respond to the modern class of anxiolytic drugs known as benzodiazepines (Fisher, 2018).[5] This may account for its calming and relaxing properties, but without the danger of addiction associated with the drug. Interestingly white blood cells also have similar receptors, possibly accounting for its effects on calming immune reactions, and also gently stimulating and strengthening white blood cell response, possibly accounting for its reputation for both treating infections and fevers whilst reducing the severity of allergic reactions.

Respiratory

The mucilaginous properties soothe the respiratory passages, making limeflower one of the prime herbs for treating irritation of the mucous membranes. The immunomodulatory flavonoids that it contains reduce the effects of allergy and inflammation. The calming effects it has on the nerves, combined with its anti-inflammatory and antispasmodic properties make it helpful in asthma and chronic cough. The warming and drying actions it has help to clear dampness and phlegm from the lungs, drying catarrh without bringing on expectoration.

Digestive

Being low in tannins it is preferable to China tea as a digestive after meals.

Doses

Tincture

1:5, 5–10 ml three times daily.

Tea

2–4g three times daily.

Combinations

Maurice Messegue's (1981) recipe for "happiness tea"[6]:

2 pinches of lime flowers
2 pinches of vervain herb
2 pinches of chamomile flowers
2 pinches of mint, all combined and infused in 1 litre of water.

Colds and flu: limeflower, elderflower, and peppermint.

For a weak stomach: limeflower, hyssop, and chamomile.

Hay fever and Asthma: limeflower, elderflower, chamomile, and thyme.

Lovage

Love-ache. Levisticum. Osha/Bear root (Native American).

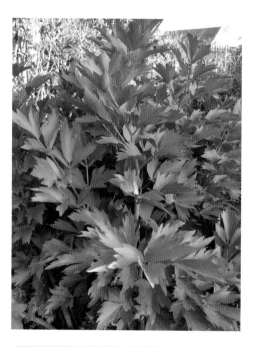

| Latin: | *Levisticum officinale* |
| Family: | Apiaceae/Umbelliferae |

Element	Fire
Planet	Sun
Humour	Choleric
Quality	Hot and dry in the second degree. Warms the stomach and digestion, cleanses and clears dampness from stomach, lungs, kidney, and bladder

Organs

Stomach
Bowels
Throat
Lungs
Kidneys
Joints
Womb

Actions

Carminative
Diuretic
Expectorant
Diaphoretic
Anti-rheumatic
Antimicrobial
Antispasmodic

Constituents

Volatile oils: butylthalide, carvacrol, ligustilide, citronellal.
Coumarins
Acids
Resin, gum

Traditional uses and humoral influences

Lovage is ruled by the sun and is warm and drying in the second degree. Nicholas Culpeper says:

"It is a herb of the Sun under the sign of Taurus. If Saturn offend the throat (as he always doth if he be the occasioner of the malady, and in Taurus is the genesis) this is your cure".

The astrological philosophy of Culpeper viewed Saturn as a cause of diseases that have a cold, blocking effect on organs. Saturn is the ruler of the cold dry earth element, and if the sickness occurred at the time when Saturn was in Taurus, which rules the neck, throat, and voice, then it will manifest as a disease of the throat. Saturn is the ruler of the melancholic humour, which has its seat in the Spleen. When the spleen becomes excessively overwhelmed with the cold aspects of this humour it leads to blockage, retention, and stasis throughout the system, stopping the humours from being correctly distributed to the organs, causing tiredness, fatigue, depression, constipation and bloating. Nicholas Culpeper says:

> "It opens, cures and digests humours ... half a dram* at a time taken in wine, doth wonderfully warm a cold stomach, helps digestion, and consumes all raw and superfluous moisture therein: it eases all gripings and pains, dissolves wind, and resists poisons and infection".

Lovage was considered to be "alexipharmic" or a resister of poison, with John Pechey in his 1706 herbal saying: "Tis Alexipharmic, and vulnerary; it strengthens the stomach and is good in Asthma ... it opens the obstructions of the Liver and Spleen; and cures the Jaundice, it is used outwardly, in baths, and cataplasms for the womb".[1]

The lungs, bowels, stomach, and womb all have a cold and moist temperament, and are prone to problems caused by excess moisture and cold building up. The gentle but warming effects of lovage help to dispel damp from these organs. When the vital heat in the body becomes dissipated, there is a risk that external heat and poisons can invade and take over the body and its organs causing infection. Excess dampness will lead to the development of putrefaction, causing internal destructive heat to develop, causing fevers. Again Culpeper comments; "It is a known and much praised remedy to drink the decoction of the herb for any sort of ague, and to help the pains and torments of the body and bowels coming from cold". Culpeper particularly recommends it for quinsy (abscess of the throat) as a gargle, for pleurisy, and for the eyes—the distilled water being dropped into them.

A traditional cordial drink of lovage, thought beneficial for the heart used to be brewed, it also included a variety of yarrow (*Achillea ligusticum*) and tansy (Grieve, 1931).[2] The young stems of lovage can be candied like angelica, whilst the leaves are often used as an addition to soups and stews.

Mythos

The name is believed to have derived from the combination of the word "love" and the fourteenth century word for parsley "ache", as its leaves resemble parsley and the plant shares the same botanical family. It may also have derived from the French "leviche", which is thought to derive from the Latin word "legusticum" due to the plant growing abundantly around the town of Leguria in Italy.

In America wild lovage is called osha or bear root, thought to be derived from the habit of bears to dig up the roots in the spring when they emerge from hibernation. The Native Americans are said to have used the root as a protection against snake bite, to help one face ones fears, and to improve communication with the nature spirits.

Emotional

A warming nourishing herb that helps us to feel cared for and safe, it will give us the ability to overcome fears and let go of feelings of inadequacy. It is helpful for when we are feeling vulnerable and anxious, enabling us to digest and break down long-term unresolved feelings of sadness, sorrow, and angst. In this way it brings us to a more optimistic and positive viewpoint. It will clear the head when we are confused about which direction to take, giving us a clearer, calmer focus.

Stomach

Having a similar warming, digestive effect as angelica and fennel, it sits somewhere between the two, and like them it is a very beneficial herb taken as a tea after food. It helps with weak digestion, bloating, nausea and for expelling flatulence. The leaves can be used fresh or the root can be added to a digestive herbal formula including chamomile flowers, rose, and sage. A combination of roasted dandelion root, chicory root, and lovage root makes a very agreeable caffeine free coffee substitute.

Lungs

It combines well with other gentle expectorants to help keep the lungs free of congestion and helps to anaesthetise the throat when it is sore or inflamed. It can be used as a gargle, or the fresh leaves or root can be chewed. It opens the airways, and simply chewing a small piece of the dried root will work as an effective broncho-dilator, making it very helpful for those with asthma, or wheezing associated with coldness and damp.

Womb and hormones

Like fennel, lovage has gentle hormonal and oestrogenic effects, it helps relieve menstrual cramps, hot flushes and night sweats. It tends to calm the emotions when they feel overwhelmed by hormonal swings and eases palpitations. Its warming effects mean that it is indicated in cold congestive conditions of the womb and reproductive organs, such as endometriosis, fibroids, and infertility, due to congestion or blockage of the fallopian tubes. A good reproductive system tonic formula is red clover, chamomile, and lovage. If one is treating menopause it helps to also add some sage leaf to the mix.

Joints

Due to its ability to both warm the digestion, activate the liver with its gentle bitter action, and to improve elimination via the kidneys, lovage is a very helpful remedy for gouty conditions and relieving stiffness and pain generally.

Doses

Tincture

5–20 ml daily.

Tea

3 g of root to a cup.

Medicinal decoction

15 g to 250 ml, brought to the boil and allowed to steep for ten minutes, drunk in divided doses throughout the day.

*Dram = 3.89g, 1/2 Dram = 1.95g (approx 2g).

Mallow

Marsh Mallow. Common mallow. Tree Mallow. Cheeses. Mortification root.
French: Guimauve
Welsh: Malws bendigaid

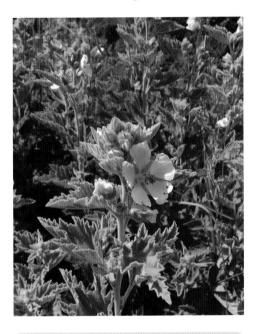

| Latin: | *Althea officinalis, Althea spp.* |
| Family: | Malvaceae |

Element	Water
Planet	Venus
Humour	Phlegm
Quality	Warm in the first degree, dry in the second, however sometimes considered cool and moist in the first degree. Mallows moisten and warm the kidneys, soften and soothe the lungs, stomach and bowels.

Organs

Stomach
Intestines
Bowel
Lungs
Kidneys
Womb
Skin

Actions

Soothing
Anti-inflammatory
Emolient/demulcent
Vulnery
Antitussive
Diuretic

Constituents

Polysaccharides
Phenolic acids; salicylic, P coumaric, caffeic acid
Coumarins
Flavonoids: kaempferol, quercertin
Pectin
Starch

Traditional uses and humoral influences

The Mallows are ruled by Venus, so are strongly associated with the Phlegmatic water humour, the lungs, the stomach, the kidneys and the womb. The mallows are considered to be warming in the first degree, and drying in the second degree. However their soothing slimy nature also gives them a softening, moistening and cleansing property. Nicholas Culpeper considers the marshmallow to be warming in the first degree, and drying in the second degree, whilst he considers other mallows to be cold and moist in the first degree.

Herbs that stop bleeding and dry up wounds are ascribed as having a drying quality or action, which doesn't preclude them from also being soothing and moistening to tissues. Culpeper says; "It not only voids choleric, and other offensive humours, but eases the pains and torments of the belly coming thereby".

Marsh mallow roots are particularly nutritious, containing 37% starch and 10% sucrose, and traditionally were made into a lozenge for sore chests and indigestion. In France these lozenges were known as "pâte de guimauve" and were the forerunner of the modern marshmallow sweets. The seed heads of common mallow were eaten by country people and were called "cheeses". In the spring the tops and leaves of all the kinds of mallows were both eaten fresh in salads and boiled and eaten like spinach.

Mythos

The generic name *Althea*, is derived from the Greek, "altho" meaning to cure. The mallow is in the Malvaceae plant family, whose name is derived from the Greek 'malake', meaning soft, this family includes hibiscus and hollyhocks. In the Greek myths it is recounted that after the birth of Althea's son Meleager, the fates appeared and said that when the last piece of wood in the hearth had burned he would die. His mother Althea grasped the last burning brand out of the fire to save him, and then buried it beneath the palace, thus keeping him

from death. This corresponds to the cooling and soothing effect of mallow as a healing antidote for conditions of choler or fire, such as inflammations, burns, fevers, and hot spasmodic digestive or abdominal pain. The Romans valued it highly, with Pliny claiming "Whosoever shall take a spoonful of the Mallows shall that day be free from all diseases that may come to him" (Fernie, 1897).[1]

Stomach and digestive organs

Marshmallow root is soothing, anti-inflammatory, and healing for the oesophagus, stomach, intestines, and bowels. It is invaluable in all inflammatory conditions of the digestive tract. When treating hiatus hernia, heartburn, and acid reflux disease, it is best prepared as a drink taken after meals and particularly before bed. For gastritis and inflammatory bowel diseases, such as ulcerative colitis, Crohn's disease, and diverticulitis, two heaped teaspoons mixed in cold water should be used on waking before food. In severe cases it should also be taken half an hour before each meal, and the same dose should be taken after the last meal before bed. Capsules make a convenient alternative when treating the stomach and bowels, however six capsules need to be taken each time to provide an adequate quantity of powder. It will reduce bleeding and help stop diarrhoea, and when used with fenugreek capsules it will also regulate bowel motions and ease constipation. Nicholas Culpeper tells the following story: "Not long since there was a raging disease called the bloody-flux; the college of physicians not knowing what to make of it, called it the inside plague, for their wits were at Ne plus ultra about it. My son was taken with the same disease, … the only thing I gave him, was mallows bruised and boiled both in milk and drink, in two days (the blessing of God being upon it) it cured him".

The leaf can be drunk as a tea, to soothe the stomach or can be added to recipes with other digestive herbs, such as chamomile and mint, to make a soothing digestive tea.

Kidneys

Traditionally the leaf has been the preferred way of using marshmallow for urinary problems. It is very beneficial as a strong infusion for interstitial cystitis and other inflammatory or ulcerated conditions of the urinary system. I combine it with horsetail herb, cleavers herb, and shepherd's purse, 15 g infused overnight and drunk the following day.

Lungs

Marshmallow root syrup calms irritating coughs and makes a very good basis for a cough linctus. Traditionally it is used in bronchitis and whooping cough as well as asthma. I combine it with elderflower, lime blossom (*Tilia europea*), chamomile, and thyme, for hay fever and respiratory irritation.

Skin

Mortification was the name given to necrosis, or the death of tissue, and marshmallow was considered a specific treatment, thus we have the name 'mortification root'. The fresh root, leaves, or flowers crushed and applied as a poultice are excellent remedies for skin inflammations, non-healing ulcers, the drawing out of splinters, and for cleansing wounds. An old Sussex lady told me that as a young girl in the 1930s she would be sent out by her mother to gather the flowering tops of the common mallows, they would then be cooked through in unsalted lard and stored in jars as an all round healing ointment for use over the year. It was considered especially helpful for dry rough skin and chafing (Chalwin, 1999).[2]

Mouth and gums

When I was first a student my teacher Christopher Hedley, a very experienced herbalist, had been extolling the virtues of marshmallow powder for drawing out poisons. He had been telling me that it was so effective that it would draw out abscesses from beneath teeth by applying the powder to the gum. That very night I had an opportunity to try it out as my mother-in-law was complaining about a tooth abscess that had suddenly flared up. Full of enthusiasm I told her not to worry as I had just learnt about the very best thing for it. I didn't have any marshmallow powder so I ground up the root in a pestle and mortar as best as I could, and told her to pack it down beside the gum next to where the abscess was. The next day she told me that she had woken in the middle of the night with a searing pain and a mouth full of what felt like sawdust. Having thought she would be giving me a telling off the next morning for causing her such a problem she went back to sleep. However it wasn't until after her breakfast the next morning that she suddenly remembered about the abscess, and realised that both the pain and swelling had completely cleared and the abscess had resolved … never again did she so readily doubt my herbal advice.

Doses

Powder

One or two heaped teaspoons taken up to three times daily in water, the powder is first mixed with cold water into a paste, then hot water is added whilst stirring vigorously, leave to stand 5–10 minutes, then drink after food and before bed.

Digestive healing powder

Marshmallow root powder, 1 part
Baobab powder, 1 part
    Cinnamon powder, 1 part
    Use a dessertspoonful mixed into food or drunk after food three times a day.

Leaf

Drink as a tea, a large pinch to a cup one to three cups daily.

Capsules

Two to six capsules after or before food, up to four times daily.

Marshmallow root syrup

Pour 1 litre of boiling water onto 50 g of dry root. Leave to stand for 8 hours. Strain, then add sugar at the ratio of 2:1 (66% sugar), or two pounds of sugar to each pint. Dissolve the sugar stirring over heat, and bring to the boil, remove from the heat when it begins to rise up the sides of the pan then allow to cool, strain through a cloth before using.

Marshmallow and elderberry winter cough linctus

Marshmallow syrup	35%
Elderberry juice	22.5%
Wild cherry bark Tr.	15%
Elecampagne Tr.	10%
Thyme Tr.	7.5%
Hyssop Tr.	7.5%
Thuja Tr.	2.5 %
	100

Marigold

Golds. Ruddes. Pot marigold.

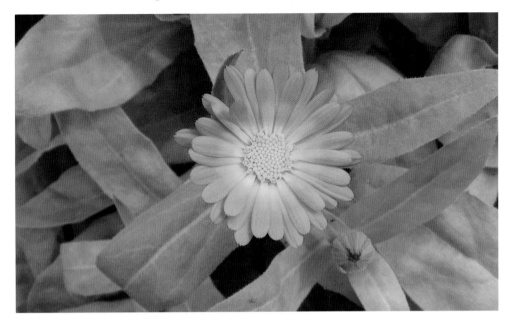

Latin: *Calendula officinalis*

Element   Fire
Planet   Sun
Humour   Choleric
Quality   Warm and dry in the first
          degree, strengthens and
          comforts the heart and
          spirits, expels poisons.

Organs

Heart
Eyes
Skin
Stomach

Actions

Anti-inflammatory
Antiseptic
Wound healing
Anti-haemorrhagic
Immune modulator
Antiviral

Constituents

Triterpenes
Flavonoids
Oils, resins
Saponins, polysaccharides

Traditional uses and humoral influences

Marigold is ruled by the Sun, and is under the sign of Leo. Culpeper said that "they strengthen the heart exceedingly, and are very expulsive" Marigold is one of the prime herbs for strengthening the vital spirit, which resides in the heart, an organ ruled over by Leo. Its name *Calendula* refers to its habit of following the sun, and the sun rules the heart, the eyes, and is the seat of the vital spirit. Congestion of blood and fluids may often be caused by coldness, so the warming effect helps to warm and soften such cold congestion, melting it away. When there has been overheating of any kind in the body, either from sickness, overwork, or stress, there is often a residue left behind, this is considered cold in nature, and is called "black bile". It tends to block and obstruct the flow of vital spirit, causing chronic illness, hard tumours, and often mental sickness. Herbs like marigold are able to gently warm, soften, and "ripen" the black bile, enabling it to then be purged from the body.

In Macer's medieval herbal, it is said that to look on marigolds would draw evil humours out of the head and strengthen the eyesight (Grieve, 1931).[1] By strengthening the innate heat or warm energy of the heart it helps to activate all of the organs and their functions, thus it activates the digestive faculty of the liver, breaking down poisons and expelling congestion helping to clear the congestion of the liver and jaundice. Its heat is considered purifying and helpful in all pestilences and fevers.

Mythos

Some say that marigold grew from the tears of Aphrodite at the death of Adonis, and in Greek custom it was the flower of fond memories and good wishes. It is protective against evil and spells, and is often associated with love charms.

In European folk medicine *Calendula* has been considered a prime medicine for cancer, and cancer like growths.

Emotional

Marigold warms and strengthens the spirits when we are feeling low and emotionally depleted. It is relaxing and comforting, soothing frayed nerves and restoring feelings of confidence and capability. It is helpful for those who get easily anxious and overwhelmed, particularly melancholic and phlegmatic personalities. It opens the heart, and helps to give us the strength to let go of anger and embrace forgiveness. A marigold bath lifts the spirits when depressed, and relaxes the whole body, reducing tension and panic. It helps us to regain lost focus and direction in life.

Heart

Marigolds contain anti-inflammatory triterpenoids, flavonoids, and antioxidants. All of these compounds will restore compromised blood vessel walls, and along with its antispasmodic effects can help to normalise blood pressure (Fisher, 2018).[2] When used as a compress, cream, or poultice, it helps the pain and swelling of varicosities.

Skin

As a wash, ointment, poultice, or cream the flowers can be used for eczema, sun burn, ulcers, phlebitis, and skin growths caused by sun damage. A poultice of the fresh or dry flowers and herb helps bruising and swellings. The wash may be used as a simple skin cleanser for the face and skin. It is helpful in fungal infections, especially as a footbath used regularly for athlete's foot. I have found it very useful in fresh poultices for slow healing leg ulcers, along with using an ointment made from the flowers. Marigold is powerfully antiviral and a poultice or compress is very effective for shingles and should be applied frequently. Regular *Calendula* baths will help clear acne and eczema, and are beneficial in psoriasis and for reducing the severity of chicken pox. The infusion is often helpful in chronic or acute skin problems, and should be drunk as a tea twice daily until improvement occurs. The ointment should be applied around open ulcers, and on small ulcerated areas it can be applied directly to them, the ointment is also essential when treating eczema, applied twice daily it stops the skin cracking and drying reducing its susceptibility to becoming infected and itchy.

Immune system

It is an immune strengthening herb, which can be used regularly for chronic problems, such as inflamed tonsils, swollen glands, and long-term inflammatory conditions. The tea or tincture can be used for treating fevers and infections, especially glandular fever. The tea may be drunk throughout the winter to protect from viruses and infections.

Reproductive and urinary system

Marigold is a useful uterine and ovarian tonic herb that helps to clear congestion from the fallopian tubes and act as an ovarian tonic, improving premenstrual symptoms and fertility.

Digestion

Marigold helps a sluggish liver and is effective as a regular infusion to help with inflammatory bowel diseases, gastritis, stomach ulcers, hiatus hernia, and also haemorrhoids, when the ointment is particularly helpful applied externally.

Eyes

It can be used daily for painful eyes and helps both blepharitis and conjunctivitis. The ointment should be applied after using a compress made by soaking a cloth in marigold infusion and leaving in place for ten minutes, with the treatment being repeated at least twice daily. A patient of mine with frequent and worsening problems with iritis eventually cured the problem with a daily calendula eye compress.

Combinations

With Echinacea for chronic congestive problems, swollen tonsils, sinusitis.

Combined with St John's wort oil to make an all healing "hypercal salve".

Doses

Tincture

1:3 in 25% alcohol. 5–10 ml one to three times daily.

Tea

2 g infused in a cup drunk up to three times a day.

Medicinal infusion

10 g to a litre, drunk over 24 hours.

Infused oil

Dry fresh marigold flowers to a leathery consistency, then steep them in olive oil in a glass jar left in the sun. Strain off when the oil takes on a bright yellow colour, usually after 10 days.

Ointment

Combine 1 oz of beeswax to each ½ pint of marigold oil (12 g to 100 ml), in a "bain marie", melt wax in the oil, then allow to cool and harden in jars.

Meadowsweet

Queen of the Meadow. Spirea. Bridewort.
Gaelic: Cneas chu chulain

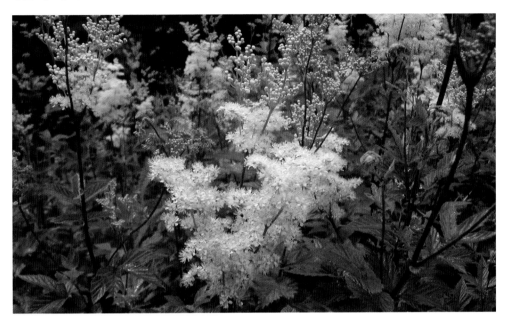

| Latin: | *Fillipendula ulmaria* |
| Family: | Rosaceae |

Element	Air
Planet	Jupiter
Humour	Sanguine
Quality	Warm and dry in the first degree, tempers heat in the liver, clears damp from stomach, bowels and joints.

Organs

Liver
Stomach
Bowels
Joints
Kidneys
Bladder
Womb
Ovaries
Skin

Actions

Anti-inflammatory
Astringent
Antacid
Anti-rheumatic
Antibacterial
Anti ulcer
Anticoagulant
Antidepressant

Constituents

Volatile oils: methylsalicilate
Glycosides
Flavonoids
Tannins

Traditional uses and uumoral influences

Meadowsweet is ruled by Jupiter, the planet that governs the sanguine or air and blood humour. It is warming in the first degree, drying and calming in nature. It is a member of the rose family, a family famed for its cooling, calming and drying properties. Meadowsweet clears heat from the liver, the stomach and the bowels. During the spring when the air element is strongest, the blood can become overwhelmed by the gathering warmth and energy. The expanding heat and moisture in the blood may bring on inflammation, swellings and spring fevers, or what we tend to call today, hay fever. The warmth of meadowsweet helps to move and clear the excess heat, and to dry the excess moisture. It is both diuretic and diaphoretic, opening the channels of elimination helping to expel the heat through transpiration or sweating, and therefore leading to a cooling of the body. Culpeper said that "the flowers are alexipharmic and sudorific, and good in fevers, and all malignant distempers; they are likewise astringent, binding, and useful in fluxes of all sorts."

Hot swollen joints, burning stomach pain, and inflamed skin irritations are all good examples of conditions that benefit greatly from meadowsweet. The salicilate compounds in meadowsweet help to bring down fevers, reduce pain, and enable good blood flow. John Parkinson, in his Theatrum Botanicum of 1640, said "it is sayd to alter and take away the fits of the quartaine agues, and to make a merry heart, for which purpose some use the flowers & some the leaves".[1]

It is a relaxing, anti-inflammatory, and astringent herb, reducing excess phlegm and swelling of mucous membranes. All the passages in the body—urinary, digestive, and respiratory—are helped by meadowsweet, which through expelling heat, cools, calms, and reduces hot wet swellings and excess phlegm.

Mythos

Meadowsweet, water mint, and vervain, were the three medicinal herbs most sacred to the druids. Jupiter, its ruler, is known as the ruler of the planets and is seen as the great protector, as well as the source of divine inspiration in the mind. The name "queen of the meadow" eludes to this royal heritage and also to its long association as a herb particularly helpful as a woman's healer, being able to stay excessive bleeding and being a beneficial herb after giving birth.

Its name meadowsweet comes from the flowers traditionally being used as a flavouring for mead, literally "mead sweet". In Gaelic the herb is called 'Cneas Chu Chullain'—the waist belt of Chu Chullain. Chullain was a royal warrior hero who was known for his terrifying battle frenzy or "riastrad". It is said in Scottish folklore that it was only meadowsweet that could calm Chu Chullain down, while another explanation is that when Chu Chullain was suffering from shingles, he wrapped the plant around his waist to heal the sores.

Emotional

Meadowsweet is calming, relaxing, and comforting. As in the story of Chullain, meadowsweet is a calming herb for emotions that have become overwhelming and frenzied or obsessive. It seems that it is the comforting effect of the herb that gives it is reputation for making the heart merry, and combining the herb with St John's wort works well when difficult emotions, such as grief and anger, have exhausted the vital spirit and saddened the heart. As a herbal bath, there are few herbs that surpass it for relaxing and calming mind, body, and spirit.

Joints

Rheum in Greek means flow, so the joints or rheumatics are strongly associated with the water element. When they are hot and inflamed, a cooling, eliminating herb associated with water, such as meadowsweet, is very helpful, especially in rheumatoid arthritis, osteoarthritis, and gout.

Urinary and reproductive system

It is a cleansing diuretic, helpful for cystitis and urinary bleeding. It makes a pleasant tea and can be drunk throughout the day. The association with female conditions as indicated by its name "queen of the meadow" points to its traditional use for benefitting menstrual pain, heavy menstruation, menstrual flooding, and to help healing after giving birth.

Skin

It is excellent when used externally as a wash or poultice, for sores and wounds.

A natural antifungal and antibacterial skin oil can be made by steeping the fresh flowers in vegetable oil and leaving in the sun. The oil can be rubbed on painful joints, and used for skin eruptions, such as shingles and eczema.

Stomach

Meadowsweet is a well-known remedy for indigestion, heartburn, gastritis, and ulceration. It is also a gentle remedy for diarrhoea, inflammatory bowel disease, and to stop bleeding. It is thought to both reduce hyperacidity and, due to its bitter properties, improve the secretion of bile, helping with digestion. It has a relaxing effect on smooth muscle, reducing intestinal colic and cramping.

Doses

Tea

One heaped teaspoon to a cup, (2–4 g) taken three times daily.

Tincture

1:3 25% Alc. 5–10 ml 1–3 times a day.

Milk Thistle & Thistles

Milk Thistle/Our lady's thistle

| Latin: | *Carduus marianus,*
Psilybum marianus |

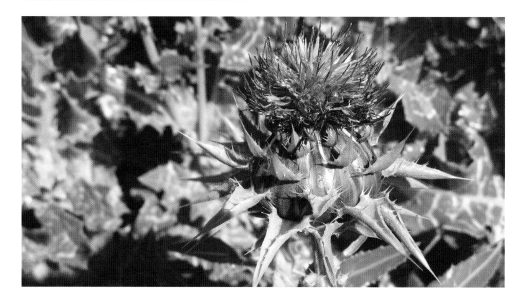

Blessed thistle/Holy Thistle

Latin *Cnicus benedictus*

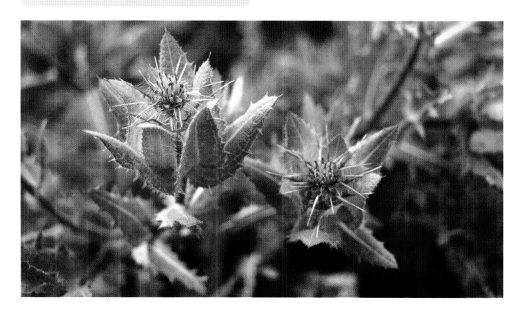

Family: Astreaceae

Milk thistle
Element   Air
Planet   Jupiter
Humour   Sanguine
Quality   Hot and dry in the first
          degree, strengthens the
          heart and liver, purges
          choler, reduces fevers

Blessed thistle
Element   Fire
Planet   Mars
Humour   Choleric
Quality   Hot and dry in the second
          degree, heats the head
          and heart, opening,
          cleansing, resists poison

Organs

Liver
Head
Womb
Stomach

Actions

Liver protective
Antiseptic
Antipyretic
Wound healing
Antiallergenic
Diuretic

Constituents

Milk thistle:
Flavolignans: silymarin, silybin
Flavonoids
Triterpenes
Bitter principles

Blessed thistle:
Lignans: arctigenin, arctiin
Volatile oil: cinnamaldehyde
Sesquiterpenes: cnicin
Polyacetalenes
Tannins

Traditional uses and humoral influences

Thistles were considered by Culpeper to be under the rulership of Mars and to be hot and dry in the second degree, with cleansing and opening properties and to powerfully resist poisons. Milk thistle was, however, placed under the rulership of Jupiter. However, Gerard (1636) says in his herbal; "Concerning the temperature and virtues of these thistles we can allege nothing at all".[1] Traditional assignations of temperature and the quality of a plant always finally comes down to a personal judgement. We all experience the world differently and it is unlikely that we will agree on everything. One of the benefits of energetic systems of medicine is that they resist rigidity and avoid trying to explain everything, allowing the personal experience of the individual to take an equal place alongside the received wisdom or opinions of others. We are always re-interpreting the world around us depending on our own experiences, remembering that nothing remains the same and that everything is impermanent. However, all thistles share the properties of being fever-reducing, blood and liver cleansing, and are liver restoratives.

According to Grieve (1931) the ancients supposed the Scotch thistle to be specific in cancerous complaints and "in more modern times the juice is said to have been applied with good effect to cancers and ulcers". When Mrs Grieve wrote her herbal in the 1930s, she says that the seeds of milk thistle were generally used for the same purposes as blessed thistle.

Blessed thistle is under the sign of Aries, which rules the head with Culpeper saying, "It helps swimming and giddiness of the head because Aries is in the house of Mars. It is a remedy excellent against the yellow jaundice and infirmities of the gall because Mars Governs Choler". He considered it to be beneficial through a similar sympathetic action to all the other infirmities associated with Mars; red faces, tetters (any itchy skin disease including psoriasis), ringworm, plague, sores, boils, itch, and the biting of mad dogs and venomous beasts. Its martian heat makes it anti-pathetic to cold or saturnine conditions, enabling it to strengthen the memory and cure deafness, while it is through its equal antipathy to the wet phlegmatic diseases of Venus that it was included in treatments for venereal disease.

Milk thistle is placed under the rulership of Jupiter, and the name is likely due to its traditional use as a nursing plant to increase milk flow. Although considered to be dry and heating like all the other thistles, milk thistle is probably not quite as hot and drying as the rest.

Culpeper states: "All thistles are good to provoke urine, and to mend the stinking smell thereof; as also the rank smell of the arm pits, or the whole body; being boiled in wine and drank, and are said to help a stinking breath, and to strengthen the stomach".

Milk thistle is considered very effective in cooling the liver and also for cooling the passions of the heart and "the swoonings thereof". In the writings of the French herbalist Maurice Messegue he suggests milk thistle as a circulatory tonic, helping to strengthen blood vessels, and to help with low blood pressure, migraines, vertigo, and low energy.

The melancholy thistle, which is most common in northern England and Scotland, is placed under the sign of Capricorn and therefore aligned to both Saturn and Mars. Its effect of ridding the body of melancholy was both by its cold dry saturnine sympathy, cooling excess heat, and its warming martial effect being antipathetical to the excess coldness of superfluous melancholy when it is found in the body.

Culpeper says of this thistle that "the decoction in wine being drank, expels superfluous melancholy, and makes a man as merry as a cricket; superfluous melancholy causes care, fear, sadness, despair, envy, and many evils besides". Culpeper goes on to advise us to let go of our cares and worries, saying "religion teaches to wait upon Gods providence, and cast our care upon he who cares for us. What a fine thing were it if men and women could live so! And yet seven years of care and fear makes a man never the wiser, or a farthing richer". Gerard (1636) wrote that the same applied to milk thistle and that "the root if bourne about one doth expel melancholy, and remove all diseases connected therewith … My opinion is that this is the best remedy that grows against all melancholy diseases".[2]

The young stems of milk thistle were traditionally considered a very useful spring tonic, steamed and eaten as a vegetable and the heads prepared like the globe artichoke.

Mythos

It is said that the word *marianus* derives from "Mary" and the belief that the Virgin Mary spilt a drop of her breast milk on the plant, which gave its leaves white veins and the property of helping nursing mothers.

The name *Carduus* is believed to refer to a Greek word indicating that the thistle could be used in the process of preparing wool for spinning, known as carding the wool.

The Scotch thistle has the Latin name *Onopordon* rather than *Carduus*. It is said to be derived from the Greek words for an ass, "onos" and "pordon" meaning "I disperse"—the species being said to be produce the dispersing of wind in asses when they forage on them.

In the Northern European traditions, thistles have been held sacred to Thor, who like Mars is a god of destruction, fire, and war. The bright colours; purples, reds, and yellows, seen in the flowers and leaves of thistles are said to correspond to the bright lightning Thor dispenses, and cultivating thistles would therefore also protect one from the destructive effects of thunder bolts.

Gynaecological

Milk thistle is haemostatic and is recommended by Messegue for heavy periods, when a herb is described as "drying" this usually indicates an ability to stop bleeding. Hormones are both produced and broken down in the liver, so the improvement of liver function is also likely to help to regulate hormonal cycles. It was also traditionally used as nursing herb, to improve milk flow.

Stomach

The bitter principles in thistles have a stimulatory effect on the digestive organs and increase the release of bile from the gall bladder. In large doses it works as a gentle emetic.

Liver

The flavolignan "silymarin" in milk thistle has been shown conclusively to protect animals from a variety of different liver toxins, in particular the toxins from death cap mushrooms. Treating animals with silymarin and silybin prior to administering death cap mushrooms gave them 100% protection from death, and giving injections of the same compounds to humans within 48 hours of ingesting the fungus has been shown to be highly effective in reducing fatalities (Williamson, 2003).[3] Silymarin is effective for treating liver cirrhosis and chronic hepatitis, it is active against the hepatitis B virus, while also lowering fat levels in the blood and helping with fatty liver (Fisher, 2018).[4]

Traditionally obstructions or blockages of the liver can be caused by an excess of heat or cold. When caused by heat it may be due to an acute disease, fevers, alcohol, excessive emotional states, or by a person having a choleric constitution. Excessive cold conditions may be caused by excess phlegm, excess Melancholy, or poor digestive heat and activity or the slow depletion from a chronic illness. The true hepatic herbs, including the thistles, have a bitter stimulating effect on the flow of bile through the liver and were thus considered to cool and open obstructions when the organ was overheated and to help to open and disperse heat throughout the organ where there was excessive coldness and dampness. Cooling herbs, such as dandelion or violets, would help in cases of excessive heat and warming hepatics, such as hyssop and gentle spicy herbs, should be given in cases of excessive cold.

Allergy

Messegue (1981) considers milk thistle in particular as a potent remedy for allergies, saying it is "the most effective of all plants in allergies of all kinds—sea sickness, car or plane sickness, hay fever, nettle rash, or asthma. None of these can hold out for long against treatment by this plant".[5] It is interesting that these conditions correspond to the martial diseases listed by Culpeper, especially the itchy eruptive skin diseases.

In Grieves' herbal (1931) she also suggests that "a decoction of the root is astringent and diminishes discharges form mucous membranes", confirming that thistles have for a long time been thought of as having a useful role in conditions such as hay fever and asthma.

Doses

Tea

The tea made from the leaves is a gentle bitter liver tonic. Decoctions can also be made from the root and seeds.

Decoction

A heaped teaspoon of ground milk thistle seeds can be decocted for ten minutes in a cupful of water and drunk in the morning, or the ground seeds can be eaten at breakfast. The ground seeds can also be taken in capsules 2–3 g a day, however the alcoholic tincture is a poor way of extracting the active constituents and shouldn't be bothered with.

Mint

Peppermint. Brandy mint. Water mint. Wild mint. Horse mint

Latin: *Mentha piperita*

Spearmint. Garden Mint. Spire Mint. Mackerel mint. Our ladies Mint. Green Mint

Latin: *Mentha spicata*

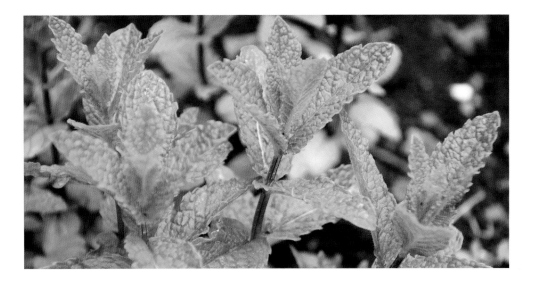

Element   Water
Planet   Venus
Humour   Phlegmatic
Quality   Hot and dry in the third
           degree, heats head, lungs,
           stomach and womb,
           binding, digestive,
           diaphoretic.

Organs

Throat
Stomach
Bowels
Head
Lungs
Womb

Actions

Stimulant
Carminative
Antispasmodic
Anti-inflammatory
Sedative
Diaphoretic
Antiseptic
Antioxidant

Constituents

Essential oils: menthol, menthone
    acetate, limonene
Flavonoids: rutin, menthoside,
    luteolin
Phenolic acids and lactones:
    rosmarinic acid

Traditional uses and humoral influences

The mints are ruled by Venus and thus have a relationship with the phlegmatic humour. They are hot and dry in the third degree. The warmth of mint clears and dries phlegmatic conditions, such as coughs and colds. The Egyptians are said to have cultivated and used mint extensively, and according to Pliny, the herb mentastrum, (horse mint) was a cure for snake and scorpion bites and an all round antidote to poison in general. He said that it regulated menstruation, cured dandruff, ear worms, jaundice, lumbago, and gout. Pliny also said that the other mints (in particular water mint) had the properties of relieving haemorrhages, excessive menstruation, intestinal disorders, ulcerations, and abscesses on the womb, liver conditions, and hiccups.

Venus rules the reproductive organs, so it is not surprising to find mint so extensively recommended for treating female disorders. According to Culpeper, "It is an herb of Venus. Dioscorides saith it hath a healing, binding and drying quality, and therefore the juice taken in vinegar stays bleeding". He also goes on to warn … "it stirs up bodily lust; but therefore too much must not be taken, because it makes the blood thin and wheyish, and turns it into choler, and therefore choleric persons must abstain from it" He is here warning against the potential of the hot quality of peppermint to overwhelm the softer cooler phlegmatic portion of the blood and to bring about scorching and irritation. This is of course what we see happening when the irritant aspects of the volatile oils such as menthol are not used judiciously.

I had a patient with a choleric temperament, who commented on how too much peppermint tea would bring on severe headaches, in this case exacerbating their hot dry temperament and overheating the brain. Conversely I discovered that the chronic bladder irritation and pain of a phlegmatic patient I treated had been caused by her drinking at least three cups of peppermint tea daily over a number of years in an attempt to relieve irritable bowel syndrome. This reminds us how important it is to pay attention to the temperaments and actions of our herbs and use them in accordance with the individuals temperament, rather than just prescribe medicinal herbs on the basis symptoms alone.

Venus also rules the expulsive faculty in the body along with the moon. The expulsive faculty resides in the kidneys, bowels, and lungs. Heat digests, moves, and expels waste, whereas cool condenses. When there is excessive cold in these organs then phlegm and dampness build up, causing congestion and stasis. The warmth of the mints allows this excessive phlegm to be broken down (digested) and then expelled. It's not surprising then to find mint being helpful in all congestive conditions of the lungs, stomach, and bowels, as they all share a cool moist temperament and are all involved in the digestion and expulsion of excess phlegm. In country medicine, mint has often been used in combination with elder flower and yarrow to treat colds and fevers.

Mythos

Menthe was a nymph and the daughter of the water god Cocytus. She was lusted after by the god of the underworld, Hades. When his wife Persephone saw what was occurring she turned Menthe into the mint plant. There was a temple built at the foot of mount Menthe in Elis in honour of Hades, and mint was used in the Greek funerary rites, possibly the sweet smell offsetting the odours of bodily decay. According to a legend from the Abruzzi mountains in Italy, Mary the mother of Jesus survived on eating spearmint after the death of her son, and so it became thought of as a sacred plant of the virgin. In Italy it took the name "erba sancta Maria" or "herba buona" (good herb) and in England "our ladies mint". The Roman poet Ovid described mint as a symbol of hospitality, telling the story of Baucis and Philemon who rubbed their serving tray with mint before offering food to Jupiter and Mercury. With these sacred associations it is not surprising that all mints have been regarded as deterrents of the devil. The smell of mint is anathema to mice and rats, and would be put in larders to keep pests away, in ancient times mice were considered a symbol of disease. According to Grieve in A Modern Herbal (1931), water mint, meadowsweet, and vervain were the three most sacred plants of the druids, and it was said to have been used in water magic in European folk tradition and be one of the magical bunch of fifteen herbs.

Emotional

Mint has a clearing effect on the mind, refreshing the brain and clarifying thought processes. It warms, comforts, and relaxes, and can help to bring the mind into focus after a shock or trauma. It helps us to get going again when we have lost our sense of momentum and gives us a renewed energy when our spirits are flagging.

Stomach and bowels

The stomach and bowels are associated with the phlegmatic humour, which is cold and wet, so these organs are prone to excess damp and cold. This excess is considered to be the main cause of cramps and also colic.

Mint warms the stomach, aids digestion, and reduces bloating. Culpeper says of the mints; "It suffers not milk to curdle in the stomach, if the leaves thereof be steeped or boiled in it before you drink it. Briefly it is very profitable for the stomach".

Spearmint is very similar in action to peppermint but is considered to be gentler and less powerful. However, this makes it a more suitable remedy for those with a sensitive stomach, and for children in particular. It was commonly made as an infusion of one ounce to a pint and given in wineglassful doses to children for fevers and inflammatory diseases. It was also thought especially helpful as "a specific for allaying nausea and vomiting and to relieve the pain of colic" and it was common to put a couple of drops of spearmint oil on a sugar lump for children's colic (Grieve, 1931).

Peppermint water made from distilled water saturated with peppermint oil is still an official medicine included in the British Pharmacopoeia and is officially indicated for intestinal colic and flatulence.

Lungs and respiratory system

As an ingredient in inhalations, steams, and baths, peppermint is very beneficial for relieving coughs, sinus congestion, clearing excess phlegm and reducing wheezing and a tight chest. It is both analgesic and antispasmodic, while also effectively opening the airways. Peppermint oil diluted in a carrier oil or added to an ointment makes an effective addition to a chest rub, and for applying to the forehead to relieve sinus pain.

Womb

The warming drying quality is considered helpful to the womb, which like the head has a cool and moist or phlegmatic temperament. It is considered able to strengthen the womb helping to regulate periods, and its drying quality makes it beneficial in excess menstrual flow. Culpeper comments, "It stirs up venery, or bodily lust; It is good to repress the milk in women's breasts, and for such that have swollen, flagging or great breasts … the often use thereof is a very powerful medicine to stay women's courses and the whites".

Head

The head has a cold and moist temperament, and therefore is prone to being affected by an excess of these qualities. Traditionally it is thought that lethargy, palsy, convulsions, and epilepsy are caused by excessive phlegm blocking the flow of the animal spirit that activates the brain and nervous system. Culpeper comments, "Applied to the forehead and the temples it eases pains in the head".

According to Mrs Grieve (1931), "In cases of hysteria and nervous disorders, the usefulness of Peppermint has been found to be well augmented by the addition of equal quantities of wood betony, its operation being hastened by a few drops of the tincture of caraway". She goes on to give a recipe for children's teething;

"½ oz peppermint herb, ½ oz skullcap herb, ½ oz pennyroyal herb, pour on a pint of boiling water, cover and let it stand in a warm place for thirty minutes. Strain and sweeten to taste, and given frequently in teaspoon doses warm." She also recommends; "The following simple preparation has been found useful in insomnia: 1 oz peppermint herb, cut fine, ½ oz Rue herb, ½ oz Wood betony. Well mix and place a large tablespoonful in a teacup, fill with boiling water, stir and cover for twenty minutes, strain and sweeten, and drink the warm infusion going to bed" (Grieve, 1931).

Joints

Warming rubs and baths made with peppermint are very helpful for joint pains. The essential oil can be added to base oils or creams and applied to painful and swollen joints.

Recipe for an arthritis cream

In 50 g base cream add the following essential oils:

    10 drops peppermint
    10 drops wintergreen
    5 drops rosemary
    5 drops black pepper
    5 drops clove

Doses

Tincture

1:3, 5 ml 3 times daily.

Infusion

5 g three times daily.

Inhalation

The herb may be used as an inhalation, use 2 tablespoons to 2 pints of boiling water, inhale with head covered over a bowl for ten minutes. The mix may be reheated and used a second time.

Mistletoe

Birdlime. Mystledene. Lignum Crucis All heal. Mistle.
French: Gui blanc
Dutch: Maretak

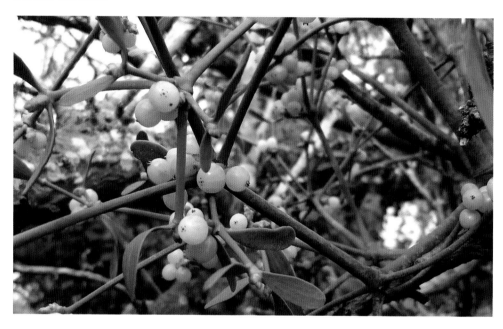

Latin: *Viscum album*
Family: Loranthaceae

Element   Fire
Planet   Sun
Humour   Choleric
Quality   Hot and dry in the second
           degree, strengthens the
           head and the animal spirit,
           calms the heart and mind

Organs

Head and nerves
Heart

Actions

Hypotensive
Nervine
Sedative
Antispasmodic
Cardiotonic
Immune stimulant
Anticancer
Heamostatic

Constituents

Polypeptides: viscotoxins
Glycoproteins
Triterpenes: oleanic, betulinic, and
    oleanolic acids
Flavonoids: quercertin, naringenin
Lignans
Polyphenols: caffeic, *p*-coumaric
    acids

Traditional uses and humoral influences

Mistletoe is ruled by the sun, with a hot and dry action. According to Culpeper, its actions may also be influenced by the planet of the tree on which it grows. When mistletoe grows on the oak, which is ruled by Jupiter it will have more influence on the blood humour and the liver, and will particularly strengthen the decision-making part of the brain as that is under Jupiter's rulership. Culpeper says;

"Both the leaves and berries of Mistletoe do heat and dry, and are of subtle parts; the birdlime doth mollify hard knots, tumours, and imposthumes; ripens and discusses them, and draws forth thick as well as thin humours from the remote parts of the body, digesting and separating them.

Using it to treat skin outbreaks (an imposthume is a swelling containing pus) is a continuation of practice coming from the time of the ancient Greek herbalists Dioscorides and Hippocrates. They recommended the birdlime, which is the sticky substance that comes from within the berries, for old boils and swellings, with the later Roman writer Pliny commenting on the birdlime having a soothing effect that can be used to make tumours disintegrate and ulcers dry out.

It was held in high regard as a herb for afflictions of the head, such as epilepsy, dizziness, and palsy, and was generally used to treat a range of conditions thought to be due to a depleted nervous system. M Grieve says; "It has been employed in convulsions, delirium, hysteria, neuralgia, nervous debility, urinary disorders, heart disease, and many other complaints arising from a weakened and disordered state of the nervous system". The animal spirit governs the nervous system, whose temperament is cold and dry and is associated with the etheric element. Mistletoe has a warming action and is associated with the element ether as it is a plant that thrives between earth and sky. This makes it particularly beneficial when the animal spirit and the nervous system has lost its heat and the vital activity of the brain has diminished.

There is also a long history of use for mistletoe in the form of an intravenous treatment for cancer, possibly due to the traditional use in treating "Hard Knots and tumours" alluded to by Culpeper.

Mythos

The name mistletoe is believed to derive from the Anglo Saxon "mist", meaning to be "different from" and "tan" meaning twig, thus it is the different twig that grows in the tree. The Latin name *Viscum* comes from the word for thick and sticky, referring to the sticky substance that constitutes the berries. The Roman writer Pliny recorded that it was one of the most revered herbs of the druids, especially that which grew on an oak, becoming a symbol of the triumph of life over death, and a signifier of the life force that descends to us from the heavens via the tree of power and strength, the oak. In this way it brings together wisdom, knowledge, light, and strength in one plant. The berries were seen as the seed of the gods and the plant was considered particularly magical because it was suspended between earth and sky. The druids believed it to be a plant that would bring fertility and rid the body of every kind of poison. They would cut it with a golden sickle and it was to be kept from touching the ground so as not to lose any of its magical potency.

Throughout time it has been a plant revered as a symbol of life and rebirth. In Greek and Roman legends mistletoe is the plant with which one can enter hell, but more especially a plant through which one can also depart the underworld. It was the key that Persephone used to free herself from the underworld each spring, and according to Virgil it was from mistletoe wood that the "golden twig" was made, which Aeneas used as a protective token when he descended into the underworld to search for his father Anchises.

In Norse myth Balder was the most beloved of the gods, being both beautiful and just. He was the Son of Odin and Frigg the goddess of magic. However, there was a divination that Balder would soon die, so to protect him Frigg got a promise from all cosmic entities that they would not harm her son. Though she thought the mistletoe to be such a small and soft plant that it could never be used for harm, so she did not ask it to take the pledge. When Loki the Norse trickster god heard of this omission he saw an opportunity for some mischief and made a dart from its wood. He tricked the blind god Hodi to throw it at Balder, who died immediately when the dart struck him, much to the distress of all the living beings and the gods themselves. From this point forward it was decreed that the mistletoe would never again be used as a weapon of war but only as a symbol of love. This developed into the custom of kissing under the mistletoe to mark the beginning of the year, and to celebrate the triumph of love and light over darkness.

There is a European belief that mistletoe protects against the magical white "she elves" of the air, they are shape shifters becoming cats, wolves, goblins, and various other creatures. They were believed to be able to jump onto people's chests, ride on plants, and be apt to cast mischievous spells. It is said that the mistletoe grows on the branches where the she elves have sat, and that a branch of mistletoe carried or hung about the house would offer protection against such threats.

Emotional

Mistletoe relaxes us, giving release from overwhelming stress. When the heart feels burdened with overwhelming darkness it opens the door to a rebirth of hope and light. A remedy for all who feel lost and without hope, mistletoe offers freedom from all that oppresses us.

Head

Mistletoe is certainly a helpful herb for the brain, having a calming and gentle sedative effect. It reduces mental tension and is particularly helpful for conditions associated with chronic stress, including headaches associated with high blood pressure. In 1720 an English physician, Sir John Colbatch published a pamphlet entitled "The Treatment of Epilepsy by Mistletoe" (Grieve, 1931).[1] He considered it a specific for the condition and was said to gather the herb from lime trees growing at Hampton court.

Heart

Mistletoe is very effective for arrhythmias and a rapid heart rate associated with stress and a weakened heart. It was considered to be an alternative to foxglove as a strengthener of the heart, particularly when that was reflected in a weak or erratic heart rate. As a cardiotonic herb, it is traditionally used for high blood pressure, atherosclerosis, and calming the heart.

Doses

Infusion of dried herb

2–6 g once or twice daily.

Tincture

1:3 2–6 ml a day.

Dried powder

0.5–1 g per day.

Motherwort

Lion's tail

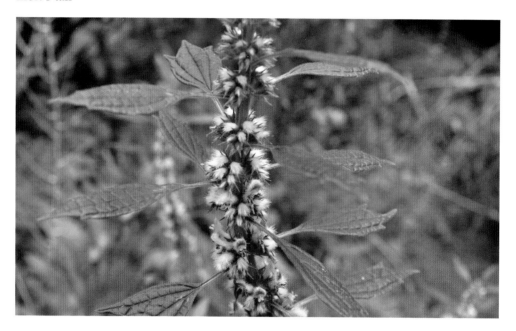

| Latin: | *Leonurus cardiaca* |
| Family: | Lamiaceae |

Element	Water
Planet	Venus
Humour	Phlegmatic
Quality	Warm in the first degree, dry in the second degree. Cleanses and dries cold humours, digests and disperses them. Strengthens the heart.

Organs

Heart
Lungs
Womb
Joints and sinews

Actions

Nervine
Antidepressant
Sedative
Heart tonic
Hypotensive
Antispasmodic
Diaphoretic
Anti-thyrotoxic
Diuretic
Birthing herb
Wound healing

Constituents

Alkaloids: stachydrine, leonurine
Iridoid glycosides: leonuride, ajugol, galiridosides
Bitter glycosides

Flavonoids: quercetin, kaempferol, apigenin
Terpenes: leocardin, ursolic acid
Tannins, phenols, terpenoids
Phenyl propanoids

Traditional uses and humoral influences

Motherwort is warm in the first degree, dry in the second, and ruled by Venus. It is under the astrological sign of Leo, the astrological sign that rules the heart and the stomach, indicating that these organs have a particular affinity with the herb. It is helpful in all damp, cold, and congested states, drying up dampness and cleansing excess cold humours from the body. Culpeper said, "It is of good use to warm and dry up the cold humours, to digest and disperse them" It has a particular affinity with the heart and the womb, strengthening both organs and helping to cleanse them of dampness. Gerard (1597) says of motherwort, "Divers commend it against infirmities of the heart: it is judged to be so forcible, that it is thought it took this name Cardiaca of the effect. It is also reported to cure convulsions, cramps, and palsies, to open the obstructions or stoppings of the intrals, and to kill all kinds of worms in the belly. The powder in wine provoketh not only urine and the monthly courses, but also is good for them that it is hard travail with child. Moreover, the same is commended for green wounds" (Grieve, 1931).[1]

In John Parkinson's 1640 herbal he includes motherwort in his entry for *Melissa* (lemon balm), doing so "for the vertues sake"[2]—both lemon balm and motherwort lift the spirits, calm the heart, and ease mental tension. Today we use both to treat an overactive thyroid gland,

the symptoms of which are a rapid or irregular heart rate, anxiety, and loose frequent bowel motions.

Mythos

The womb was often referred to as the "mother", indicating that motherwort was considered particularly helpful for female reproductive issues and was specifically indicated as a birthing herb. The Latin name *Leonurus cardiaca* can be translated as the lion heart, although it is also said that it may have been given the name Leonurus as the leaf shape has a similarity to a lion's tail. In either case it is considered to be a powerfully protective herb, used for the heart, the lungs, and in fevers. The protective properties were also believed to extend to the energetic and spiritual realms, with Maude Grieve (1931) saying, "In Macers herbal we find 'Motherwort' mentioned as one of the herbs which were considered all-powerful against 'wykked speryts'".

Emotional

It is a relaxing and calming herb, which helps to soften the grip of painful emotions on the heart. It is particularly helpful to reduce the feelings of tension that come with stressful situations, allowing a feeling of acceptance to replace emotions of panic. It is helpful for panic attacks, premenstrual irritability and depression, and to support those having to endure long periods of grief, sadness, and loss.

Heart

Culpeper says: "It is held to be of much use for the trembling of the heart, and fainting and swooning; from whence it took the name Cardiaca" Studies have shown it to have both a relaxant effect on arteries and an inhibitory effect on pulsating cardiac muscle,[3] which may account for its helpful action in high blood pressure, palpitations, and arrhythmia. The alkaloid leonurine in particular has been shown to be vaso-relaxant, an action that is enhanced by the phenyl propanoids, such as verbascoside, which it also contains. Extracts of the whole herb demonstrate antioxidant activity, which we know will help protect blood vessels from inflammation and the development of atherosclerotic plaques and the blockages that they cause (Fisher, 2018).[4]

Nicholas Culpeper also attested, "There is no better herb to take melancholy vapours from the heart, to strengthen it, and make a merry, cheerful, blithe soul than this herb". Melancholy vapours are cold in nature, and arise from the spleen—the seat of the melancholic humour. As the spleen sits beneath the heart and stomach, its cold vapours are prone to rise up, block and dampen the innate heat flowing from the heart. This has a depressing and depleting effect on the vital spirit, bringing on feelings of weakness and loss of hope and positivity. Cold obstructions to the free flow of the innate heat and vital spirit may also cause an irregular, interrupted, or even rapid heart rate.

Lungs

Although motherwort is not usually placed in the category of lung herbs, in the sixteenth century we find Culpeper repeating Parkinson's recommendation that Motherwort; "Clenseth the chest of cold flegme oppressing it".[5] This may well be referring to it being helpful to clear the fluid that accrues in the lungs as a result of heart failure, through the improvement of heart function.

Digestion and stomach

Its bitter action stimulates appetite and helps to clear wind. The antispasmodic effects on smooth muscle will help to relieve colic and intestinal spasm. The older herbalists such as Culpeper also recommended it to "kill worms in the belly". Its bitter properties increase bile flow; these combined with its relaxant effects on smooth muscular passages make it helpful for flushing gall stones and reducing spasm in the bile ducts.

Womb

Motherwort is a traditional labour herb, recently it has been shown to contain oxytocic alkaloids, such as stachydine, which will help with labour and stimulate the let down reflex. There is debate about how water soluble these compounds are, so there seems to be sense in Parkinson's recommendation to take "the powder thereof to the quantity of a spoonefull drunke in wine," commending it as "a wonderful helpe to women in their sore travels".[6] Motherwort is, however, considered safe to take in pregnancy, and it is also helpful for painful periods, delayed periods, and when there is light or absent bleeding. As a remedy for premenstrual syndrome it combines well with vervain herb and valerian root.

Bladder and kidneys

Although it is not often listed in modern herbals as a diuretic, Culpeper and others considered it to "provoke urine". It is particularly helpful in relaxing the urinary passages, making it a prime herb to use in cases of benign prostatic hypertrophy and to aid in the passing of kidney stones.

Doses

Tincture

1:5, 2–10 ml three times daily.

Tea

2–4 g one to three times daily.

Capsule

400 mg 1–3 daily.

Tincture mix for PMS

Motherwort	40%	
Vervain	30%	100 ml, 5–10 ml as needed
Valerian root	30%	

Mugwort

Mugwort. Felon herb. St Johns plant. Flea bane. Bulwand. Wormit

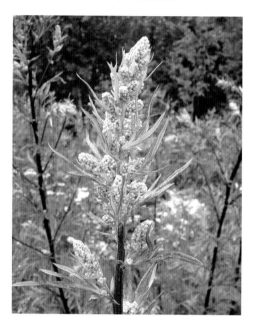

Latin:	*Artemisia vulgaris*
Family:	Asteraceae

Element	Water
Planet	Venus
Humour	Phlegmatic
Quality	Hot and dry in the second degree, heats the womb, strengthens the nerves, allays fatigue

Actions

Emenagogue
Nervine
Bitter stomach tonic
Diuretic

Organs

Stomach
Womb
Head

Constituents

Volatile oils: Linalool, cineole, thujone
Sesquiterpene lactones
Flavonoids: quercetin, kaempferol
Coumarins

Traditional use and humoral influences

Mugwort is ruled by Venus and is hot and dry in the second degree. Venus is associated with fertility, love, affection, and nurture. Venus also rules food, from which energy is drawn into the body, it is the substance of food that forms new tissues through growth and regeneration. She is thus connected to the process of generation, birth, and the activity of the womb.

Nicholas Culpeper says; "This is an herb of Venus, therefore maintains the parts of the body she rules, and remedies the diseases of the parts that are under her signs, Taurus and Libra" Taurus and Libra rule the throat, neck, kidneys, and loins.

Mugwort has a stimulating tonic action, especially good for countering fatigue and exhaustion, it was customary to place the leaves in the shoes to ensure that one didn't tire, a practice said by the Roman writer Pliny to have originally been utilised by Roman soldiers on long marches. Culpeper commented;

"A Decoction made with Chamomile and Agrimony, and the place bathed therewith while it is warm, takes away the pains of the sinews and the cramp". Venus also rules the procreative spirit, which resides in the testes of men and in the womb and the ovaries of women. It is the spirit behind the energy of reproduction and produces in us the desire to procreate. It is warm and moist in character and when fertility is compromised by cold conditions, mugwort can provide the warmth to reinvigorate its activity. The procreative spirit is strengthened by Venus and the herbs that work in sympathy with her, whilst it is diminished and dulled by the cold drying effect of Saturn and the earth humour, and weakened by Mars and the choleric or fire humour.

Its warming effects make it useful in colds and chills, and its diaphoretic action makes it useful in fevers, enabling a good sweat to be produced, thus breaking the fever cycle.

Mythos

Mugwort is known in Christian folklore as one of the "St John's worts" because it flowers around the time of the feast of John the Baptist, the 24th of June. It was one of the herbs burnt on the midsummer fires to bring protection and cleansing. It was gathered along with other flowers, such as elecampagne, yarrow, and St John's wort herb to make bunches that were used in the festivals around assumption day, the 15th of August. These bunches were consecrated in church and then hung up in the rafters to afford the house protection from demonic forces, and to provide health and wellbeing for the body and soul. Throughout Europe mugwort's special protective powers against spells, demons, lightning, and plagues was well known, and it was known throughout Europe as mater herbarum—mother of herbs.

The Latin name comes from Artemis, the Greek goddess who at her own birth helped to deliver her twin, Apollo the sun god, leading to her becoming the goddess of childbirth, whilst she remained chaste and childless herself. She is the protectress of nature and is the nurturing goddess of fertility. Venus, mugwort's ruling planet, promotes love, romance, dreams, the flow of emotions, and is the embodiment of the water or phlegmatic humour.

The compacted down from the underside of the leaves of mugwort make a traditional incense used in Chinese medicine called moxa. It is burnt in small cones placed over acupuncture points in which a blockage has been detected. It is seen to have a dissolving effect on these blockages and their removal allows the "Chi" to once again flow unhindered along the meridian channels.

Emotional

Mugwort is protective and strengthening, a wash made with the fresh leaves and rubbed into the limbs will clear any feelings of negative contamination. It has always been considered an important dreaming herb, sleeping with a sprig under the pillow will help give dreams of direction and clarity. It can be used as a night time tea with valerian root and rose petals. It makes a protective and cleansing herbal bath and steam especially if one feels overcome by the negativity of others, like using moxa, it will help to disperse lingering and difficult emotions and stuck energy.

Gynaecology

In the French Salernitan herbal, written in the 12th Century,[1] mugwort is recommended to counter sterility caused by dampness, but warns that if the problem is due to dryness it will worsen the condition. The herbal advises using a hot compress of the leaves over the area of the womb, a treatment that was also suggested a thousand years previous by Dioscorides. Massaging with the oil or using a decoction in the bath with the addition of bay leaves, was also recommended. Infertility in women may sometimes be caused by congestion of the fallopian tubes, a condition considered to be one of cold damp congestion. Other conditions where there is thought to be an element of dampness or congestion affecting the reproductive system, such as polycystic ovarian syndrome and endometriosis, can also benefit from its use as a tea, or combined with other herbs such as motherwort and yarrow as a tonic medicine.

It has also traditionally been used in French folk medicine as a strong infusion (30 g to ½ litre) to help with period pain, and it works well in this case combined with chamomile flowers. As an emenagogue it may well help with light and scant periods. Combined with pennyroyal it can help with a stalled labour, and was very likely to have been used as a traditional birthing herb.

Head

Mugwort has been traditionally valued in palsy, fits, and epilepsy. Gerard says "Mugwort cureth the shakings of the joints inclining to palsy" (Gerard 1636).[2] This may well be referring to it being helpful in tremors. The head and the animal spirit, which resides in the brain, are often prone to cold obstructions, these can interfere with the flow of the animal or "animating" spirit to the muscles to produce movements, thus causing weakness, tremors, and paralysis of limbs. The warming aromatic nature of mugwort enlivens the mind and the animal spirit, enabling the messages to once again flow unhindered.

Stomach

Mugwort is a warming aromatic bitter herb capable of stimulating the appetite and helping to ease bloating and wind. It has a long tradition of being used alongside wormwood as an antiparasitic herb.

Doses

Tea

The herb can be taken as a tea, 2–3 g twice daily.

Tincture

1:3 2–5 ml twice daily.

Medicinal infusion for period pain

15 g to 500 ml, drunk over 24 hours.

Myrrh

Sanskrit: Bola. Daindhava

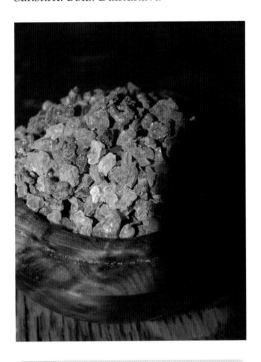

Latin:	*Commiphora molmol*
Family:	Burseraceae
Element	Fire
Planet	Mars
Humour	Choleric
Quality	Warm in the first degree, dry in the second. Resists poisons, opens, cleanses, and expels damp congestion, moves stagnant blood.

Organs

Stomach
Liver
Heart
Lungs
Womb

Actions

Digestive tonic
Stimulant
Expectorant
Antispasmodic
Healing, astringent
Antiseptic
Emenagogue
Anti-inflammatory
Antithrombotic
Antifungal
Vulnery

Constituents

Volatile oils, furanosesquiterpenes, heerabolene, eugenol
Bitters
Resins, commiphoric acid
Gum

Traditional uses and humoral influences

A cooling, bitter astringent herb. In Arabic "murr" is the word for bitter. In Ayuvedic medicine, it is considered to clear impurities in the blood, heart, and uterus and to strengthen the heart, clear coughs, digest toxins, and cure diseases originating in the blood. It clears impurities from the blood and clears stagnation in tissues and organs. Mars rules the hot part of the blood, which is needed to thin the blood to enable it to move through the smaller vessels. The cooling action of Myrrh comes from its cutting and cleansing action helping to allow heat to be moved and dispersed.

Traditionally it is used in sacred incense, and for embalming by the ancient Egyptians. It is currently considered to be a powerful lymphatic tonic, increasing the number of white blood cells. It is a prime remedy for inflammation of the throat, mouth, gums, and for mouth ulcers.

It is extremely helpful in the treatment of external ulcers, boils, and wounds. It staunches bleeding and can be used as a first aid remedy directly on cuts to disinfect and stop bleeding, either the 90% tincture or a weaker 20% tincture can be used or the powdered resin may be used directly.

It is able to clear phlegm from the lungs and helps with sinusitis and inflammation of the ears, nose, and throat. The resin itself can be used orally to reduce pain and swelling in the throat and will clear up chronic inflammation of the tonsils. The resin can be used in this way or as a mouth wash to treat gingivitis, tooth abscesses, and gum disease. It is considered helpful for breaking down the stagnation when blood pools, especially in the lower abdomen and in the uterus and reproductive organs, it has a gentle emmenagogic action helping in amenorrhoea.

Its antimicrobial components are active against herpes infections, including chickenpox, cold sores, and herpes, and it is very beneficial for intestinal infection and reducing parasitic infections. There is also evidence of anti-mutagenic properties (Williamson, 2003).[1]

Doses

Tincture

The tincture or essential oil can be applied directly externally. The tincture being either made in 90% alcohol or 25% alcohol are both effective to treat open cuts, grazes, wounds, and ulcers.

Mouth wash or gargle

Can be made by dissolving the resin in hot water, or by diluting 5 ml of the tincture in a glass of water.

Nettle

Common nettle. Stinging nettle.

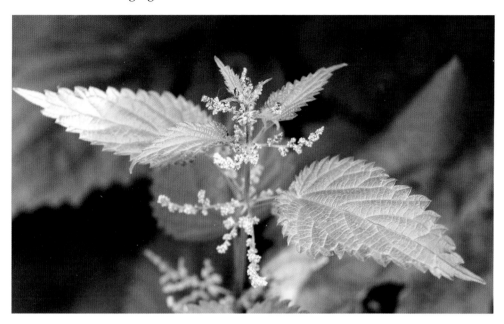

| Latin: | *Urtica urens/dioca* |
| Family: | Urticaceae |

Element	Fire
Planet	Mars
Humour	Choleric
Quality	Hot and dry in the third degree, heats the lungs, kidneys, bladder, and womb. It is opening, astringent, diuretic, and dissolves stones

Organs

Lungs
Kidneys
Womb
Skin
Joints

Actions

Anti-inflammatory
Astringent
Antiallergenic
Diuretic
Antilithic
Blood cleansing

Constituents

Flavonoids
Triterpenes
Lectins, lignans
Glycoprotein
Indoles: serotonin, histamine
Vitamin C, iron

Traditional uses and humoral influences

Nettles are ruled by Mars and are hot and dry in the third degree. They are opening, cleansing, and astringent, and clear phlegm, dampness, and cold melancholic blockages from the blood and the organs. Nicholas Culpeper says:

"This is also an herb Mars claims dominion over. You know Mars is hot and dry, and you know as well that winter is cold and moist; then you know the reason why nettle tops eaten in the spring consume the phlegmatic superfluities in the body of man, that the coldness and moistness of winter hath left behind."

Nettles are cleansing and activating, their diuretic effect complements the traditional blood purifying properties, ensuring that the waste products released into the blood are then flushed out through the kidneys. They are high in trace elements including iron, and their use as a traditional spring tonic was customary in all country areas, reflected in the old country saying:

"If they'd eat nettles in March,
And Mugwort in May,
So many fine maidens,
Wouldn't go to the clay"
(De Cleene & Lejeune, 1999)[1]

Nettle's strong martian energy helps them to stimulate phlegmatic temperaments into action, and as the brain is also cold and moist in temperament, they can help to clear mental lassitude, indecision, and confusion. I have found that taking a juice or infusion of the tops to be a perfect herbal antidote for patients suffering from "chemotherapy brain". When there is an excess of either heat (choleric humour) or cold and wet (phlegmatic humour), diuretics are used to expel the excess from the body, and we find nettle being used to clear hot inflammatory conditions as well as cold congestive conditions. It has always been a valued country medicine with Hilda Leyel, the founder of the Society of Herbalists, in 1927 proclaiming; "No plant is more useful in domestic medicine!" (Bartrum, 1995).[2] Indications for its use include gout, fevers, fatigue, and debility. The tea or fresh juice would be taken at the onset of a fever, to help cleanse the body. The infusion, tincture, and fresh juice is considered helpful to stop bleeding, both externally in cuts or haemorrhages, as well as internally, both from the lungs when there is coughing of blood or in the bowels when there is blood in the stool and diarrhoea.

Nettle seeds were considered an antidote for the bites of snakes, dogs, and scorpions, while flailing the skin with nettles was considered helpful for gout, sciatica, and rheumatism. It is said that the Romans introduced a variety of nettle called *Urtica pilulifera*, and in the work "Britannica" published in 1586 the historian William Camden wrote; "The soldiers brought some of the nettle seed with them, and sowed it there for their use to rub and chafe their limbs, when through extreme cold they should be stiff or benumbed, having been told that the climate of Britain was so cold that it was not to be endured" (Grieve, 1931).[3] The variety they brought is said to be only found in the east of England. It has smooth leaves, globular flowers, and stings that are considerably more painful than the common nettle. For pain relief it was a common country remedy to strike the areas with fresh nettles, and this was recorded being used up until fairly recent times as a cure for rheumatism. It was considered aphrodisiac, and the leaves were said to stimulate desire if applied to the genitals, especially for women.

Mythos

The common name of the nettle is thought to be derived from the Anglo Saxon word "noedl", meaning needle, it shares an ancient indo European root, "ne", a verb meaning to bind, sew, or spin. This may well be in relation to its usefulness as a fibre for weaving. Nettle can be woven to make material as rough as sacking or as fine as silk, and in the early 1900s there was much exploration of its potential as a crop rivalling cotton. The early Germanic peoples dedicated the nettle to Thor or Donar, the gods of thunder, fertility, and marriage, and it was a common belief that nettles would keep lightning away. Pliny the Elder (77AD) wrote that many regarded the nettle as a sacred plant, which was eaten to remain in good health all year round. Similar to other plants with stings, thorns, and prickles, nettles have been eaten as remedies against demons. In the Flemish herbal of 1554, Rembert Dodoens says:

"He who has nettles on him, together with a few leaves of cinquefoil (*Potentilla reptans*), will be free of all spirits and apparitions which frighten man; for they take away all fear from man, as we are assured by some".[4]

It was common to use, jump over, or to hang nettles over thresholds on various saints days throughout Europe as protection against evil and bad fortune.

Witches were said to use nettles in their potions, and they were said to grow at the crossroads where witches would meet.

Emotional

Nettles restore and re-awaken a tired and despondent mind and spirit. They clear confusion and help in overcoming indecision, having a refreshing and uplifting effect on the whole body. They help to embolden us when our boundaries are being disregarded by others and restore a sense of self worth when we are suffering from self doubt.

Lungs

Nettle is antiasthmatic, Mrs Grieve says "The juice of the leaves, mixed with honey will relieve bronchial and asthmatic troubles, and the dried leaves burnt and inhaled will have the same effect". Asthma is considered a cold condition of the lungs, so the hot cutting effect of nettle is helpful to clear the damp cold congestion.

Skin

Nettle tea has always been a well known remedy for eczema, urticarial, and all minor skin maladies. In William Fernie's Herbal Simples published in 1897, a wash or tincture of fresh nettle is recommended for burns, by applying on wet cloths, diluting the tincture with an equal amount of water.

Kidneys

As a powerful but gentle diuretic, nettle leaf, seed, and root are all used.

Traditionally nettle is used to help reduce the formation of kidney stones and to dissolve them when present. This has always been considered part of the reason that it is such an effective blood purifier and spring tonic herb. Research reported to me by the herbalist David Winston that he undertook at his clinic in America, has shown that nettle seed tincture may be helpful in low or failing kidney function. It has been suggested in recent times that the root may be useful in benign prostate enlargement.

Joints

There is a long tradition of the fresh herb being used for rheumatic complaints, especially as a country remedy used in the spring. It is also helpful for gout and arthritis, drunk as a tea, a fresh tincture, or fresh juice. From personal experience the fresh juice can be an effective treatment for rheumatoid arthritis as well as helping the pain of osteoarthritis. It is believed that nettle is able to dissolve the uric acid crystals and other deposits that build up in joints triggering inflammatory pain.

Doses

Tea

Maria Trebben, in Health Through God's Pharmacy (1980),[5] recommends drinking three cups of tea a day made from fresh nettles for the first 4 weeks of the spring.

The tea can also be made with 3–5 g of dried herb to a cup.

Fresh Juice

20 ml, up to 3 times daily.

Tincture

5 ml 1–3 times a day.
A useful infusion recipe for gout is:

Nettle	15 g
Couch grass	10 g
Fennel	15 g
Peppermint	10 g
Elderflowers	10 g

Drink 15 g of the mixture a day.

Plantain

Common plantain. Broad leaved plantain. Waybroad. San-Lus. Ploughman's wound-wort. Psyllium
Welsh: Llydan y Ffordd

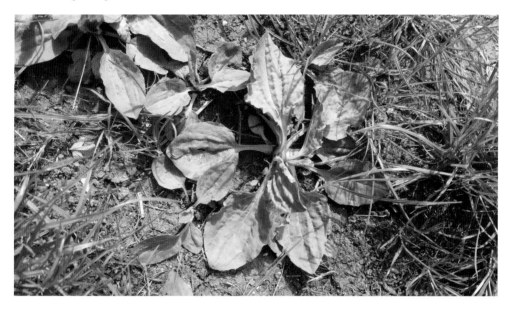

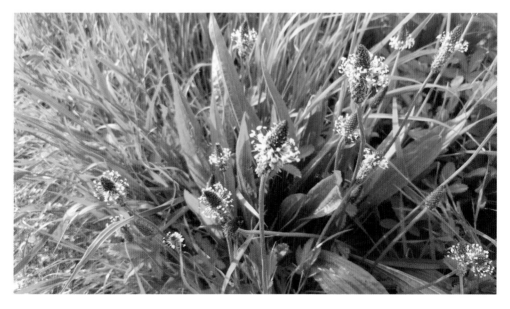

Latin: *Plantago major, Plantago lanceolata, Plantago ovata*
Family: Plantaginaceae

Element   Water
Planet   Venus
Humour   Phlegmatic
Quality   Cold and dry in the second degree, cools head, lungs, bowels and kidneys. Cleansing, astringent, glutinating

Organs

Head
Lungs
Stomach, bowels
Kidneys
Womb
Skin

Actions

Astringent, drying
Anti-inflammatory
Healing
Diuretic
Antimicrobial
Anticatarrhal

Constituents

Iridoids: aucubin, asperuloside, verbenalin
Phenylethanoids
Flavonoids: luteolin, apigenin
Triterpenes based on oleanolic and ursolic acids
Mucilage, tannins, polysaccharides,
Fatty acids, zinc, potassium, silicon

Traditional uses and humoral influences

Both the broad-leafed and narrow-leafed plantain have very similar properties and indications. Culpeper says;

"It is under the command of Venus, and cures the head by antipathy to Mars, and the privities by sympathy to Venus; neither is there hardly a Martial disease but that it cures". Martial diseases are conditions of heat, including fevers, inflammations, and all diseases of choler, such as carbuncles, shingles, anger, and sudden pain. Mars is antipathetic to the kidneys and bladder, causing inflammation, pain, and blockage and is also antipathetic to the cool temperament of the brain causing frenzy, fury, and hot migraines.

With its cooling and drying actions, plantain cleanses and clears heat, and with its softening or glutinating action it soothes, protects, and tonifies mucous membranes throughout the body. This means it has been used to treat all mucous containing passages including the sinuses, lungs, intestines, urinary, and the reproductive passages. Culpeper says: "The juice of the plantain clarified and drunk for divers days together, … prevails wonderfully against all torments or excoriations of the bowels, helps the distillations of rheum from the head, and stays all manner of fluxes, even women's courses, when they flow too abundantly".

Plantain is anti-inflammatory and immune protective, helping to reduce allergic reactions both externally and internally. Its drying properties mean that it helps to reduce bleeding, both externally and internally. It has particularly been held in high regard for the coughing up of blood and for helping with lung conditions in general. Of its drying properties Culpeper says; "It is good to stay spitting of blood and other bleedings at the mouth, or the making of foul and bloody water, by reason of any ulcers in the reins or bladder, and also stays the too free bleeding of wounds".

Emotional

Calming and centring, plantain gives a sense of being nourished and supported, promoting a feeling of well being. It helps when feeling overextended and dispersed, enabling one to feel rooted and connected with where one stands in the world. It reduces feelings of agitation and impatience, helping us to release tension and anxiety.

Mythos

One of the nine sacred herbs mentioned in the Anglo Saxon Lacnunga, plantain has been praised since ancient times as a potent healing plant. Its Scottish Gaelic name San-Lus, means "all heal". Pliny (23–79 AD) states on "high authority" that if "it be put into a pot where many pieces of flesh are boiling it will sodden them together".[1]

The name comes from the Latin word for foot, planta, as it is able to both withstand being walked on and tends to flourish on paths and tracks. In the new world, as the seeds were spread with the colonists, it appeared where they had walked and was given the name white man's footprint. When the leaves are opened up there are long elastic sinews within them, this is said to be a sign according to the doctrine of signatures that it would strengthen sinews and bring

back their suppleness. It was considered by the Native Americans to be a specific cure for snake bites, and the Chippewa tribe would carry the root with them as a charm against being bitten.

Head

When conditions of heat (particularly in fevers and respiratory infections), cause hot vapours to rise up from the body, as they encounter the cool temperament of the head, they condense and produce catarrh and excess mucus, called "distillations of rheum" by Culpeper. He also says, "The juice mixed with oil of roses, and the temples and forehead anointed therewith, eases the pains of the head proceeding from heat, and helps lunatic persons very much".

Lungs

According to Culpeper, "It is held an especial remedy for those that are troubled with the phthisic, or consumption of the lungs, or ulcers of the lungs, or coughs that come from heat".

Plantain is a very helpful remedy for excess mucus anywhere in the respiratory system, from the lungs to the sinuses. It therefore helps in allergies and other conditions that cause rhinitis, coughs, and swelling or pain of the nasal passages, and is a valuable remedy for chronic weakness of the lungs.

Stomach and bowels

It was common to recommend the root for treating complaints of the bowels. However, an infusion of the leaves also works well; a traditional remedy to treat diarrhoea and piles is to use one ounce of dried leaves to a pint of boiling water, leave to cool for twenty minutes then drink in wineglass-full doses three or four times a day. In the same way that Culpeper recommended its use for "excoriations" of the bowels, plantain has continued to be used for treating peptic ulcers, colitis, and is likely to be helpful in most inflammatory bowel diseases. The seeds of *Plantago ovata*, also known as psyllium seeds, are very beneficial for inflammatory bowel disease, irritable bowel, and diverticulitis; a desert spoonful soaked in water should be taken three times a day after meals.

Kidneys

With its soothing and anti-inflammatory actions, plantain is a helpful remedy for urinary pain, inflammation, infections, and chronic cases of instial cystitis. It is safe to use over long periods and can be combined with other urinary remedies, such as couch grass, cleavers, shepherd's purse, and horsetail.

Womb

Its association with the planet Venus indicates the traditional use of the herb for complaints of the reproductive system. Culpeper recommends it for excess menstruation and any conditions associated with heat and dryness. This could include conditions such as endometriosis and ovarian and uterine pain associated with inflammatory conditions.

Externally

The wash, juice, or an ointment made from the leaves is particularly good at healing inflammations, cuts, or ulcers. The leaves crushed into a paste and applied in a poultice will help in chronic ulcers, especially varicose ulcers of the legs. I had a diabetic patient who enjoyed gardening but was often getting small cuts on her legs that would ulcerate. She always kept a patch of plantain growing in the garden and found that simply applying a leaf to the wound or ulcer would quickly heal it up.

Doses

Infusion

2–4 g three times daily.
    Medicinal strength: 15 g of herbs infusion infused in 500 ml per day.

Tincture

5 ml three times a day.

Anti allergy and catarrh tea

Equal parts of elderflower, lime blossom, chamomile, thyme, and plantain.

Rose

Rose. Red rose. Damask rose. White rose. Apothecary's rose. Field rose. Dog rose. Sweet briar. Wild rose

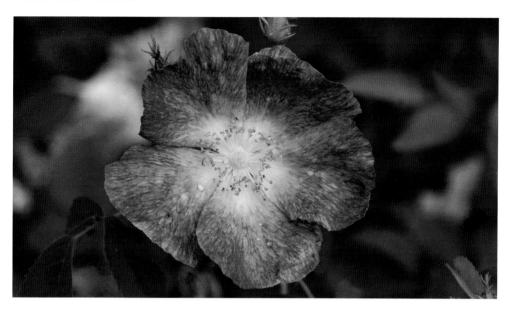

Latin:	*Rosa damscena, Rosa gallica, Rosa centifolia*
Family:	Rosaceae
Element	Damask rose: Water Red roses: Air
Planet	Damask rose: Venus and moon. Red rose: Jupiter
Humour	Damask rose: Phlegmatic Red roses: Sanguine
Quality	Cooling in the first degree, drying in the first or second, clears heat, strengthens, and consolidates.

Organs

Head
Heart
Lungs
Stomach
Liver
Womb

Actions

Anti-inflammatory
Astringent
Stops bleeding
Antidiarrhoeal
Sedative
Euphoric

Constituents

Volatile oils (ninety-five compounds
    identified)
Phenols: tannins, gallic acid
Flavonoids: quercertin, rutin,
    kaempferol, myricetin
Anthocyanins

Traditional uses and humoral influences

Nicholas Culpeper tells us; "Red roses
are under Jupiter, Damask under Venus,
white under the Moon … The white and
red roses are cooling and drying and yet
the white is taken to exceed the red in
both the properties, but is seldom used
inwardly in any medicine".

Roses have been in use as medicine
since the earliest of times, with evidence that roses were being cultivated in
Sumaria and China over 5000 years ago.
The ancient Greek herbalist Dioscorides
tells us that they cool and contract. Culpeper agreed with this 2000 years later,
stating that they "mitigate the pains
that arise from heat, assuage inflammations, procure rest and sleep". He went
on to say, "Red roses do strengthen the
heart, the stomach and the liver, and the
retentive faculty." The retentive faculty
resides in the spleen, it is the seat of the
melancholic humour, which is cold and
dry. Roses share this property, and will
therefore both help to reduce heat, and
with their drying action help to retain
nourishment in the body.

The twelfth century mystic Hildegard
Von Bingen, said that a person who is
"inclined to wrath" should make a "powder of sage and rose, less sage than rose,
and take as snuff, for the sage eases the
wrath, and the rose cheers" (Throop, 1998).[1]

The rose can be used in foods, as
tea, as distilled water, as tincture, in
baths and washes, and as a powder. It
is always soothing, cooling, calming,
and anti-inflammatory. Cold cream was
so named because it had rose water as
its main ingredient. Other external uses
include drying and healing wounds and
ulcers. The distilled water helps all hot
inflammations of the skin and eyes, and
can be freely used as a wash.

Mythos

From ancient times the rose has been
considered the first and foremost symbol
of love. It was dedicated to Aphrodite,
her son Eros, the three graces, Dionysus,
and Juventus, the god of eternal youth. It
is associated with fertility and the spring
and was used in all the ancient festivals,
especially those associated with love and
fertility, such as the feast of Hymen, the
god of marriage. There are many ancient
stories as to the genesis of the rose. One
myth says that like Aphrodite, the flowers arose out of the foam of the sea and
were originally white, but became red
when Eros, the god of love, accidentally
spilt some nectar on them while dancing. Another story recounts that when
Aphrodite's lover Adonis, was gored
by her husband Aries (who had transformed himself into a wild boar) her
tears became the first roses when they
fell on the ground and as the blood of
Adonis seeped into the earth the flowers
then turned red.

The five petals of wild roses were
considered by Aristotle to refer to the
constant and recurring cycle of the cosmos, which consists of five elements.
Along with the return of its blooms in

spring each year this made it a power-ful emblem of the cycles of rebirth and death, in fact Hecate the goddess of the underworlds was often depicted with a crown of five-petalled roses, and graves were strewn with the flowers and pet-als. In the nineteenth century it was still customary in Wales to place white roses on the grave of unmarried women repre-senting purity and chastity, and red roses on the graves of those noted for their kindness and generosity.

Emotional

There is no other plant that has the power of roses to uplift the spirits and release negativity and emotional dis-tress. It helps in states of grief, despair, and also anguish, cooling, and calming our emotions. It brings back a rosier view of the world when we feel overwhelmed by darkness and makes the spirit sing once again. It helps release tension and enables us to feel open and relaxed. For states of grief a combination of red or wild rose petals, hawthorn, and lemon balm works particularly well.

Head

From the earliest records of the ancient Greek herbalists, we find roses being recommended for headaches, ear aches, and sore eyes. It has always been said that rose will help to relieve all pains and afflictions of the head that come from heat. It was even considered that vinegar of roses applied to the temples would help headaches caused by too much sun. The brain has a cool wet phlegmatic temperament, which is why we still talk about needing to "chill out" when we are stressed and anxious, and we also think that we make better decisions when we are "cool, calm, and collected".

Rose helps us to let go of stress and to calm an agitated mind, clearing troubling thoughts and calming excessive mental activity. The seventeenth century, herb-alists Gerard, Parkinson, and Culpeper all considered roses helpful to "brin-geth sleep". The petals can be added to a herbal tea, or taken as a distilled water or tincture. A favourite combination that I often recommend for a sleep tea is vale-rian root, rose petal, and sage leaf.

Heart

The heart is the seat of the vital spirit, and the soul is said to reside within it. The vital spirit is a combination of innate heat and the radical moisture. The innate heat activates and energises the body, the organs, and the faculties, while the radical moisture provides lubrication enabling the heat to circulate. If inter-nal heat becomes too great it dries and scorches the organs causing burnt cho-ler or black bile to accumulate, leading to blockages and obstructions. As the heart is the seat of the emotions, when they become extreme or overheated they damage the heart and have a depressing effect on the vital spirit. Rose is one of the main antidotes to the damaging effects of excessive heat, and is considered one of the main cordial herbs, which calm, cool, and protect the heart. The strengthening effect of rose was also considered capa-ble of reducing the trembling or palpita-tions of the heart.

John Gerard in his herbal of 1597 summed up the properties of rose on the heart saying, "The distilled water of

Roses is good for the strengthening of the heart, and refreshing of the spirits, and likewise for all things that require a gentle cooling".[2] It was also recommended by Nicholas Culpeper that the decoction of red roses made with wine, with the roses left in, "is profitably applied to the region of the heart to ease the inflammation therein

It was a tradition when making a medicine that it should contain at least one constituent that will nourish the heart, as it is the seat of the divine spirit in the body. These additions to medicines would either be red in colour, associated with the sun, or have a particular affinity with the heart. Adding roses to any medicine is a good way of doing this, and always adds to its overall benefit.

Lungs

A syrup of roses or rose honey is very soothing for irritating coughs and a sore throat. Rose water can be combined with honey to make a very pleasant cough suppressant. Rosehip syrup helps coughs, bronchitis, and asthma. It is also antibacterial, rich in vitamin C, and anti-inflammatory bioflavonoids, it soothes and calms inflamed respiratory passages.

Liver and stomach

The whole rose flower including the stamens have a bitter quality, gently encouraging the digestive process, liver activity, and bile secretion. Culpeper said, "Red Roses do strengthen the heart, the stomach and the liver, and the retentive faculty … being dried they have then a binding and astringent quality". Rose is also gently astringent, calming and cooling for all of the digestive system, helping to stop diarrhoea and settle an upset stomach.

Doses

Rose petals can be added to tea mixes, or drunk on their own.

Tincture

The tincture can be made by steeping fresh rose petals in brandy. Then 5 ml taken 1–3 times daily.

Floral water

5–10 ml as needed.

Sleep tea

Rose petals	40 g	
Sage	40 g	160 g
Valerian root	80 g	

Rosemary

Polar plant. Compass weed. Coronaria. Rosa marinus

French: Incensier

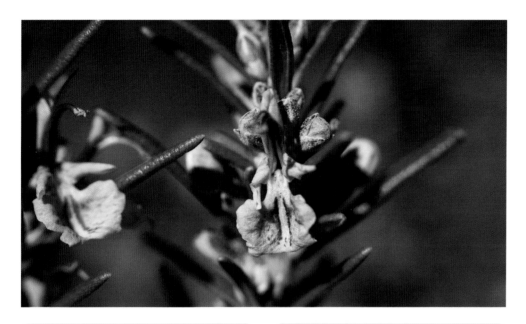

| Latin: | *Rosemarinus officinalis* |
| Family. | Laminaceae/labiatae (mint family) |

Element	Fire
Planet	Sun
Humour	Choleric
Quality	Hot and dry in the second degree, heats and dries the heart, head, stomach and liver, carminative, helps the memory

Organs

Heart
Brain
Liver
Spleen
Stomach

Joints
Womb

Constituents

Flavonoids: apigenin, diosmin
Rutin
Volatile oils: borneol, linlool, camphor
Polyphenols: rosmarinic acid, caffeic acid
Diterpenes, triterpenes

Actions

Anti-inflammatory
Antiseptic
Carminative
Stimulant
Antidepressant

Traditional uses and humoral influences

From a 1607 sermon by doctor of divinity, Roger Hacket.

"Speaking of the powers of Rosemary, it overtopeth all the flowers in the garden … it helpeth the brain, strengtheneth the memorie, and is very medicinable of the head. Another property of the Rosemary is, it effects the Heart. Let this Rosemarinus, this flower of men, ensigne your wisdom, love and loyaltie, be carried not only in your hands, but in your hearts and heads" (Grieve, 1931).[1]

Rosemary is ruled by the sun and is in Aries. It is hot and dry both in the second degree. Aries rules the head and all structures above the first vertebrae of the neck. As a traditional remedy it is used in headaches, and migraines, a tea being made from the fresh sprigs. A traditional combination would be to combine it with lavender. Its warming influence on the head corresponds with the ancient association of rosemary for remembrance, with the eyes also considered to be strengthened by it. As a country remedy it was commonly used for any kind of pain in the body. The stimulating and reviving effect on the vital spirits of the heart and the animal spirits of the brain mean that it is an uplifting herb, protecting against depression and low mood.

Rosemary was always the first port of call in country medicine for treating pain, especially if the pain was considered to be coming from a cold cause. Fresh sprigs of rosemary as an infusion was particularly recommended for headaches, rubs made from the oil were applied to aching muscles and joints, and rosemary baths were considered particularly good for relieving pain and reviving the spirits.

Mythos

Rosemary was traditionally burnt as an incense and left on the altars of Greek and Roman divinities. Used as an emblem of love, fidelity, and remembrance, and given to guests at both weddings and funerals. The name comes from the Latin "ros", meaning dew, and "marinus", meaning sea, alluding to it growing abundantly on Mediterranean coasts and having silvery undersides to its leaves, like dew being reflected in the sun. It was customary for women to make garlands and crowns from it, as it was often included as a symbol of love in songs of the medieval troubadours. It is a herb considered to be a powerful protection against pestilential fevers, which along with being an emblem of remembrance motivated the habit of giving mourners a sprig of rosemary in the belief that smelling it would be a powerful defence against any morbid "effluvia" from the corpse, which may carry disease.

The herb was burnt with juniper as incense in hospitals to clear disease, a practice said still to have been in use in France up until the early 1900s. In Spain and France it was traditionally considered a powerfully protective herb against witches and evil influences.

Emotional

Rosemary will bring back a clearer vision when we are feeling confused or unsure. The focus that it provides will help us to have a more open and generous attitude to ourselves and others. When we are feeling worn down by continual worry or sadness it is a wonderful herb to bring back a strong a sense of possibility, enabling us to once again face up to the challenges that have been over-whelming us.

Head

"The decoction of Rosemary in wine, helps cold distillations of rheums into the eyes, and other cold diseases of the head and brain, as the giddiness and swimmings therein, drowsiness, the dumb palsy, or loss of speech, the leth-argy, the falling sickness, to be both drank and the temples bathed there-with" (Culpeper).

It is traditionally used in head pain, especially those coming from a cold cause. Migraines in particular were often considered to be caused by an excessively cold brain, so the warming and activating effect of rosemary on the brain and circulation has always been considered very helpful. The brain has a cold and dry temperament and was described as containing an etheric wind, which moved with the animating spirit around the body, passing thoughts and sensations throughout the body and mind. In Galenic medicine, the back part of the brain is considered to be the area of memory and retention of ideas. As the retentive faculty throughout the body is ruled by the earth or melancholic humour, which is also cold in nature, any increase in cold is especially likely to obstruct the free movement of ideas out of the area of memory and therefore be responsible for dull wits and memory loss. The warmth of rosemary helps to activate the brain and the movement of memories, bringing them back into the forebrain and once again into the mind's eye.

Heart and circulation

The heart is ruled by the sun, and a solar herb like rosemary that has warming strong effects is particularly useful when the heart is weakened and has lost its innate heat and activity. If the innate heat weakens, it allows the watery side of the circulation to build up and overwhelm the arterial or fire aspect of the heart. This was considered to be the cause of dropsy or the swelling that occurs when the heart begins to fail. This can arise from physical weakness, old age, or the overwhelming effects of excess cold and dampness building in the body.

When the heart is weak rosemary will help to regulate the heart rate, improve palpitations and reduce arrhythmia, especially if the pulse is thin, deep, short, or slow. Rosemary sustains the spirits and improves blood flow both to and from the heart. It is considered a power-fully protective and strengthening herb when the heart is affected by cold mel-ancholic vapours and is one of the herbs that cherish and refresh the vital spirit. Nicholas Culpeper lists it as a strength-ening cordial herb along with balm, bor-age, citron peel, and spices in general.

The polyphenol rosmarinic acid has anti-inflammatory effects, it reduces spasm and has anticonvulsant effects on smooth and cardiac muscle. Inflam-mation is recognised as the triggering mechanism for the development of ath-erosclerosis and the cholesterol plaques that obstruct blood flow through arter-ies. It is therefore helpful for most cardiac complaints, including angina, arrhyth-mia, and cardiovascular disease in gen-eral. It reduces the formation of thrombi or clots in the vascular system and the flavonoid diosmin has been shown to be effective for reducing capillary fragility (Fisher, 2018).[2] When peripheral neuralgia is caused by poor circulation, rosemary hand and footbaths are an excellent remedy, even when the pains in the feet make them feel like the feet are burning, rather than feeling cold.

Stomach, liver and spleen

Rosemary is a warming herb that clears excess cold and phlegm from the stomach. It is useful when the appetite is poor and there is bitter belching and distension.

Nicholas Culpeper says;

"It is very comfortable to the stomach in all the cold maladies thereof; helps both the retention of meat, and the digestion, the decoction being taken in wine. It is a remedy for the windiness in the stomach, bowels, and spleen, and expels it powerfully. It helps those that are liver-grown, by opening the obstructions thereof".

The antispasmodic effects, alongside the gentle digestive stimulating effects of its bitter aspects, make it very helpful when the digestion is overloaded or weakened leading to bloating, colic, and cramps.

Hair loss

Rosemary has always been a traditional remedy for thinning hair and hair loss, used as a rinse made from fresh rosemary infusion, or by using the spirit of rosemary.

Doses

Tea

Rosemary tea may be made from infusing a sprig of fresh rosemary in a cup.

Dried herb 1–3 g infused in a cup, drunk up to 3 times a day.

Capsule

400 mg, 1–4 daily.

Tincture

1:3 25%: 5–10 ml, 1–3 times daily.

Baths

Use 50 g of dried herb, or ten 10 cm sprigs of fresh tops, infused in 1litre of hot water, leave to steep for ½ an hour then add to a full bath. Alternatively the liquid can be reheated and used as a footbath or hand bath for 10 minutes twice daily.

Sage

Garden Sage. Red sage. Broad leaved Sage. White Sage. Salvia salvatrix

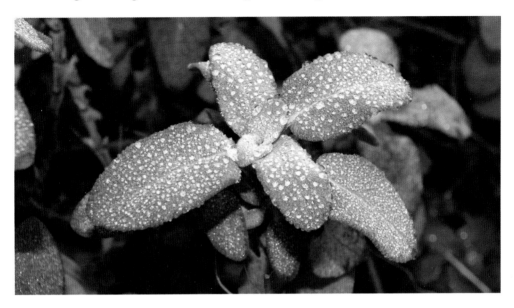

Latin:	*Salvia officinalis*
Family:	Lamiaceae/Labiatae
Element	Air
Planet	Jupiter
Humour	Sanguine
Quality	Hot and dry in the second degree, heats the head, stomach, liver, spleen, womb, and joints, is astringent, diuretic, and an emenogogue

Organs

Head
Stomach
Throat
Lungs
Liver
Spleen
Womb

Actions

Digestive tonic
Carminative
Diuretic
Relaxant
Antiseptic
Astringent
Antispasmodic
Anti-inflammatory

Constituents

Volatile oils: thujone, camphor, cineole
Terpenes: ursolic and oleanolic acids
Diterpenes
Phenolic acids: rosmarinic, caffeic, and gallic acid
Tannins
Flavonoids: apigenin and luteolin

Traditional uses and humoral influences

Sage is ruled by Jupiter and is hot and dry in the second degree, astringent, diuretic, and warms the head, liver, stomach, spleen and joints. In Culpeper we read: "Matthiolus saith, it is very profitable for all manner of pains in the head coming of cold and rheumatic humours: as also pains of the joints, whether inwardly or outwardly, and therefore helps the falling sickness, the lethargy, such as are dull and heavy of spirit, the palsy, and is of much use in all defluxions of rheum from the head, and for diseases of the chest or breast".

The word "rheumatic" in this case refers to excessive water and dampness overwhelming the humours and organs, causing stagnation and blockage, manifesting in catarrh, phlegm, swellings, and stiffness of joints.

Nicholas Culpeper also tells us that sage is "good for the liver and to Breed blood". This belief was so prevalent that we find Maurice Messegue three centuries later advising, "It is contra indicated for people of a Sanguine temperament: outgoing, red faced etc. It can only increase their fullness of blood. Rather it is indicated for bilious people, for melancholy people, for apathetic people. It can set them up".[1]

The liver and spleen are warmed and cleansed by the stimulating action of sage. The spleen is the seat of the earth or melancholic humour, making it prone to becoming blocked with the cold dry build up of melancholic humours. This build up of melancholy leads to cold vapours rising up and overwhelming the heart, blocking the flow of vital spirit around the body. Without the vital spirit stimulating the activity of all the organs, the body feels lethargic and feelings of sadness, fearfulness, and depression arise. Sage clears congestion, removes stasis in the liver and other organs, and clears damp from the system wherever it arises.

A medieval name for the plant is "salvia salvatrix" meaning "sage the saviour", as it was thought to protect against pestilence and plague. In recent times the essential oil has been shown to be anti-mutagenic, and the rosmarinic acid it contains is anti-inflammatory, antiviral, antibacterial, and antioxidant.

Mythos

> "He that would live for aye, must eat sage in May."—English saying (De Cleene & Lejeune, 1999)[2]

The name of the Genus, *Salvia* derives from the Latin "salvere", meaning to be saved. The traditional beliefs in its healing properties are reflected in the Latin saying; "Cur moriatur homo cui salvia cresit in horto?"—Why should a man die whilst sage grows in his garden?

As a country remedy for ague (fevers) it was customary in Sussex to chew fresh sage leaves for nine consecutive mornings while fasting. In the Jura region of France, sage is used to mitigate grief, and this belief seems to have been common in England as well, with Samuel Pepys saying, "Between Gosport and Southampton we observed a little churchyard where it was customary to sow all the graves with Sage".[3]

Emotional

When we are feeling burdened down by difficult emotional states that we can't release, sage will bring back a sense of lightness. Its calming effects gently infuse themselves into the heart and the mind, restoring a sense of everything being back in its right place. It clears the mind, giving us a brighter vision of what we are having to face, enabling us to emerge from under the cloud of dark and depressive thoughts. It will help us to have a more restful sleep, enabling us to wake free of anxious thoughts and with renewed vigour.

Head

Jupiter not only rules the liver, but also the mid part of the brain, the part that was considered to be concerned with judgement and discernment. In the same way that the liver differentiates poisons from nutrients in food, and makes healthy blood, the mid part of the brain differentiates between unwholesome irrational thinking and rational correct thinking; in the same manner that the liver creates good blood the mid brain cultivates good ideas. Gerard says,

> "Sage is singularly good for the senses and memory, strengtheneth the sinews, restoreth health to those that have the palsy, and taketh away shakey trembling of the members".[4]

Its restorative actions on the nervous system have been praised throughout time; Maurice Messegue (1981) assures us that "They increase the circulation of the blood and are a wonderful help to the nervous system. I particularly recommend it for people who are under stress-whether the mental and nervous stress of academics and students studying for

examinations, or the stress of anaemic people, convalescents, neurasthenics, depressives".[5] Any issues of the nervous system coming from a cold cause may be helped by the warming effect of sage on the brain. Nervous weakness, impaired memory, depression, and poor concentration are all helped by sage. It has been shown that the flavonoids and diterpenes in sage reduce anxiety and induce relaxation via GABA binding activity. Extracts of the essential oil have been shown to reduce the breakdown of the neurotransmitter acetylcholine, the compound responsible for sending signals from nerves to muscles (Fisher, 2018).[6] Theoretically this could be the reason why sage may be so effective in increasing cognitive function, and as Gerard recommended, helpful for trembling and shaking.

Recent research has confirmed that sage improves mood as well as cognitive function, in a 4-month study it was also shown to improve cognitive function in Alzheimer's patients with no evidence of side effects (Fisher, 2018).[7] All of these effects were so aptly summarised by Nicholas Culpeper over three centuries ago; "Sage is of excellent use to help the memory, warming and quickening the senses". A treatment for headache from Hildegard von Bingen written in 1170: "If a depression conditioned by various fever attacks cause a person headaches, he should take mallow and twice that amount of sage, crush these into a pulp in a mortar and pour a bit of olive oil on it. If he has no oil, a little vinegar will do. He should then apply it over the skull from the forehead to the neck and wrap a cloth over it. He should do this for three days. During these three days he should add fresh olive oil or fresh vinegar in the evening and continue this until he gets better. For mallow juice releases the bile; however, the sap of the sage dries it up, the olive oil anoints the afflicted head, and the vinegar draws out the bitterness from the bile" (Throop, 1998).[8]

Stomach

The gentle bitter taste of sage improves digestive function, with the antiseptic properties helping to eliminate pathogenic organisms, such as *E coli*, and *Helicobacter pylori*. This makes it useful in gastroenteritis, indigestion, colic, wind, and diarrhoea. The tea can be drunk throughout the day or taken in smaller strong doses as a tincture.

Antiseptic

Its powerful antimicrobial actions make it helpful externally as well as internally, gargles work well for gingivitis and sore throats, and washes help with cuts, wounds, and ulcers.

Gynaecological

It will help to dry up breast milk after lactation and reduces hot flushes and night sweats. It can help with hormonal balance, tending to strengthen and increase menstruation when light or absent. It is an effective uterine and ovarian tonic, especially in cases of pelvic congestion, and reduces vaginal discharge.

Doses

Tincture

1:3, 5 ml, three times a day.

Wine

From Maurice Messegue (1981)[9]:

"As a fortifying agent, a restorative: put 2 handfuls into a bowl, add a litre (1 ¾ pints) of boiling red wine; let it infuse for a quarter of an hour; strain; sweeten to taste. (A glassful at meals and before going to bed.)".

Tea

Sage tea is traditionally made with 30 g dried herb to 500 ml boiling water. It can also be drank as a simple tisane with a teaspoon (3 g) to a cup.

The "old-fashioned" recipe from M. Grieve's herbal for sage tea:

"Half an ounce (15 g) of fresh sage leaves, one ounce (30 g) of Sugar, the juice of one lemon, or a quarter ounce (7 g) of grated rind, are infused in a quart (2 pints/1136 ml) of boiling water and strained off after an hour".

Sleep tea

Valerian root: 2 parts,
Sage leaf: 1 part,
Rose petals: 1 part,
Infuse 1–2 large teaspoonfuls for 10–15 minutes, drink in evening.

Hormonal balance tea

Equal parts of:
Sage leaf, chamomile flowers, rose petals, red clover flowers.
Drink 2–3 cups daily, 1 heaped teaspoonful per cup.

St John's wort

Balm of warrior. Rosin rose. Touch-and-heal
French: Fleur de Notre-Dame

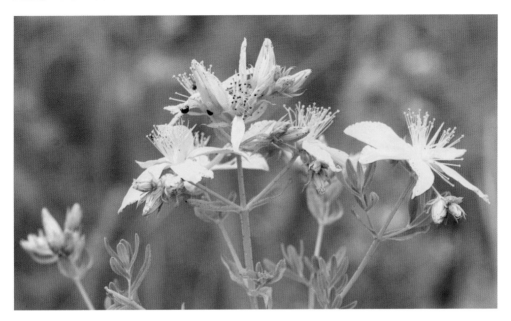

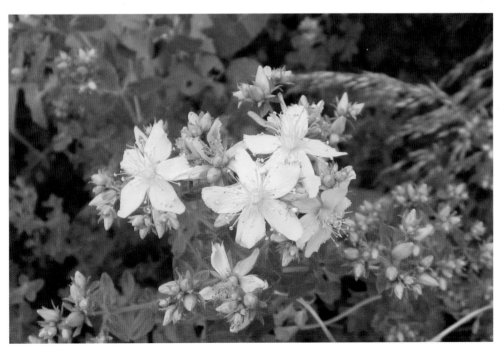

Latin: *Hypericum perforatum*
Family: Cluciaceae

Element   Fire
Planet   Sun
Humour   Choleric/vital spirit
Quality   Warm and dry in the
            first degree, expels cold,
            strengthens the spirits,
            warms and dissolves
            swellings, and loosens
            thick or congealed phlegm

Organs

Heart
Liver, Blood
Stomach
Brain, Nerves
Bladder, Womb

Actions

Warming
Cleansing
Anti-inflammatory
Anti-heamorrhagic
Antimicrobial to both viruses and
    bacteria
Antiseptic
Anxiolytic
Antidepressant
Cancer protective

Constituents

Essential oils
Flavonoids: hyperoside, rutin,
    quercetin
Naphthodianthrones: hypericins
Volatile oils, tannins

Phenols, serotonin, melatonin
Vitamins A, C, iron, calcium,
    magnesium, zinc, copper

Traditional uses and humoral influences

St John's wort is ruled by the sun and is under the astrological sign of Leo, the astrological sign that rules the heart and the stomach. St John's wort flowers on Midsummer's Day, and perfectly encapsulates the sun's vital essence. The sun is the source of life, its light and heat radiating out to all living beings, regenerating and sustaining them. In a similar way the heart is the source of innate heat and vital spirit in the body and is therefore likened to the sun of the body, or the "sol corporalis". It is the innate heat within the vital spirit that activates the various faculties of the body; the digestive, procreative, retentive, and expulsive faculties. The sun also rules the eyes and St John's wort is both helpful to use as an eye wash for inflammation but also for helping us to clarify our mental vision and focus.

It is considered the herb best able to protect the vital spirit from the congesting effects on the blood and the spirits of excess melancholy. The seat of melancholy is the spleen and when there is excess cold and dry melancholic humour accumulating in it, vapours rise up and overwhelm both the heart and the head, obstructing the flow of vital spirit and the dulling the senses. These cold melancholic vapours tend to block and obstruct the movement of innate heat, thus reducing the healthy activation of all the organs and bodily faculties.

It is a gentle warming herb, which is specific in drying excess phlegm in the stomach and the liver. When we have had excess heat or choler in the system as is the case with excess stress and severe sickness, then there is a residue called black bile or atribilis left behind. St John's wort is one of the prime remedies used to soften this black accumulation and enables the body to expel it. We can then use herbs that expel excess choler, such as feverfew to complete the return to normal.

Mythos

The red juice produced by squeezing the flowers was considered in Germany to be the blood of Balder, god of nature, summer, and light. When this tradition became Christianised it became St John who was associated with the plant, and thus the red pigment in the juice became known as the blood of St John. The botanical name comes from the Greek words "hyper" and "eikona", meaning above and image. This refers to the tradition of hanging the plant over sacred images and shrines as a protective offering, drawing on its ability to drive away evil and negativity. A similar belief was that if one sleeps with a sprig of St John's wort under the pillow on the 24th of June it will protect one from an untimely death in the following year. To confer protection against lightning one should hang in the house or throw it on the roof on St John's day. Planting it in the four corners around a house or field would bring protection from any form of dark energy and putting a sprig under the pillow would ward off night mares. In his "Miscellanies" the English Antiquary, natural philosopher and author wrote; "A house (or chamber) somewhere in London was haunted; the curtains would be rashed at night, and awake the Gentleman that lay there. Henry Lawes to satisfied did lie with him, and the curtains were rashed so then; and the Gentleman grew lean and pale with the Frights. One Doctor gured the house of this disturbance ... the principal ingredient was Hypericon or St Johns wort put under his pillow" (De Cleene & Lejeune, 1999).[1]

It has a long tradition of being a female herb, with it being known in many European countries as one of the ladies' bedstraws, indicating that it was thought to be a helpful herb for improving fertility and treating uterine or menstrual problems. In France one of its common names is "Fleur de Notre Dame"—our ladies flower.

It was the emblematic herb of the Knights Templars during the crusades, both alluding to the fact that they were also called the Knights of St John and that the plant was considered to be one of the most important "vulnerary", or wound-healing, herbs.

Emotional

There cannot be a better herb for helping us through difficult emotional situations. It gives us back a feeling of positivity and resilience, enabling us to brush aside all dark thoughts and feelings. When the brain becomes excessively affected by the cold restrictive and retentive effects of melancholy, we lose our ability to look forward and are cut off from exploring new possibilities. By clearing the melancholy, we help to once again sharpen the senses and open our mind to new ideas, enabling ourselves to look forward rather than become consumed by excessive or dark thoughts. In this way it is mentally clarifying and puts the world around us back into perspective. Its traditional use as a protective herb for sacred images points towards the protective nature of the herb for the sacred within us, the heart. It also helps to lift us emotionally as well as mentally, making us feel better as well as being able to think more positively.

Brain and nerves

It is a very helpful herb in states of sadness, depression, and low spirits, as well as being specific for breaking cycles of insomnia (Fisher, 2018).[2] A single dose of 5–10 ml St John's wort tincture in a little water before bed is very effective at correcting lost sleep patterns. A small regular dose of 10 ml a day of the tincture or juice will help to regenerate an exhausted nervous system and may be used over a period of months if necessary. It can be used to reduce the withdrawal effects from conventional antidepressants and isn't habit forming. It is considered to be a strengthener and healer of the nerves with the oil being used externally for damaged nerves, and the herb taken internally for conditions such as shingles, nerve pain, and palsy.

Formerly it was considered helpful for epilepsy. I have found that it calms nervous ticks and is very helpful in agitation and ADHD states. It is safe to give to children, up to 5 ml of tincture twice daily, or one to two capsules daily depending on age.

The forebrain is considered to be the place where we apprehended new ideas. This is the area that is considered to be most active and having the greatest heat and therefore is most connected to the sun energy and the plants that it rules. It is also the place where the mind opens and expands and is the traditional site of the third eye where the consciousness connects with and receives divine enlightenment. However, the brain was always considered to be susceptible to too much wind stirring the thinking process up and stopping the mind from remaining stable and able to make correct judgements. The mentally strengthening effect of St John's wort also enables the brain to focus when there is too much stimulation, either due to excessive thinking, mental overload, or hyper stimulation.

Bladder and urinary system

It is a general urinary tonic, it is helpful in all inflammatory conditions, chronic cystitis, urinary pain, urethritis, epididymitis, and traditionally also for bed-wetting.

Gynaecology

The herb is traditionally used to help regulate menstruation and to reduce excessive bleeding or menhorragia, as well as haemorrhage. Its ability to arrest haemorrhage makes it particularly helpful after giving birth, and it is useful in the menopause to ease mental distress, emotional swings, palpitations, and anxiety.

Skin and wounds

"It is a singular wound herb; boiled in wine and drank, it heals hurts or bruises; made into an ointment, it opens obstructions, dissolves swellings, and closes up the lips of wounds" (Culpeper, 1652).

It is very effective used as a fresh herb poultice applied to non-healing leg ulcers. I use the herb as a wash for burns and as a poultice for shingles and chicken pox. St John's wort oil, made by infusing the freshly collected flowers in olive oil takes on a bright red colour and was formerly known as the "blood of St John" (De Cleene & Lejeune, 1999)[3] it is very effective at healing wounds and treating burns. Combining the oil with marigold cream and lavender makes the all-round salve often also used in homeopathy called HyperCal.

It may cause a photosensitive rash if you go out in the sun when taking it internally, so avoid sunbathing as a precaution especially when you first start using it. In many years of prescribing it the only times I have seen skin reactions is when someone mistakenly took an excessive dose, and the severe itchy rash that ensued quickly subsided once they discontinued taking it. In the other case the patient went on a Mediterranean beach holiday the week after commencing treatment and a skin rash occurred, which also subsided quickly when the herb was discontinued.

Liver and stomach

"Two drams of the seed of St. John's Wort (4g approx) made into a powder, and drank in a little broth, doth gently expel choler or congealed blood in the stomach" (Culpeper).

This traditional use would have helped gastritis and other inflammatory conditions of the stomach and digestive system. I have found it very helpful for any inflammatory conditions of the gut, the bowels, and for gastritis, for which I usually prescribe it as a tea or juice.

St John's wort is an activator of liver function and stimulates the cytochrome P450 enzyme pathway in the liver. This is one of the major metabolic routes for clearing pharmaceutical drugs from the system, potentially weakening their effect, and therefore it is often labelled as being contraindicated when taking pharmaceutical drugs. However, it seems clear that although this is a potential risk, there are other many variables at play which means that often no interactions with pharmaceutical drugs are observed. To be safe it is wise to seek the advice of a qualified herbalist prior to taking *Hypericum* alongside other medications. In my practice I have not found interactions with St John's wort to be as significant as feared by pharmacists in general. However, this does confirm its ability for eliminating waste products and other accumulations, which may disrupt liver function. This supports its traditional use for gout and rheumatic pain and for clearing melancholy and other cold congealed blockages.

Cancer

Laboratory in vitro studies into St John's wort have shown it to be inhibitory to bladder cancer, prostate cancer, and leukaemia (Fisher, 2018).[4] Both hyperforin and hypericin have been shown to be active against a number of cancer cell lines and to be able to kill cancer cells. It has also been shown that the plant inhibits the CYP enzyme conversion of procarcinogens into their active forms.

Doses

Infusion

3–5 g a day

Capsule

1–2.5 g as a powder or in capsule form daily.

Tincture

5–10 ml of 1:3 daily.

Juice

10–20 ml of fresh juice daily.

Thyme

Mother of thyme. Running thyme

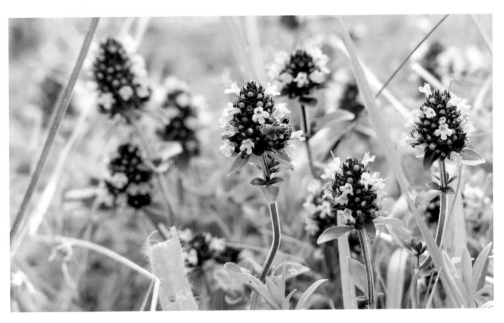

Latin:	*Thymus vulgaris*, *Thymus serpylum*
Family:	Lamiaceae
Element	Water
Planet	Venus
Humour	Phlegmatic
Quality	Hot and dry in the third degree. Heats the head, lungs, stomach, kidneys, bladder, and womb.

Actions

Antispasmodic
Expectorant
Anti-tussive
Carminative
Antiseptic
Astringent
Diuretic
Diaphoretic
Emenegogue
Anthelmintic

Organs

Lungs
Stomach
Kidneys
Womb
Head
Joints

Constituents

Volatile oils (1–2.5%)—up to 97 oils identified, including: thymol, carvacrol, thujene, camphor
Flavonoids: apigenin, luteolin.

Phenolic acids: caffeic, gentisic,
    p-coumaric.
Tannins
Vitamins: B complex, C, and E

Traditional uses and humoral influences

Thyme is ruled by Venus and is hot and dry in the third degree, giving it a sharp burning taste, with a cutting, cleansing action. It is a warming, diaphoretic herb that helps to cleanse any excess of humours, especially when they are the result of excess damp and cold conditions. Thyme's drying action is particularly helpful in cleansing the body of thin watery humours, such as catarrh and mucous, and to draw out and cleanse the body of the vapours that arise when there is a blockage leading to overheated organs. From the 1640 herbal by Parkinson we read; "Tyme … doth helpe somewhat to purge phlegm … the decoction is good for those that are troubled with shortnes or straightnesse of breath".[1]

Thyme's hot sharp cleansing action makes it helpful in all cold or congested conditions of any of the phlegmatic organs (lungs, kidneys, stomach, intestines, brain). In these phlegmatic organs coldness is prone to become excessive and to thicken the humours, blocking the flow of vitality, thus undermining the organs' function. The cutting and cleansing action of such a hot and penetrating herb purges and cleanses these cold blockages. Thyme is also capable of purging choler and any hot choleric swellings, such as gout.

The warmth of thyme increases vitality, especially after a period of weakness, and it is particularly helpful when used as a steam or as a bath. The warming effect of thyme is said by Culpeper to help a hardened spleen, which is seen as an indication of an excess of the cold dry melancholic humour. If the tongue is blue or purple, often with swollen sides, and the pulse is deep and slow, this is also a sign of excess melancholy and coldness blocking the movement of healthy blood and keeping it retained in the spleen. This kind of blockage causes the cold melancholic vapours to rise up from the spleen and overwhelm the heart and then also block the flow of the vital spirit. From this, melancholy, fearfulness, palpitations, breathlessness, and depression follow. Thyme's warming effect will draw out and soften the cold hardness of the spleen, purging the blood, enabling free movement and the transportation of the nutrients around the body.

Mythos

"I know a bank where the wild thyme blows, Where oxlips and the nodding violet grows, Quite over-canopied with luscious woodbine, With sweet musk-roses and with eglantine". (Shakespeare, 1564–1616)

From A Midsummer Night's Dream, Oberon, Act 2, Scene 1, describing the abode of the queen of the fairies.

It is said the name thyme is a derivative of the Greek word for fumigation, due to its pungent smell, and its traditional use as a herb burnt for cleansing. Alternatively, it may come from the Greek word "thumus", signifying courage—the plant being held in great regard in ancient and medieval days as a source of invigoration with its cordial heart strengthening qualities. It was said that the medieval ladies of the court would embroider a bee flying over a thyme flower on the scarves that they gave their knights to inspire courage.

Pliny tells us that when burnt it puts to flight all venomous creatures, and in ancient Greece to comment that someone had the "smell of thyme" was a way of admiring their elegance and style (De Cleene & Lejeune, 1999).[2]

Emotional

By clearing feelings of fearfulness, thyme is able to restore ones feeling of courage and hopefulness. It brings back a sense of joyfulness when the world seems to have lost its colour. It is helpful for depression that is associated with exhaustion, long-term sickness, and insomnia.

Stomach

Thyme is a gently bitter, warming, relaxing, carminative, and digestive herb. It is helpful for treating bloating and wind and for those with a weaker digestion. In Parkinson's herbal of 1640 he says that it "is of good use in meates and brothes, to warm and comfort the stomacke, and to helpe to breake wind as well for the sicke as the sound".[3] Its bitterness stimulates the secretion of bile acids, which help break down fats. Traditionally we find it added to heavy stews and to dishes with cheese and thick creamy sauces.

Lungs

Nicholas Culpeper said, "a noble strengthener of the lungs, as notable a one as grows, it purges the body of Phlegm and is an excellent remedy for shortness of breath". Thyme gently stimulates the movement of mucous up and out of the lungs, helping to clear and expectorate without irritation. Parkinson (1640) recommends that thyme should be "taken with hony, licoris and aniseede in wine, it helpeth a dry cough".[4] For asthmatics, drinking it regularly as a tea is helpful especially when combined with chamomile, elderflower, lime flower, and plantain.

It is particularly good as an inhalation for coughs, congested sinuses, and blocked ears; 30 g of equal parts thyme and chamomile flowers are brought to the boil in 1 ½ litres of water and then the steam inhaled for ten minutes. The inhalation can be re-used twice more before it loses its strength. Asthmatics should use the inhalation once or twice daily when they feel the chest tightening or becoming congested with phlegm. To treat a sore throat, use an infusion of 30 g dried herb to 500 ml of water, sweeten with honey and take in regular doses. If you have it growing fresh in the garden, chewing a sprig will both deaden the pain of a sore throat and disinfect the tonsils, adenoids, and sinuses. The levels of the hot antiseptic oils are highest in young plants and when the flowers are in full bloom.

Kidneys

Thyme is a warming kidney antiseptic, traditionally used to help clear kidney and urinary stones. If taken as a strong infusion it can quickly clear an attack of cystitis. To make this, 15 g may be infused overnight in a pint of hot water to get the best strength and it is then drank over the following day. Even a 20-minute steep-ing of the herbs will make an adequately strong medicine. When steeping the herb it is best done in a sealed vessel, so that none of the essential oils are lost.

Head and nerves

Thyme is a warming and stimulating herb for the head. The seventeenth century herbalist Gerard recommended it for headache, also for sciatica, presumably thinking of it using it as a rub on the limbs and back. While Culpeper suggested that; "if you make the vinegar of fresh thyme and anoint the head with it, it presently stops the pains thereof. It is excellently good to be given either in phrenzy and lethargy, although they are contrary diseases". His contemporary, Parkinson recommends applying the distilled water with the vinegar of Roses to the forehead to help with "the rage of frensye, & expeleth Vertigo that is the swimming or turning of the braine."[5]

The Austrian folk herbalist Maria Treben (1980) also considers it to be an excellent herb for the nerves and head. She suggests making a herb pillow from thyme, yarrow, and chamomile and using it for facial neuralgia. The pillow is warmed in a pan with a little water, and regularly applied to the affected part. She also suggests drinking 2 cups of thyme tea (one heaped teaspoon of dried herb to each cup) in regular sips throughout the day. In her herbal she also recommends rubbing weak limbs and the limbs of those with MS with thyme tincture and using a thyme bath for people who suffer nervous overstimulation or depressions. She also recommends this bath for nervous children who do not sleep well.[6]

I have also found that using the respiratory inhalation of thyme and chamomile before bed not only stops a persistent night time cough but also induces a deep restful sleep. The combined relaxant effects of the chamomile and the thyme enhance one another increasing the overall effectiveness of the inhalation when suffering from insomnia.

Joints

Thyme has often been applied externally to treat joint pain and swellings. It can be used as a poultice, added to the bath, or made into an aromatic massage oil. It contains many warming, anti-inflammatory volatile oils and was also considered helpful taken internally for inflammatory forms of arthritis, such as gout.

Gynaecology

It is a warming herb that helps to bring on a period when it is dragging on, with its anti-spasmodic action a strong infusion 30 g to 500 ml can be drunk for period pains, while also being used as a compress (a cloth is soaked in the infusion and applied to the abdomen with a hot water bottle placed on top).

In pregnancy, the tea can be used for a stalled labour, in a similar dose as above, and also to use as a bath by the mother after delivery, to ease pain, heal any tears, and restore energy.

Healing

I once treated a patient suffering with severe athlete's foot, he came to me when both feet had lost most of the skin, they were wet and raw. I gave him a footbath of thyme and marigold flowers and told him to steep the herbs with oats, then strain and use the liquid twice daily as a foot bath, within a week the feet were healing, and within three weeks the feet had a covering of completely normal healed skin again.

Doses

Tincture

1:3 5 ml 1–3 times daily.

Tea

One teaspoon to a cup, two cups daily.

Medicinal infusion

30 g to 1 pint, infuse overnight, drink in equal divided doses over 2 days.

Bath

Infuse 200 g herb in 1 litre, leave to stand until cool, add to bath.

Inhalation

10 g Thyme herb, 10 g Chamomile flowers, 5 g juniper berries, bring to boil in 2 pints of water steam for 10 minutes, once or twice daily. The mix may be reheated once or twice more.

Valerian

All heal. Setwall. Amantilla. Phu. Spikenard

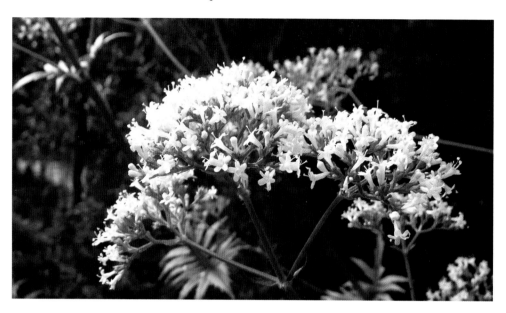

Latin:	*Valeriana officinalis*
Family:	Valerianaceae

Element	Ether
Planet	Mercury
Humour	Etheric/animal spirit
Quality	Hot in the first degree, dry in the second. Heats the heart, bowels, and head, astringent, diuretic, and emmenagogue.

Organs

Heart
Head
Bowels
Kidneys

Actions

Nervine
Sedative
Stimulant
Antispasmodic
Carminative
Hypotensive
Anodyne

Constituents

Volatile oil: valerenic acid, eugenol
Iridoids: valepotriates
Alkaloids: actinidine, valerine, chatinine
Gamma aminobutyric acid (GABA)
Tannins, flavonoids, sterols

Traditional uses and humoral influences

Valerian is ruled by Mercury, is hot in the first degree and dry in the second degree. Culpeper calls valerian "temperately hot"—temperate herbs being the ones that don't themselves heat organs up, but rather bring them into the correct temperament.

Mercury is associated with the etheric element (cold and dry) and is the activator of the animal spirit, the brain, and the nerves. Valerian's gentle warming aromatic action allays any diminution of heat within the nervous system, particularly when it comes from exhaustion. There is no better herb for nourishing a weakened and depleted nervous system. It repairs the nervous function after shock, trauma, and extreme over-worrying.

It is a relaxing tonic, helpful to bring airy types (sanguines) back down to earth, and helps with overthinking. Valerian warms and strengthens the head and heart in those with cold constitutions who have become mentally depleted or emotionally exhausted.

> "It is excellent against nervous affections, such as headaches, trembling, palpitations, vapours, and hysterical complaints"
> —(Culpeper)

Its country name "all heal" attests that it has had a great domestic reputation, and traditional uses have included: migraine, colic, irritability, sleeplessness, muscle cramps, menstrual pain, menopausal restlessness, confusion, smokers cough, convulsions, excitability, and wound healing.

As my herbal teacher and mentor Christopher Hedley used to say "valerian is not just a tranquiliser!".

The tincture was widely prescribed during the world wars to reduce the damaging effects on the nervous system from air raids and shell shock without adversely effecting mental activity and vital functions.

Emotional

Valerian is very helpful for deep, stuck feelings, especially when those feelings produce an underlying sense of tension and anxiety. It is helpful when we have a foundational sense of anxiety, one which just seems to be there, sitting quietly intransient beneath everything else that we feel. Perhaps we can have an inkling that those emotions have been set in motion far in the past. Although we have no memory of the actual events that caused the emotions, we experience a sad familiarity with this background feeling. When this long term feeling of being uncomfortable and on edge is constantly present, valerian can be most helpful. These states of stuck or retained feelings are a good example of "melancholia". It is an emotional state that is not of the head, nor even really of the heart, but it profoundly effects the thoughts and feelings we have. These stuck emotions become like the cold hard residue left behind after the fire of trauma has passed, this is the "atra bilis" or dark bile that Culpeper described as being a potential root cause of chronic illness, madness, and hard tumours or possibly even cancer. Valerian helps because it grounds us without constricting the emotions, it allows us to once again send our roots down to a deep place of nourishment and tranquillity, allowing us to release ourselves to a deeper, quieter place where we can release the pain of long-term emotional distress.

Mythos

The name most likely derives from the Latin "valere", to be in health, although it was referred to by Galen and Dioscorides as "phu", a name associated with the common reaction to its smell, which can often be disagreeable. Its Middle Eastern relatives have a more enticing aroma and were often used in perfumes, the most well-known is spikenard. In the gospels, John 12 1–8: "Mary therefore took a pound of expensive ointment made from pure nard, and anointed the feet of Jesus and wiped his feet with her hair. The house was filled with the fragrance of the perfume".

In Gerard's herbal originally published in 1597 he tells us that the country people so valued the herb they would not cook a dish without including it, and consequently there was a country rhyme;

"They that will have their heal,
Must put setwall in their keale".[1]

According to the nineteenth century herbal of William Fernie (1897),[2] in German folklore imps were thought to be afraid of it.

Head

Valerian is a powerful nervine, taken consistently it reinforces the nervous system, helping depression associated with anxiety. Its stimulant action strengthens nervous weakness, or "neurasthenia", and is particularly indicated for panic attacks with palpitations, when it combines well with hawthorn.

Studies show that it improves the quality of sleep and reduces the time taken to fall asleep. The valepotriate compounds that it contains have been shown to have sedative effects on the central nervous system as well as potentiating the sedative neurotransmitter GABA, which the plant also contains (Fisher, 2018).[3]

In states of general anxiety, it can be used to settle and calm. I have found it useful in Alzheimer's disease and in dementia patients to reduce tension and mental agitation, in which case I give a 400 mg capsule three times a day after food. It does not interact with other sedative medicines.

Heart

In The Model Botanic Guide to Health by William Fox (1891),[4] valerian is included in a recipe for inflammation of the heart, along with marigold, tansy, vervain, and hart's tongue. The symptoms would include heart pain, feelings of suffocation, and great anxiety. He also suggested combining valerian and scullcap in equal parts to make up his "soothing drops", which were considered ideal for children as well as adults.

It combines well with other herbs, such as mistletoe and lime flower, for high blood pressure, and with hawthorn and motherwort for arrhythmia, a fast heart rate, and palpitations.

Bowels

It is carminative, relieving intestinal spasm and colic. The bowels are considered to be susceptible to cold conditions, as they have a cold wet temperament, so the aromatic warming effects of valerian help to reduce bloating and spasmodic pain. A helpful combination for treating IBS. is equal parts of valerian root, chamomile flowers, and aniseed, 15 g combined in a pint, steeped overnight and drank throughout the following day.

As well as the traditional use for colic, it is a bowel relaxant for constipation associated with tension.

Muscle pain

The relaxant effects are very beneficial in chronic back pain and other forms of muscular spasmodic pain. The tincture or tea can be used; 5 ml of the tincture three times a day or 10 g steeped overnight and drunk in two divided doses, morning and evening.

Kidneys

It was considered a helpful herb by Culpeper for "Provoking Urine, and help[ing] the strangurary". He was probably referring to its antispasmodic effect helping to relax the urinary passages and facilitate a better flow in conditions such as prostate enlargement.

Doses

Tincture

5 ml one to three times daily.

Capsules

400 mg, one to three times a day.
Combine with scullcap, chamomile, and lemon balm for anxiety, and with hawthorn for palpitations.

As tea for promoting sleep

3 parts valerian root, 1 part sage, 1 part rose petals.
As a mix for panic attacks: 40% valerian, 30% motherwort, 30% vervain.

Vervain

Divine weed. Enchanter's weed. Colombine. Berbine. Herb of the cross. Holy wort. Pigeons grass. Isis tears. Simpler's joy
Celtic: Fer faen.

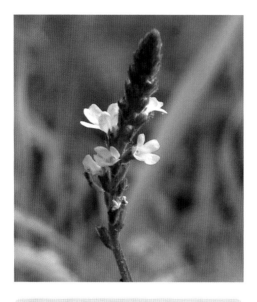

Latin:	*Verbena officinalis*
Family:	Verbenaceae

Element	Water
Planet	Venus
Humour	Phlegmatic
Quality	Hot and dry both in the second degree, heats the head, kidneys, and womb, is opening, cleansing Healing, and strengthening.

Organs

Head
Lungs
Liver

Spleen
Kidneys
Joints
Womb

Actions

Anti-inflammatory
Calming
Sedative
Digestive
Diuretic
Diaphoretic

Constituents

Iridoids: verbenalin, aucubin
Phenylpropanoids: verbascoside
Flavonoids: luteolin, apigenin, kaempferol quercetin
Volatile oils: limolene, citral
Sterols: dauscosterol, β-sistosterol
Triterpenes: ursolic and oleanolic acids
Fatty acids

Traditional uses and humoral influences

Vervain is ruled by Venus, it is a bitter herb, which is hot and dry in the second degree. In 1640 John Parkinson described it in the following way: "Vervaine is hot and dry, bitter and binding, and is an opener of obstructions, clenseth and healeth; for it helpeth the yellow jaundies, the dropsie and the goute, as also the defects of the Reines and Lungs and generally all the inward paines and torments of the body".[1]

Vervain has a calming action on the nerves and brain and a strengthening action on digestion and elimination. Being associated with the phlegmatic humour its warming tonic action strengthens all organs with a cold and moist temperament, which include the brain, the stomach, the intestines and bowels, the lungs, and the urinary system. Its cleansing action helps to clear swellings of the joints, with its bitterness increasing bile flow and elimination of toxins.

Bitter herbs like vervain are often classed as having a cooling action, potentially causing some confusion as while Culpeper and Parkinson say that it is hot and dry, their contemporary Gerard suggests that it is cooling in temperament. However, like the other extremely bitter herb wormwood, vervain is considered to clear heat via its ability to open obstructions, allowing blocked heat to dissipate. The heat in the herb also has a rarefying action, potentially dispersing and thinning out excessive fire in the body, again leading to a cooling action.

Vervain also has a diaphoretic action making it especially beneficial in fevers, helping to quickly bring the temperature down. The herb is now known to have anti-inflammatory actions, and the essential oils are antibacterial and antioxidant, confirming its reputation for being helpful to use both externally and internally for hot inflammations. Poultices were often recommended as an application, they tend to stain the skin red, which was believed to show that they brought warming blood to the surface clearing coldness and dampness, but also potentially dispersing excess heat.

Culpeper said that it "doth wonderfully cleanse the skin, and takes away the morphew (skin blemish), freckles, fistulas, and other such like inflammations and deformities of the skin in any parts of the body".

It is a good wound herb, reducing bleeding and increasing the rate of healing in ulcers and skin inflammations. There are records of it being used externally in Spain for inflammatory skin conditions and in Sicily for psoriasis (Fisher, 2018).[2]

Emotional

Vervain sweeps away confusion and distraction. It allows those things that are truly important to be differentiated from superficial concerns and worries. It helps mental focus and liberates the mind from stagnant and suffocating thoughts and emotions.

Mythos

The Greeks and Romans named vervain "hiera botane"—the sacred herb. Pliny the elder (77AD) said that the Romans revered no plant more than vervain, using it to sweep and cleanse the altars of Jupiter. The annual festival of Verbenalia was held in its honour, and the herb itself was dedicated to Venus, the goddess of love and fertility, with garlands of the flowers being worn at weddings. It was revered as a plant that would aid in the settling of disputes and was an emblem of justice. Roman envoys of peace were known as the Verbenarii and they would travel carrying sprigs of vervain as a signifier of peace. Celtic poets crowned themselves with vervain to bring on divine inspiration, and the druids were said to use it in making divinations. Vervain is traditionally gathered during the time when the dog star Sirius is rising, and when there is no moon or sun in the sky—this occurs in the months of July and August when the plant is also in flower. Incantations such as this one from Lancashire were to be said on gathering:

"Hallowed by thou, vervain,
If though growest on the ground".

If this ritual was followed and appropriate offerings made to the earth when gathering the herb, it would protect from all evil and harm, confirmed by the old English saying; "Vervain and dill hinder witches from their will" (De Cleene & Lejeune, 1999).[3]

Head and nerves

The brain itself has a cold moist temperament and is prone to imbalances caused by an excess of the phlegmatic humour. John Pechey in his herbal of 1706 said of vervain; "'Tis Cephalic … 'Tis reckon'd a specific for pains of the head, from whatever cause they proceed. The distilled water is applied outwardly to the head; and four ounces are taken inwardly with four drops of spirit of salt. Forestus says, he knew two who were cured of the head-ach, only by hanging the green herb about their necks when many other medicines were used to no purpose".[4]

In 1640, Parkinson said that when applied to the temples with the oil of roses and some vinegar, vervain would; "helpeth to ease the inveterate paines and ache of the head, and is good for those that are fallen into a frensy".[5] This reputation for calming the nerves and relieving frenzy is still acknowledged by present day herbalists, who particularly value it for reducing anxiety

and for its sedative action. I once had a young patient who was suffering from insomnia as a withdrawal effect of long term cannabis use, he had heard about vervain and came to get some to take. Despite its bitter taste he drank it as a tea before bed and found it to be very effective, it helped him with insomnia and also reduced his mental agitation. In fact, he found it so useful that he continued to return for some time to buy it. It is often used in mixes for treating depression and melancholy. Messegue (1981)[6] includes it in his tea of happiness along with lime flower, chamomile, and mint.

I have often found it very beneficial for M.E. and similar debilitating conditions such as fibromyalgia and recurrent migraines. Thomas Bartram (1995) also recommends it for "Post viral fatigue syndrome, ME. Nervous exhaustion from prolonged physical exertion".[7] Some of my ME patients have found the most useful way to use it is as a daily footbath.

The kidneys

The Celtic name ferfean comes from "fer"—to drive away, and "faern"—a stone, indicating that it was a popular remedy for kidney stones and bladder problems. With its cleansing, anti-inflammatory and astringent properties, it makes a good addition for infusions used for strengthening the urinary tissues. In Parkinson's herbal (1640) he recommends it for "defects of the reines and the bladder, to cleanse them of that viscous and slimy humour which ingendreth the stone, and helpeth to break it being confirmed, and to expel the gravel".[8]

Womb

Nicholas Culpeper said that it would help all problems of the womb coming from a cold cause, this can include scant or absent menstruation, period pains, and infertility. Modern research has shown vervain to have strong oestrogen and progesterone receptor binding properties, probably accounting for it often being used to help with menopausal symptoms including hot flushes, emotional sensitivity, palpitations, and insomnia. A combination of vervain, valerian, and motherwort makes a very helpful premenstrual tension mixture.

Liver and spleen

All bitter herbs have good effects on the digestive system. Vervain has always had a reputation for treating digestive problems with Nicholas Culpeper saying that it "strengthens as well as corrects the diseases of the stomach, liver and spleen".

Doses

Tea

One teaspoon per cup, up to three cups daily.

Tincture

1:3 5 ml three times a day.

Digestive tonic

6 drops of tincture directly on the tongue, or 10 drops in a little water taken 10 minutes before food.

PMT mix

Vervain 30%
Valerian root 30%
Motherwort 40%

Take 5 ml of the tincture as needed, up to 4 times a day.

Violets

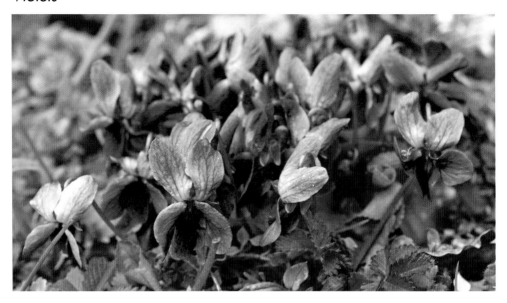

Sweet Violet. Apple leaf. May Violet

Latin: *Viola odorata*

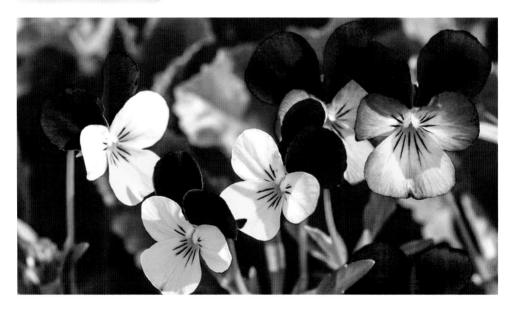

Heartsease. Wild pansy Pansies. Love lies bleeding. Love in idleness. Love idol. Cuddle Me.

Latin: *Viola tricolor*

Family: Violaceae

Element   Water
Planet   Venus
Humour   Phlegmatic
Quality   Cold in the first degree,
           moist in the second
           degree. Cools head, lungs,
           heart, and stomach.
           Cleansing, cooling,
           cordial, purges choler.

Organs

Lungs
Stomach
Joints
Skin
Heart
Head

Actions

Anti-inflammatory
Emollient
Demulcent
Expectorant
Antirheumatic
Cordial
Anticancer

Constituents

Polysaccharides: mucilage up to 18%
Flavonoids: rutin, apigenin
Saponins
Alkaloids
Phenolic acids: salicylates
Essential oils
Cyclotides

Traditional uses and humoral influences

The violets are cooling and moistening, with their copious mucilage giving them a softening and lubricating action. "All Violets are cold and moist while they are fresh and green, and are used to cool any heat, or distemperature of the body, either inwardly or outwardly" (Culpeper).

Culpeper considered sweet violet to be ruled by Venus, but he says of heartsease; "The herb is really Saturnine, something cold, viscous and slimy However, both plants have had similar uses as cooling moistening herbs for the head, heart, stomach, lungs, skin, joints, kidneys, and womb. Sweet violet has always been considered a very useful herb in treating the effects of excess heat and choler in the body, which can manifest as fevers, carbuncles, frenzy, poor sleep, anger, and hot itchy skin problems. Choler or the fire humour is antipathetic to those organs with a moist cold temperament, such as the brain, lungs, stomach, bowels, kidneys, urinary system, and the womb, making the cooling effect of violets beneficial in any conditions of heat or dryness in those organs. Culpeper says: "The dried leaves or flowers of Violets, but the leaves more strongly, doth purge the body of choleric humours and asaugeth the heat if taken in a draught of wine or other drink".

The violets are considered helpful for jaundice and dry obstructions of the liver, Culpeper states:

> "It is good also for the liver and the jaundice, and all hot agues, to cool the heat, and quench the thirst., but the syrup of violets is

of most use, and of better effect, being taken in some convenient liquor".

The Italian physician Pietro Mattioli writing in 1554 says; "Fresh Violets thus cool, easing hot pains in the manner of narcotics, extinguish all inflammations, soothe the trachea and lungs, purge yellow bile and extinguish its heat, and ease headache from a hot cause, they bring sleep" (Tobyn et al., 2011).[1]

Mythos

The sweet violet is dedicated to Persephone, the Greek goddess of the spring, fertility, and the underworld. The Greek name for violet is "ion", it is said that Zeus took Io as a lover, and to hide her from his wife Hera he turned her into a heifer and created violets to feed her. Another story is that Aphrodite asked Cupid who was more beautiful, herself or a group of young maidens standing close by. Undiplomatically he told her that he preferred the maidens, so in anger she struck them turning them purple. In sympathy, Eros then turned them into violet coloured flowers. Ever since the sweet violet has been considered a symbol of purity, chastity, and modesty.

Emotional

The violets are cooling and calming, helping with long-term anxiety states and panic attacks. They generally help with extreme or deep-seated worry, steadying those who feel overwhelmed by stress and emotional overload. They gently move the mind towards serenity, comforting and nourishing the spirit, and bringing a sense of ease into the body.

The medieval mystic Hildegard Von Bingen said; "Anyone oppressed by Melancholy with a discontented mind, which then harms his lungs, should cook violets in pure wine. He should strain this through a cloth, add a bit of galingale, and as much liquorice as he wants, and so make a spiced wine. When he drinks it, it will check the melancholy, make him happy and heal his lungs" (Throop, 1998).[2]

Stomach

The roots and seeds are an emetic if taken in strong doses and the whole herb has a gentle laxative effect. If the leaves are taken in stronger doses, they act as a purgative. Maurice Messegue (1981)[3] suggests using a handful of leaves in a litre of water, and to drink 2 cupfuls daily for a gentle laxative effect, and for treating the stomach and respiratory system use half a handful of the herb to a litre. This roughly equates to 15 g to a litre for the half handful and 30 g to a litre for the stronger dose.

Heart

The temperament of the heart is a fine balance of heat and moisture, with hot and agitated emotions having the capacity to dry and scorch the heart. Venus rules the moist cold part of the circulation, which we still today call the venous circulation. It is what moves and clears heat from the heart protecting it from the potential damage caused by overwhelming or agitated and angry emotions. Culpeper assigns it as one of the cordial herbs, saying; "The dried flower of Violets are accounted amongst the cordial drinks, powders and other medicines, especially where cooling cordials are necessary".

Gerard (1597) also says of violet: "it has power to ease inflammation, roughness of the throat and comforteth the heart".[4] The five cordial herbs according to Culpeper are: rose, violet, melissa, borage, and bugloss.

Excess heat in the heart may bring on a more rapid, erratic, or irregular heartbeat. It can be associated with feelings of panic and anxiety. Often the pulse feels tighter and harder, floating and rapid. Both sweet violet and heartsease calm, steady, and cool the heart, reducing agitation and tension. The rutin and the salicylates that they contain are anti-inflammatory and reduce capillary fragility, along with the other flavonoids they are also antioxidant, all of which helps to strengthen the circulatory system and protect against degeneration of blood vessels.

Reproductive and urinary system

The soft moist quality of violets gives them a sympathy with the reproductive and urinary system. Historically they have been prescribed for heavy menstrual bleeding, especially if associated with conditions of heat or excess yellow bile. The cooling demulcent properties make both kinds of violets useful in urinary pain, with the anti microbial properties being especially beneficial for cystitis and urinary infections in general.

Lungs

The cooling moist properties of violets have been made use of in asthma, coughs, pleurisy, bronchitis and to soothe respiratory irritation in general. Treating the lungs with violet was a common recommendation.

John Gerard aptly says; "The floures are good for all inflammations, especially of the sides and lungs, they take away the hoarsenes of the chest, the ruggedness of the windpipe and jawes".[5]

The Italian physician Mattioli wrote in 1554; "Violets carry off inflammations of the throat, pleurisy and other hot swellings of the lungs".[6] They are considered to help dry and painful lung conditions, having both a gentle soothing effect, as well as encouraging gentle expectoration. A syrup of the flowers was a traditional way of using the herb, but a tea or decoction is equally effective.

Head

The Greeks placed violet flowers on their foreheads to induce sleep and prevent headaches and hangovers. They also valued them for calming anger and to cheer the heart, a use also recommended by Culpeper:

> "it likewise easeth the pains in the head caused through want of sleep, or any pains arising of heat". He suggested applying a poultice of the leaves or flowers to the head itself with oil of roses.

As a tea both heartsease and violets calm and cool the brain, allowing worries to be gently washed away, giving a sense of mental ease and freedom from nervous stress. The violets certainly benefit sleep, and drunk before bed help to restore broken sleep patterns and allow the mind to awaken refreshed the following day.

Joints

The anti-inflammatory compounds in the violet family related to salicylic acid are very helpful to reduce aching joints, muscles, and bones. Along with herbs, such as meadowsweet, rosemary, and horsetail they can make a very beneficial anti-rheumatic tea.

Skin

The leaves were considered helpful to make a poultice, wash, or compress to apply to any inflammations or swelling on the skin. Grieve in her herbal (1931) says of heartsease that "a strong decoction of the herb and flowers was recommended by older herbalists for skin diseases", with her contemporary, Hilda Leyel (1943), advising its use in "moist cutaneous eruptions in children".[7]

There is no doubt that it works well externally as a wash, bath, compress, or poultice for inflammatory skin conditions and healing wounds. It is high in salicylates and both kinds of violets have been shown to have broad antiseptic activity. As an infusion to drink for skin problems, such as eczema, it combines well with chamomile flowers, red clover flowers, and fennel seed.

Cancer

In 1902, a bulletin in Potter's National Botanic Pharmacopeia reported a case in which a malignant throat tumour was healed by the application of a fresh infusion of violet leaves as a poultice. It then became a popular treatment for throat and lung cancers throughout the early 20th century. Recent research has investigated the cyclotides that occur in both kinds of violet. They have been shown to be cytotoxic to a number of cancer cell lines, with the cyclotides in heartsease showing specific activity against myeloma and lymphoma cell lines.[8]

Doses

Infusion

2–4 g per cup, up to 3 daily.

Tincture

1:3 2–4 ml three times daily.

Eczema tea

Equal parts of heartsease, chamomile, red clover, and fennel seed.
Heart tea to soothe, calm, and lift the spirits:
Equal parts of rose, lemon balm, violets/ heartsease, and borage.

Willow

White Willow. Sallow tree. Osier. Withy
Ogham:Saille
Ancient
Greek: Helice

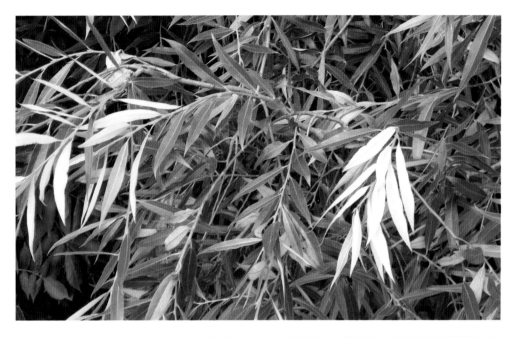

Latin: *Salix alba, Salix spp.*
Family: Salicaceae

Element   Water
Planet   Moon
Humour   Phlegmatic
Quality   Cold and dry in the
           second degree, astringent
           and cleansing.

Organs

Head
Joints
Stomach
Eyes

Actions

Analgesic
Haemostatic
Anti-inflammatory
Fever reducing
Tonic
Anaphrodisiac

Constituents

Phenolic glycosides: salicin, salicylic
    acid, triandrin
Tannins
Flavonoids
Coumaric acid

Traditional uses and humoral influences

Willow is ruled by the moon, is cold and dry both in the second degree, and is cleansing and astringent.

The moon governs the phlegmatic or water humour, which is the element that rules the joints, the brain, and the stomach and intestines. Nicholas Culpeper calls it "a fine cold tree, which both the flowers and the bark have an admirable faculty in drying up humours, being a medicine without any sharpness or corrosion".

The cold and drying effect of willow is contrary to the warmth and moistness of the procreative faculty of the body, this was thought to account for its ability to reduce the sexual drive, especially in men but also in women.

It is also due to this drying effect that Culpeper suggests that it will "staunch the bleeding of wounds, and at mouth and nose, spitting of blood, and other fluxes of blood in man or woman, and to stay vomiting and provocation thereunto".

The strengthening effect of willow on the phlegmatic humour, and the expulsive faculty associated with the moon and water element, means that it is also recommended to drink to help "provoke urine, if it be stopped" (Culpeper).

Mythos

The word willow has derivations from the Anglo Saxon word "welig", meaning supple or curved. Willow also has an ancient Indo-European linguistic root "weik" meaning to bend, which is also associated with the words wicker and withy. There may also be a link to the old English word for wizard, derived from wicca, which also gives the root for wise, wicked and witch.

The willow was sacred in Greece to Hecate, Persephone, Circe, and Hera, all of whom are death aspects of the triple moon goddess. It is the tree that loves water most and was honoured as the tree of enchantment, fertility, and rebirth. The Ancient Greek name for willow, Helice is the name of the nymph who nursed Zeus, and a willow tree representing her grew outside the cave in Crete in which he was born. According to Pliny, the earth goddess Hera turned Helice into a bear out of jealousy because of the love that Zeus showed his nurse, but then Zeus transformed her into the constellation of Ursa Minor giving her immortal life.

The name also connects the tree to Helicon, the sacred abode of the nine muses, the orgiastic priestesses of the moon goddess herself. The Roman name "salix" means to leap forward, evolving into the English verb "sally" as in "to sally forth". This is clearly associated with its ability to grow fast and shoot up in the spring.

"Saille" is also the name for willow in the druidic tree alphabet of Ogham: it is the fifth tree of the Ogham year, five being the sacred number of the goddess, and the month in which the birds nest. The willow's connection with birds is also apparent in the ancient Irish druidic song of Amergin with the line for willow reading "I am a hawk on a cliff" (Graves, 1948).[1] Birds are closely connected to the sacred goddess of old Europe, with the willow being the nesting place of the Wryneck, a bird in the woodpecker family that twists its neck and hisses like a snake. Snakes were also sacred to the ancient white goddess, and they are often to be found lying in pools and by rivers during the heat of the day, loving water as does the willow. Ancient oracular sites were placed by springs and streams, and the divinatory powers of the oracles were strongly associated with water, snakes, and sacred birds, and thus also the willow tree.

At the entrance to the underworld there was said to be a grove of black poplars and willow. When Orpheus journeyed through the underworld he was guided and protected by taking a willow branch with him. It is said that Hermes used his staff made of willow to separate two fighting snakes, from whence it became the emblem of peace and harmony, the well-known caduceus. Hermes became the patron of travellers and pilgrims and the willow staffs their symbol, a sign of someone travelling in peace.

The head

"It helps to stay thin, hot, sharp salt distillations from the head upon the lungs causing consumptions" (Culpeper) Since the head is the highest organ in the body, it is often effected by hot vapours arising from overheated organs. This may bring on insomnia, headaches, sinus congestion, and phlegm. Willow helps to dry and cool the heat and excessive temperature, and it can be used with sweet smelling remedies, such as rose, a cooling remedy whose sweet smell strengthens the animal spirit that resides in the brain.

Fever is an example of excessive heat in the organs producing vapours, which become a hot cause of headaches. The cooling effect of willow makes it a perfect antidote to these hot conditions, and like the modern use of aspirin, it reduces aches and pains and relieves headaches, while helping to reduce a high temperature. There are also records of it being used as a folk treatment for insomnia and nervousness in Europe.

Pain

The pain relieving properties have been praised since the time of the Egyptians who recommended chewing on a piece of bark for fevers and headaches, with Matthioli the C16 herbalist regarding it as an opiate.[2]

I had a patient with severe leg ulcers who experienced extreme pain and took constant pain killers. After prescribing a 15 g daily decoction of the root, the daily use of pain killers became unnecessary and were only taken once before bed. Interestingly, after six months of the treatment the ulcer that had been non-healing for many years began to resolve and finally healed completely. The amount of exudate from the ulcer had dried considerably over the period of treatment, and healing had then spontaneously occurred. Perhaps it would be incorrect to claim that the healing of the ulcer was triggered by the use of the willow bark, but it seemed very likely at the time to both the patient and myself that the two were indeed connected.

Occasionally a high dose, such as a decoction of 15 g per day, can cause some looseness of stools and abdominal discomfort. When this happens reducing the dose by half, or using the herbs as a footbath which seems to be equally effective for reducing pain, will resolve the problem of the abdominal discomfort and diarrhoea.

Joints

There is a long tradition for willow being used to treat rheumatism, gout, and painful joints. The word rheum comes from the ancient Greek meaning "flow", and the willow's association with the water element particularly aligns it with the rheumatics and the joints. Willow dries up the moisture in swollen joints, reducing pain and stiffness. It is both analgesic and anti-inflammatory. It was recommended as far back as Hippocrates (460-377BC) for treating rheumatic pain. For the pain of gout, or plantar fasciitis, a footbath made from 20 g willow, and 20 g comfrey leaf should be made up as an infusion in 1 pint of hot water and left to steep overnight. It is a very effective remedy when the feet are bathed in it for 10 minutes twice daily.

Stomach

Aspirin is a synthesised form of salicylic acid, but it has the disadvantage of being irritant to the stomach wall. Unlike aspirin, or pure salicylic acid, willow bark tends to be fairly well-tolerated by the stomach, it contains a large number of salicylate compounds working synergistically to provide both analgesic and anti-inflammatory actions without causing irritation. Infusions made from the bark were often prescribed for diarrhoea and stomach cramps, and Culpeper says; "the leaves crushed with some black pepper, and drunk in wine, helps much the wind cholic".

Eyes

Since the earliest times, willow has been recommended for treating the eyes. Nicholas Culpeper suggested that the sap taken from the tree when it flowers is "very good for redness and dimness of sight or films that grow over the eyes, and to stay the rheum's that fall into them". He is probably referring here to cataracts (films) and floaters (rheum's).

Doses

Tincture

10 ml of 1:3 tincture twice daily.

Infusion

5 g leaves or bark drunk 3 times a day.

Decoction

15 g bark infused in a pint and drank over 24 hours.

Wood avens

Herb Bennet. Goldy star of the earth. Colewort. City Avens. Clove Root. The Blessed herb. Herba benedicta

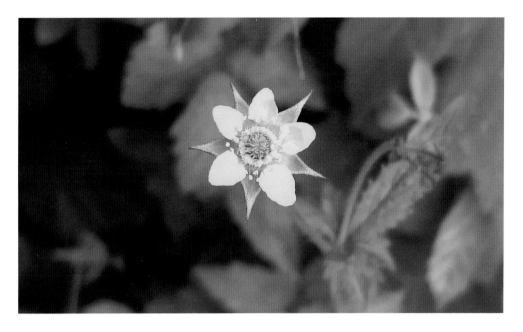

Latin:	*Geum urbanum*
Family:	Rosaceae

Element	Air
Planet	Jupiter
Humour	Sanguine
Quality	Warming and drying in the first degree, dries excess phlegm, clears cold obstructions, especially from the liver and digestive passages.

Organs

Liver
Intestines
Head

Heart
Lungs

Actions

Astringent
Anti-diarrhoeal
Stomachic
Antiseptic
Styptic

Constituents

Tannins 1.5 %
Phenols: eugenol, vicianose

Traditional uses and humoral influences

Nicholas Culpeper tells us "is ruled by Jupiter, and that gives hopes of a wholesome healthful herb". Jupiter has its seat in the liver, it is also associated with the breast, ribs, the sides, and the inhalation of breath. It controls the digestive faculty in the body and has a warm moist temperament. The liver is both the seat of the sanguine humour and the natural spirit. The natural spirit is the physical manifestation of vitality in the body and gives us a feeling of physical health, in the same way that a strong vital spirit provides us with a strong and healthy emotional state.

It is famed as a warming, protecting herb, which helps to clear any dampness that may be affecting moist phlegmatic organs, such as the brain, the lungs, and the stomach. It contains eugenol, the same oil that gives cloves their distinctive aroma and taste. When the roots are lifted fresh from the ground, there is a distinct aroma of cloves. Unsurprisingly, we find one of its country names is clove root.

Its reputation as a cordial for the heart, a tonic for the brain, and strengthener of the stomach and liver is also praised by Culpeper: "The decoction also being drank comforts the heart, and strengthens the stomach and a cold brain, and therefore is good in the springtime to open obstructions of the liver".

It was also revered as a protective herb against poisons, sickness, and even the plague itself, with Culpeper proclaiming that wood avens "is a good preservative against the plague, or any other poison".

It has been principally used for "catarrhs" or "fluxes of the belly". Along with other members of the rose family, it is an effective astringent for the intestines, being high in tannins, and is often prescribed as a gentle anti-diarrhoeal. In her herbal of 1931, Maude Grieve lists many uses including; "leucorrhoea, sore throat, ague, chills, fresh catarrh, intermittent fevers, chronic and passive haemorrhages gastric irritation and headache".

Mythos

The botanical name *Geum* is thought to have derived from the Greek "geno", meaning to produce an agreeable fragrance, referring to the gentle sweet clove like fragrance that it emanates when freshly dug up. The name "avens" is likely to have derived from the Latin word "avencia", meaning to advance.

The plant is connected with many stories of protection, healing, and the power of good to overcome evil. The name "advance" may well be an association with these qualities, or it may be in reference to its habit of quickly colonising fresh ground, with the new seedlings appearing to advance rapidly across the ground. The 1491 herbal Hortus Sanitatis states: "where the root is in the house, Satan can do nothing and flies from it, wherefore it is blessed before all other herbs, and if a man carries the root about him no venomous beast can harm him" (Grieve, 1931).[1]

Its name country name, Herb Bennet derives from it being associated with St Benedict, the founder of the Benedictine order. It is said that a monk once tried to kill St Benedict by giving him a poisoned chalice, however Benedict's holiness was so great that when he blessed the chalice before putting it to his lips, the poison—being somewhat like a devil—leapt out with a scream and the chalice shattered into a thousand pieces. The leaves and flowers often feature as carved emblems in churches. The three lobed leaves are said to correspond to the holy trinity and the five petals of the flower correspond to the five wounds of Christ. Both of these numbers have earlier resonances with the old European sacred tradition of the white goddess, with three representing the triple goddess herself and the five being the number of the etheric element, creation, and the mother goddess, Venus.

Emotional

Wood avens is considered a sacred plant for good reason; it brings hope when hope is lost, it revives the spirits when we have become dejected and feel emotionally exhausted. It brings the mind into a state of calm clarity, relaxing mental tension, removing doubt, and restoring self confidence and optimism. It is a specific herbal remedy for panic attacks, especially when the underlying state is one of feeling blocked and trapped, with no way forward.

Liver, spleen, and intestines

"It helps indigestion, and warms a cold stomach, and opens obstructions of the liver and spleen" (Culpeper).

The liver and spleen are particularly vulnerable to cold obstructions, especially those associated with the melancholic or earth humour. These are also likely to be particularly problematic in the spring after the cold congestive effects of the cold and damp winter. It was, therefore, customary in the spring to take tonics to purify the blood of these cold "crude" humours. A decoction of avens was considered especially helpful in this regard. Its gentle heating action is very beneficial for the liver, which being a warm but moist organ is very susceptible to being overwhelmed by excess dampness. We now know that the aromatic oil, eugenol, contained in avens induces the production of detoxifying enzymes in the liver, supporting this ancient belief in its blood cleansing and liver activating capabilities.

Avens has carminative actions, relaxing the smooth muscle of the intestines, helping to reduce colic and digestive spasm. Its tannins and antimicrobial actions make it a very beneficial herb in diarrhoea and any stomach or intestinal infection. Culpeper recommends it in this regard saying; "it is good … to expel crude and raw humours from the belly and stomach".

Heart

Jupiter rules the blood, and avens strengthens the blood through warming and nourishing the liver. When the blood is healthy, the heart is tonified and protected. It is now known that eugenol, the essential oil that avens contains, relaxes smooth muscle—helping to improve blood flow, and is anti-inflammatory—helping to reduce damage to blood vessels and the formation of cholesterol plaques.

John Pechey in 1706 was already extolling avens for these very same effects, saying, "it chears the heart and removes obstructions",[2] an observation previously made by Culpeper recommending avens as a comfort to the heart.

Head

Wood avens has a gentle relaxing effect on the brain and nerves. It gently warms the head, improving mental function and memory. In John Pechey's herbal (1706) we read; "tis cephalic and cordial and resists poisons".[3] Nicholas Culpeper agrees, saying that it is particularly helpful for a "cold brain". We know that the oil has anodyne, pain relieving actions, as well as relaxant properties.

Lungs

Nicholas Culpeper stated: "It is good for the diseases of the chest or breast, for pains, and stitches in the side". With its smooth muscle relaxant, pain relieving activity and antiseptic properties, we can understand why avens was considered so helpful for the chest. It was also recommended for treating fevers and infections, making it particularly helpful in respiratory infections, colds, coughs, and chills.

Doses

Tea

1 teaspoon (3 g) to a cup, three times a day.

Decoction

Root; 10 g to a cup decoct gently 3-5 mins, up to 3 cups daily.

Tincture

5 ml 1:3 tincture, up to four times daily.

Capsule

400 mg, Two capsules three times daily.

Wood betony

Bettonica, bishopswort, byscopwyrt
Celtic: Bew ton

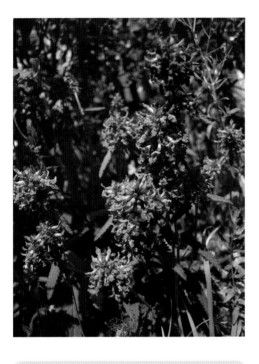

Latin:	*Stachys officinalis*
Family:	Lamiaceae
Element	Air
Planet	Jupiter
Humour	Sanguine
Quality	Hot in the first degree, and dry in the second degree. Warms head, lungs, kidneys, and stomach, dries the heart, opens obstructions.

Organs

Head
Heart

Lungs
Liver
Stomach
Womb

Actions

Sedative
Nervine
Bitter tonic
Astringent
Diuretic

Constituents

Alkaloids: stachydrine, betonicine, trigonelline
Polyphenols
Phenolic acids: caffeic acid
Flavonoids: apigenin, quercetin, coumarins
Tannins, volatile oils, terpenols

Traditional uses and humoral influences

Wood betony is ruled by Jupiter, and is hot in the first degree and dry in the second. It is also under the astrological sign of Aries, which rules the head and all structures above the first vertebrae of the neck.

John Pechey, in his Compleat Herbal of 1707, says: "'Tis hot and dry, acrid and bitter. It discusses, attenuates, opens and cleanses. 'Tis Cephalick, (H)epatick, Splenetick, Thoracick, Uterine, Vulnery and Diuretic, 'Tis used frequently, inwardly and outwardly, efpecially in difeafes of the Head".[1]

Jupiter rules the digestive faculty, the mid brain, and is the seat of the natural spirit in the body. Betony clears, opens, and cleanses cold congestion and obstructions in all the organs associated with the air element, Jupiter, and the sanguine humour. Thus we see it being recommended for helping the liver and digestion, the lungs, the brain, and for clearing dampness and congestion in the heart, the womb and the kidneys. It was considered a general tonic and restorative, with Culpeper commenting: "A dram (3.6 g) of the powder of Betony taken with a little honey in some vinegar, does wonderfully refresh those that are over wearied by travelling".

Mythos

The Roman physician Antonius Musa who attended to the needs of Emperor Augustus in 63 BC, extolled betony, listing forty-seven separate uses. It was claimed to be a panacea for all ills, evidenced by the ancient Italian saying; "sell your coat and buy betony".[2] The fifth century writer Apulius said, "It is good whether for the man's soul or for his body: it shields him against visions and dreams",[3] as in addition to its medicinal virtues it was considered to be protective against evil spirits, often being put into amulets or worn around the body.

Betony was extensively cultivated in physic gardens and monasteries and, as its protective properties extended to holy and sacred places, it was frequently planted around religious buildings, churches, and graveyards, possibly accounting for the name biscopwyrt or bishopswort. The botanical name *Stachys* comes from the Greek word for spike, and the ancient Greek herbalist Dioscorides calls it "kestron", also a reference to its sharp spike of flowers.

He provides the earliest recommendation for it being helpful for the head and nerves, suggesting its use for epilepsy and insanity, with the Celtic name deriving from the words "bew" and "ton" meaning head and good.

Emotional

Betony steadies the mind. It helps us to put things into perspective and brings the head into balance with the heart. It helps us to keep on a straight course mentally, even when it seems that everything around us is in flux and chaos. In this way it improves concentration, focus, and clarity of vision, it empties and frees the mind from distractions, making it a perfect herb to enhance meditation.

Head

Jupiter has a direct correspondence with the midbrain. This is the part traditionally said to be the area of judgement, where we differentiate ideas and thoughts in a similar way to the liver differentiating between nutritious substances and waste products and toxins. The brain itself was also considered to be susceptible to wind, as thoughts were considered to be transported around the ventricles by a mental wind. An excess of this mental wind would cause an unquiet mind, frenetic thinking and even insanity. Betony is able to cleanse and steady this wind, helping to bring balance and stability back to the mind. From earliest times it was also recommended for healing cut nerves and broken sinews, as well as being a helpful treatment for head injuries as a wound herb, but also taken internally to help heal brain injury.

From Nicholas Culpeper, we get the following recommendations: "It helps the jaundice, falling sickness, the palsy, convulsions, or shrinking of the sinews, the gout and those that are inclined to dropsy, those that have continual pains in their heads, although it turn to phrensy". All of these actions are attributable to Betony's warming and drying actions, and in particular the falling sickness, palsy, headache, and phrensy are often considered to be due to cold obstructions to the flow of the animal spirit, or nervous energy. In the 1766 herbal, Medica Britannica, it says; "I have known the most obstinate headaches cured by daily breakfasting for a month or six weeks on a decoction of betony".[4] Its main reputation today is based on its ability to help vertigo, dizziness, and headaches, and it is frequently also recommended for tension and anxiety. In A Modern Herbal by Maude Grieve (1931), she says; "Betony was once the sovereign remedy for all maladies of the head, and its properties as a nervine and tonic are still acknowledged … it is useful in hysteria, palpitations, pain in the head and face, neuralgia and all nervous affections".

In my experience it seems to be beneficial for vertigo associated with older people who potentially suffer from reduced blood flow to the brain, a condition that would be typical of one coming from a cold cause.

Liver and stomach

Nicholas Culpeper said; "It preserves the liver and bodies of men from the danger of epidemical diseases, … it helps those that loath and cannot digest their meat, those that have weak stomachs and sour belching, or continual risings of the stomach". Betony does this by opening the liver and spleen, clearing cold and damp congestion, and increasing bile flow. Culpeper goes on to say; "The decoction thereof made in wine and taken, kills worms in the belly, opens obstructions both of the spleen and liver; cures stitches, and pains in the back and sides, the torments and griping pains in the bowels, and the wind cholic; and mixed with honey purges the belly".

Lungs

"The powder mixed with pure honey is no less available for all sorts of coughs or colds, wheezing, or shortness of breath, distillations of thin rheum upon the lungs which causes consumptions" (Culpeper).

Womb

Betony was considered to help with congestive problems with the womb, easing menstruation, reducing cramps, and specifically helping during labour. Culpeper said that it "causes an easy and speedy delivery of women in childbirth". The alkaloid stachydrine that it contains has been shown to have oxytocic effects, with oxytocin being one of the important hormones associated with the let down reflex and the opening of the birth canal.

External healer

Betony is one of the traditional herbs to use for slow or non-healing wounds, as well as bruises and injuries. Culpeper attests: "The green herb bruised, or the juice applied to any inward hurt, or outward green wound in the head or the body, will quickly heal and close it up; as also any vein or sinews that are cut, and will draw forth any broken bone or splinter, thorn or other things got into the flesh. It is no less profitable for old sores or filthy ulcers, yea, tho they be fistulous and hollow".

Doses

Infusion

3–5 g one to three times a day.

Tincture

5 ml 1–3 times a day.

Powder

400 mg capsule, 3 daily.

Wormwood

Absinth. Felon. Old woman. Wormwod

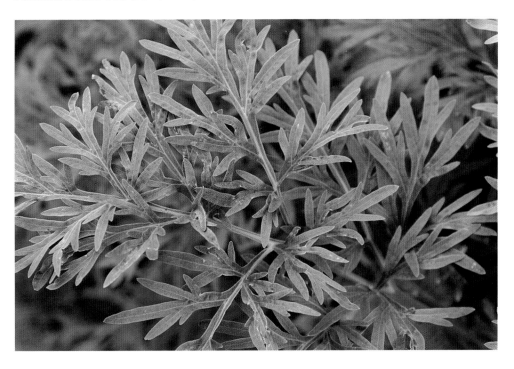

Latin:	*Artemisia absinthium*
Family:	Asteraceae/compositeae

Element	Fire
Planet	Mars
Humour	Choleric
Quality	Hot and dry in the first degree. Cleansing and strengthening, purges choler and phlegm, heats stomach, liver, and spleen

Organs

Head
Liver
Stomach

Kidneys
Womb

Actions

Bitter digestive tonic
Choleretic (increases bile flow)
Anti-inflammatory
Antidiarrhoeal
Antiseptic
Antimicrobial
Vermifuge

Constituents

Essential oils: thujones, linalool,
    chamazulenes

Bitter sesquiterpene lactones:
    absinthin, matricin, santonin
    artemisinin
Terpenoids, flavonoids,
    hydroxycoumarins
Polyacetalenes
Tannins, resin, amino acids
Manganese, potassium, silicon

Traditional uses and humoral influences

Wormwood is hot and dry in the first degree, it is ruled by Mars, the planet of fire, heat, and war.

"It is hot and dry in the first degree, viz. Just as hot as your blood and no hotter. It remedies the evils choler can inflict on the body of man by sympathy. It helps the evils (of) Venus … by antipathy; and it does something else besides. It cleanses the body of choler" (Culpeper).

Its ability to cleanse both heat and dampness, especially from the liver, makes it a prime remedy for aiding the digestion and improving the appetite. The heat it brings into the stomach improves the appetite (working in sympathy with the hot apprehensive quality needed to draw out the elements from food, and to stimulate the appetite) and its opening and cleansing warmth is antipathetical to dampness. Its bitter stimulation encourages the flow of the hot bile from the gall bladder into the intestines to cleanse the gut wall, to warm and stimulate the bowel, and to increase peristalsis, aiding both digestion and elimination through defecation. Culpeper believed it to be one of the best herbs for jaundice, and to strengthen the body through increasing the "breeding of blood" in the liver through the process of the concoctions. In medieval

Europe, there were few herbs that were more highly valued, with Hildegard Von Bingen, the twelfth century Benedictine abbess from Rhineland saying "Wermuda is very hot and has much strength. It is the principal remedy for all ailments" (Throop, 1998).[1] It was used for treating fevers and infections, and recent research has shown that the sesquiterpene lactone artemisinin is active against plasmodium falciparum, the micro-organism responsible for malarial infection. In laboratory tests it was also shown to have antiviral properties, reducing invasion by the herpes, cytomegalovirus, and Epstein Barr classes of virus.

Wormwood was recommended for clearing melancholy, which is caused by an excess of the earth humour building up in the spleen. The heat of wormwood is capable of cleansing the spleen of any excess of the cold earth element, restoring the natural temperament of the body, and clearing any cold melancholic blocks to the flow of vital spirit.

Mythos

Artemis, from which its traditional Latin name derives, is the Roman name for the Greek goddess Diana, the goddess of hunting and war. It is said that she gave wormwood as a medicine to the centaur Chiron the healer, who passed on the knowledge of its use to physicians through instructing Asclepius, the god of healing. It was considered protective against evil spirits, and to cure bites from venomous creatures and mad dogs as well as resisting all kinds of poisons. It was also used in love charms with it being said that if a girl slept with some of the herb beneath her pillow she would dream of her future husband. In country lore it was believed that if you carried the plant with you it would protect from tiredness and prevent the hands or other parts of the body from becoming too hot.

Emotional

When we are stuck in a trough of depression, lacking the motivation and inspiration to make the necessary changes, wormwood can give us the kick start that we need. With its ability to clear heat as well as dampness it will help to bring out and cleanse suppressed feelings of anger and resentment, and help us to move on from such damaging and depleting emotional states.

Stomach

N. Culpeper states; "it causes appetite to meat, because Mars rules the attractive faculty in man".

By warming the stomach through increasing the secretion of gastric juices, wormwood improves digestion and clears wind. Its antimicrobial properties also protect the stomach from any dysbiosis and reduces the activity of *Helicobacter pylori*, the bacteria linked to the formation of stomach ulcers. It has also been shown to have antimicrobial effects on *E.coli*, *Staphylococcus aureus*, *Salmonella*, and *Candida* organisms (Fisher, 2018).[2] By stimulating bile secretion, the heating affect also extends to the intestines, clearing excess dampness, which is the cause of wind, bloating, and colic.

It has often been used in combination with cloves and walnut husk as an anti-parasitical treatment. However, due to concerns about the potential toxicity of walnut, I now use a combination of wormwood, cloves, and thyme herb in a capsule to treat digestive infections or parasites. Giving two capsules made with this combination three times a day for up to ten days works well for worms and yeast overgrowth. I also use it for treating food poisoning and gastric infections.

Liver

"The Sun never shone on a better herb for the yellow jaundice than this" (Culpeper) We know that strong bitter herbs stimulate the digestion and activate liver function through a reflex action on the tenth cranial nerve or the vagus nerve. They trigger the parasympathetic response in the autonomic nervous system, which reduces the tone of smooth muscle, brings blood to the liver and digestive organs and neutralises the effects of adrenaline, thus calming us down. The blood is made in the liver during the process of the second concoction, so the activation of the liver in this way increases the removal of waste products and dead blood cells, and increases the production of new fresh blood.

Kidneys

Wormwood is an effective but gentle diuretic, it warms the kidneys, disinfecting and relaxing the urinary passages.

Head

Culpeper dramatises the effects of wormwood by saying; "The moon was weak the other day, and she gave a man two terrible mischiefs, a dull brain and a weak sight; Mars laid by his sword, and comes to her. Sister moon, said he, … I will with my herb wormwood cure him of both infirmities by antipathy". When the energy of the moon, which governs the temperament of the brain and is one of the luminaries governing the sight, has become diminished, then excess moisture, (moisture is also ruled by the Moon) will build up. This excess cold and dampness will then lead to mental dullness, memory loss, confusion, migraines, and a dulling of the sight. The warming and drying properties of wormwood make it an appropriate antidote to these problems with its martian energy also being able to cut through and cleanse the mistiness in the eyes. Wormwood was traditionally used for poor memory, and due to the presence of a number of compounds including choline it is likely to have an activating effect on neuronal and mental activity.

Womb

The essential oil thujone is known to have an irritant effect on the uterine lining, stimulating menstruation and also potentially working as an abortifacient.

It has been used for helping both absent or delayed menstruation and for warming and clearing excess phlegm, dampness, and congestion from the reproductive organs and helping to strengthen and stimulate the contractions of labour.

Do not use during pregnancy.

Doses

Infusion

Herb taken as an infusion 1-2 per cup up to three times a day.

Tincture

1:3 5 ml twice daily.

Capsule

400 mg 1–3 times daily.

Digestive capsules for gut infections

Equal parts wormwood, cloves, and thyme, in a 400 mg capsule, given as a dose of two capsules three times daily for up to ten days.

Yarrow

Milfoil. Herbe militaris. Bloodwort. Sneezewort
Gaelic: Earr-thal-mainn (tail of the earth), Lus na Fala (herb to stop bleeding)

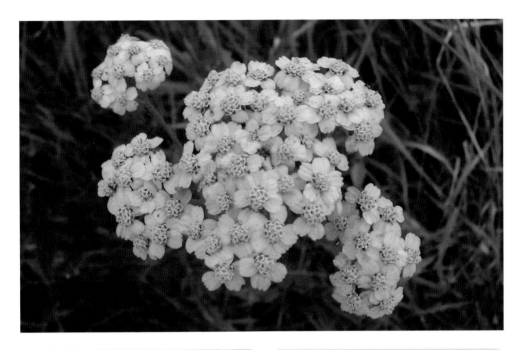

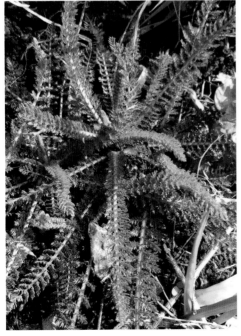

Latin:	*Achillea millefolium*
Family:	Asteraceae/Compositae
Element	Water
Planet	Venus
Humour	Phlegmatic
Quality	Warm and dry in the first degree. Cools kidneys and bladder, astringent, healing, cleansing, diuretic.

Organs

Joints
Skin

Blood
Stomach
Womb
Ovaries
Urinary system

Actions

Antipyretic – anti-fever
Anti-inflammatory
Heamostatic
Anti-hypertensive
Diuretic
Diaphoretic

Constituents

Volatile oils: chamazulenes, camphor,
    eugenol
Sesquiterpenes
Flavonoids
Alkaloids
Coumarins

Traditional uses and humoral influences

Yarrow is ruled by Venus, is warming and drying in the first degree, and has a retentive influence. Nicholas Culpeper doesn't indicate a temperament for yarrow other than saying that it is drying. However, Hildegard Von Bingen suggests that it is "a little bit hot and dry" (Throop, 1998)[1] putting yarrow into the same category as other gentle herbs used in fevers and chills, such as lime flower, elderflower, and chamomile.

Venus rules the phlegmatic humour, or water element in the body, so it is a drying herb that is indicated in any condition where the water element has become excessive. This will apply to swellings of the joints, and any cold conditions of the stomach, lungs, intestines, or urinary system. Venus rules the wet or watery side of the circulation, what today we still call the "venous" circulation. The blood in the veins is blue like water, and it flows slowly like water rather than with the strong forceful and hot action of the arterial circulation. The veins were considered to be the channel of the humours, taking the nourishment to the organs. When there was an excess of the phlegm humour, it was considered to result in swellings, oedema, and congestion in the veins, in which case a drying and cleansing herb of Venus, such as yarrow would be indicated.

Yarrow is certainly a powerful, cleansing, and relaxing herb, particularly helpful for clearing any excess dampness in any of the passages. It clears the sinuses and respiratory passages, the reproductive and urinary passages, and also the digestive passages of dampness, drying and opening them. It has traditionally been thought to be a powerful blood cleanser able to expel illness and toxins from the body. At the onset of a chill it was recommended that one take a yarrow bath or a footbath and then go to bed to sweat it out. The activating effect on the innate heat would help to resolve the fever and cleanse the body of any infection or poison. It is a useful diaphoretic along with lime flower, elderflower, and peppermint.

Gerard in 1597 wrote "The leaves of Yarrow doe close up wounds, and keep them from inflammation".[2] Country use continued this practice up until recent times as the herb is so effective for treating wounds and slow healing ulcers.

Mythos

Yarrow was named *Achillea millefolium* by Linnaeus in 1753. The genus name is based on the idea that Achilles, Spartan hero and demigod in the Iliad of Homer, used yarrow to heal wounds. Its medieval name "herba militaris" is in recognition of its blood-staunching, antiseptic, and wound-healing properties.

Traditionally it was known as a herb used by country-wise women and midwives, for helping in childbirth, and for women's problems generally. This has meant that it was a herb often associated with witches.

In the traditional Chinese divinatory system, the "i ching", it is yarrow stalks that are cast to determine the various hexagrams that form the divinatory symbols.

Yarrow and its North American varieties were used in traditional Native American herbal medicine by tribes across the continent. The Navajo considered it to be a "life medicine", they chewed it for toothaches and poured an infusion into the ears for earaches. The Miwok in California used the plant as an analgesic and head cold remedy. The Pawnee used the stalk for pain relief and the Chippewa used the leaves for headaches by inhaling it in a steam. The Cherokee drank a tea of common yarrow to reduce fever and aid in restful sleep.

Gyneacological

The reproductive system is considered warm and moist in character, so the drying effect of yarrow is very helpful in damp congestion in the reproductive system and organs. Thus it may be helpful when there is premenstrual water retention, swollen breasts, or in cystic ovarian conditions.

Yarrow is an effective ovarian tonic, both used in weak or erratic menstruation, painful periods, and excessive bleeding. In cases of menstrual flooding, a strong infusion (30 g to 500 ml) can be drunk over 24 hours, or until the bleeding subsides.

It is very helpful in polycystic ovarian syndrome, endometriosis, and fibroids, as well as helping hot flushes during the menopause and easing other symptoms, such as aching joints. For fibroids, a regular daily bath with yarrow alongside its daily internal use is considered helpful and a decoction used as a wash is specific for itching in the vagina and urinary passages.

Urinary

It is a very helpful herb in cystitis and urinary bleeding. Described as a gentle diuretic, yarrow tea was recommended by the folk herbalist Maria Treben (1980) for sluggish kidneys,[3] as well as it having a traditional use in the treatment of urinary stones.

Circulatory

The chamazulenes in yarrow are known to be amongst the most powerful anti inflammatory compounds in the plant world, and these alongside its antispasmodic actions make it a very helpful herb for circulatory disorders, especially angina, claudication and reynauds syndrome. Together with its heamostatic actions, the coumarins that yarrow contains also aid blood flow and reduce the "stickiness" of platelets in the blood.

Stomach and bowels

"Inwardly taken it helps the retentive faculty of the stomach" (Culpeper). Herbs that strengthen the retentive virtue of the stomach were called "stomachics" and were considered to help with lack of appetite and an inability to digest food properly. Yarrow is a gentle digestive bitter, which enables it to stimulate the release of digestive juices, bile from the liver, and enzymes from the pancreas aiding the breakdown of proteins and fats helping with flatulence, liver disorders, and also regulating the bowels.

Rheumatics

With its anti-inflammatory actions and its ability to improve circulation and elimination, yarrow has a reputation as a helpful herb for joint pain, especially when caused by poor elimination and depleted liver function, such as is the case with gout.

Doses

Tincture

1:3 5 ml 1–3 times a day.

Tea

For micro-circulatory conditions; combine yarrow, hawthorn and lime flower, as a tea or in tincture form.

For colds and flu: yarrow, elderflower, lime flower, thyme and chamomile as a tea mixture.

CHAPTER TWENTY

Herbal formulary

Allergy: chamomile, burdock, elder flower, lime flower, marigold, meadowsweet, milk thistle, plantain.

Bleeding: cleavers, meadowsweet, mallow, nettle, plantain, St John's wort, willow, yarrow.

Blood:
Stagnation: angelica, myrrh, rosemary, wormwood.
To breed: sage.
To cool: meadowsweet, rose, willow, violets.
To purify: cleavers, dock, nettle, myrrh.
To clarify: borage, burdock, dandelion.

Bones:
Broken: comfrey, wood betony.
Osteoporosis: clover, comfrey, horsetail.
Pain: willow bark, chamomile, rosemary.

Cancer: birch, cleavers, clover, dock, myrrh, St John's wort, sweet violet.

Catarrh: bay, elder, thyme, lime flower, plantain, sage.

Circulation:
Poor: angelica, elder, guelder rose, hawthorn, hyssop, juniper, yarrow, rosemary, thyme, yarrow.
Reynaud's syndrome: angelica, elder, guelder rose, hawthorn, rosemary, sage, yarrow.
Varicosities: marigold, St John's wort, yarrow.

Chickenpox: marigold, myrrh, St John's wort.

Cramps: angelica, lovage, hyssop, geulder rose, motherwort, mugwort, rosemary.

Digestion:
Acidity: mallow, meadowsweet.
Bitters: angelica, elecampagne, hops, myrrh, vervain, wormwood, yarrow.
Bloating: angelica, bay, fennel, hops, lavender, lemon balm, lovage, mint, mugwort, sage, wormwood.
Diarrhoea: dock (seeds), hawthorn (berries), meadowsweet, wood avens, mallow. plantain, rose, willow, wood avens, yarrow.
Diverticulitis: comfrey, mallow, plantain, yarrow.
Colic: angelica, fennel, lavender, lemon balm, lovage, meadowsweet, mint, motherwort, rosemary, sage, wood betony, wormwood.
Constipation: angelica, bay, fenugreek, dock, elder (bark), fennel, fenugreek, hops, plantain, violets, wood betony.
Cramps: chamomile, fennel, guelder rose, hyssop, meadowsweet, mint, mugwort, wormwood.
Gastritis: chamomile, mallow, meadowsweet, violets.
Inflammatory bowel diseases—Crohn's, colitis: chamomile, marigold, mallow, meadowsweet, plantain, sage, willow, wood betony.
Nausea: angelica, fennel, hyssop, lovage, mint, rosemary.
Reflux and hiatus hernia: fenugreek, mallow, plantain.
Parasites: angelica, elecampagne, mugwort, myrrh, wormwood.
Stomach ulcers: chamomile, comfrey, liquorice, mallow, meadowsweet, willow.
Vomiting: mint, sage.
Weak digestion: angelica, elecampagne, fennel, feverfew, juniper, lovage, rosemary, sage, wormwood, yarrow.
Wind: fennel, hops, juniper, lavender, lovage, motherwort, mugwort, rosemary, sage.

Drawing things out: hawthorn, mallow, plantain, wood betony.

Ears:
Congestion: bay, plantain, thyme.
Pain: chamomile.
Tinnitus: lemon balm, plantain, vervain, wood betony.

Exhaustion: angelica, elecampagne, mugwort, nettle, sage, St John's wort, wood betony.

Eyes:
Blepharitis: chamomile, elder, marigold, rose, St John's wort.
Conjunctivitis: bay, chamomile, elder flower, rose, St John's wort.
Iritis: marigold, rose.
Styes: chamomile, rose.
Macular degeneration: juniper, marigold.

Fevers: birch, borage, cleavers, elder, feverfew, lime flower, lovage, marigold, meadowsweet, nettle, rose, St John's wort, vervain, violets, willow, wood avens, Wormwood, Yarrow.

Gall bladder: dandelion, hops, wormwood.

Grief: hawthorn, lemon balm, rose.

Gums: mallow, myrrh, sage, thyme.

Haemorrhoids: comfrey, St. John's wort.

Haemorrhage: mallow, myrrh, nettle, plantain, willow, yarrow.

Hair loss: nettle, rosemary.

Hay fever: chamomile, elderflower, feverfew, lime flower, milk thistle, plantain, thyme, yarrow.

Heart:
Angina: angelica, hawthorn, lemon balm, lime flower, yarrow, guelder rose.
Failure: angelica, birch, broom, juniper, mistletoe, rosemary.
High blood pressure: cowslip, guelder rose, hawthorn, lemon balm, lime flower, marigold, mistletoe, motherwort, rose, valerian, wormwood.
Irregular beats: broom, motherwort, mistletoe.
Low blood pressure: angelica, broom, juniper, mistletoe, rosemary.
Palpitations: broom, mistletoe, motherwort, lemon balm, rose, violet.
Stimulant: angelica, broom, rosemary, thyme, yarrow.
Weakness: birch, broom, cowslip, elder, marigold, meadowsweet, mistletoe, thyme, vervain, wood avens.

Immune system:
angelica, elderflower, lime flower, marigold, mistletoe, myrrh, sage, wood avens.

Infections:
Bacterial: angelica, birch, elecampagne, juniper, lavender, marigold, myrrh, rosemary, sage, thyme, vervain, wood avens, wormwood.
Fungal: bay, juniper, lavender, marigold, myrrh, thyme.
Viral: angelica, elderflower, elecampagne, juniper, lemon balm, lavender, lime flower, marigold, myrrh, vervain, wormwood.

Joints:
Fibromyalgia: angelica, birch, chamomile, elder, feverfew, hyssop, thyme.
Gout: angelica, burdock, clover, cowslip, dandelion, lovage, mints, nettle, vervain, yarrow.
Pain: birch, chamomile, dock (poultice), feverfew, guelder rose, lavender, nettle, rosemary, sage, thyme, valerian, willow, yarrow.
Osteo arthritis: chamomile, comfrey, cowslip, juniper, willow.
Rheumatoid arthritis: angelica, burdock, birch, borage, nettle, hyssop, willow.
Sprain: comfrey, willow.
Swelling: birch, nettle, willow, thyme.

Liver:
Cholesterol lowering: fenugreek, lime flower, marigold, wormwood.
Jaundice: hops, hyssop, lavender, lovage, marigold, mints, vervain, wood betony.
To clear obstructions: angelica, bay, dandelion, hops, sage, violets, wormwood.
Weakness: borage, burdock, fennel, hyssop, lime flower, lovage, milk thistle, St John's wort, vervain, wood avens, wood betony.

Lungs and respiratory system:
Asthma: angelica, elecampagne, fennel, guelder rose, lime flower, lovage, milk thistle, mint, nettle, thyme.
Bronchitis: borage, burdock, elecampagne, mallow, plantain, thyme, violets.
Congestion: bay, guelder rose, juniper, lavender, myrrh, thyme.
Cough: cowslip, lime flower, elder (flower to soothe), mallow, plantain, rose, violets.
Coughing blood: borage, comfrey, mallow, nettle, plantain, willow, wood betony, yarrow.
Expectorant: angelica, elder (berry), juniper, mint, myrrh.
Infection: angelica, bay, juniper, lime flower, mint, mustard (poultice), myrrh, thyme, wood avens.
Pleurisy: angelica, borage, lime flower, lovage, plantain, violets.
Phlegm: bay, elder, lime flower, thyme, vervain.
Sinusitis: chamomile, elder flower, lime flower, mint, myrrh, thyme.
Wheezing: lavender, lovage, feverfew, guelder rose, juniper, mint.
Whooping cough: chamomile, clover, guelder rose, lime flower, thyme.

Lymphatics: burdock, cleavers, clover, marigold.

Melancholy: angelica, bay, borage, dandelion, elecampagne, feverfew, lemon balm, meadowsweet, milk thistle, rosemary, rose, St John's wort, violets, wood betony.

Menopause:
Depression: angelica, chamomile, feverfew, rose, St John's wort, wormwood.
Hot flushes: angelica, fenugreek, feverfew, clover, hops, lemon balm, lovage, rose.
Palpitations: angelica, chamomile, motherwort, St John's wort, vervain.

M.E: angelica, elder, elecampagne, juniper, lime flower, marigold, St John's wort, wood avens, wood betony.

Negativity: bay, cowslip, lemon balm, lovage, marigold, motherwort, rose, St John's wort, violets, wood avens.

Nervous system:
ADHD: chamomile, sage, St John's wort, valerian, vervain.
Anxiety: chamomile, cowslips, feverfew, hawthorn, hops, lavender, lemon balm, lime flower, meadowsweet, mistletoe, motherwort, rose, sage, violets, vervain, wood betony.
Convulsions: mint, mistletoe, motherwort, mugwort.
Dementia: hyssop, juniper, lavender, mint, rosemary, sage, St John's wort, valerian, wood betony.
Depression: borage, lemon balm, meadowsweet, mint, motherwort, rose, sage, St. John's wort.
Fainting: angelica, bay, hyssop, lavender.
Headache: chamomile, cowslip, lavender, lime flower, mint, rose, vervain.
Insomnia: cowslips, roman chamomile, lemon balm, lavender, lime flower, hops, rose, St. John's wort, thyme, valerian, violets.
Neuralgia: rosemary, thyme, vervain.
Memory: lemon balm, rosemary, sage, St. John's wort, wormwood.
Migraine: angelica, bay, cowslip, feverfew, lavender, lime flower, sage, vervain.
Panic attacks: chamomile, guelder rose, motherwort, hops, rose, St. John's wort, valerian, vervain, wood avens.
Palsy: angelica, bay, cowslip, feverfew, lavender, mint, motherwort, mugwort, rosemary, sage, St. John's wort, vervain.
Parkinsonism: fennel, lavender, mugwort, nettle, sage.
Relaxant: chamomile, hawthorn, lemon balm, hops, lime flower, marigold, rose, valerian, wormwood.
Sedative: chamomile, cowslip, hops, lavender, lemon balm, lime flower, mistletoe.
Stroke: lime flower, sage, valerian.
Vertigo: angelica, cowslip, lavender, lemon balm, milk thistle, mint, sage, rosemary, thyme, wood betony.

Pessimism: angelica, lavender, rose, sage, St. John's wort, wood avens.

Protection: angelica, bay, juniper, thyme, wormwood.

Purification: bay, mint, myrrh, vervain, thyme.

Reproductive system:
Endometriosis: chamomile, elder, elecampagne, violets, yarrow.
Epididymitis: St. John's wort.
Fertility: clover, marigold, mugwort, plantain.
Fibroids: angelica, bay, elecampagne, feverfew, yarrow.
Lactation—to increase: aniseed, fennel, fenugreek, milk thistle, nettle.
Lactation—to decrease: sage, mint.
Labour—stalled: fenugreek, feverfew, mint, motherwort, mugwort, wormwood, wood betony, yarrow.
Pelvic congestion: angelica, Bay, elecampagne, feverfew, mint, mugwort, thyme, wormwood, yarrow.
Pelvic pain: angelica, feverfew, lavender, guelder rose, hawthorn, meadowsweet, mugwort, rosemary, St John's wort, vervain, willow.
Polycystic ovary syndrome: angelica, clover, mugwort, yarrow.
Post-partum haemorrhage: shepherd's purse, St John's wort, wood betony, yarrow.
Miscarriage—threatened: burdock, clover, guelder rose.
Premenstrual tension: chamomile, motherwort, mugwort, St John's wort, vervain.
Periods:
Absent: angelica, bay, juniper, mugwort, wormwood, yarrow.
Heavy: cleavers, horsetail, marigold, meadowsweet, milk thistle, mint, nettle, plantain, shepherd's purse, St John's wort, violets, willow, yarrow.
Irregular: angelica, mint, yarrow.
Painful: angelica, bay, chamomile, feverfew, guelder rose, lavender, lemon balm, meadowsweet. mint, mugwort, sage, St. John's wort, thyme, vervain, wood betony, wormwood.
Vaginal atrophy: clover, fenugreek.

Sadness: chamomile, borage, lemon balm, lime flower, meadowsweet, St John's wort, violet.

Shingles: chamomile, hops, lavender, lemon balm, St John's wort.

Skin:
Acne: bay, birch, rose, marigold, nettle.
Abcesses: marigold, mallow, myrrh, plantian, thyme, wood betony.

Bites: chamomile, lavender, mallow, marigold, meadowsweet.

Boils: burdock, dock, marigold, mallow, plantain, wood betony.

Burns: chamomile, lavender, meadowsweet, nettle, St John's wort, violet.

Cold sores: lemon balm, marigold, wood avens.

Dermatitis: chamomile, dock, marigold, meadowsweet, violets, yarrow.

Eczema: bay, borage, burdock, chamomile, cleavers, clover, elecampagne, elder, lavender, marigold, milk thistle, nettles, violets.

Itching: dock, chickweed, elecampagne, hops, meadowsweet, milk thistle.

Psoriasis: burdock, chamomile, cleavers, clover, marigold.

Rosacea: bay, elder, feverfew, lemon balm, marigold, violets.

Sunburn: chamomile, cleavers, marigold, rose, St John's wort.

Ulcers: burdock, cleavers, clover, comfrey, lemon balm, plantain, St John's wort, violet, wood betony, yarrow.

Urticaria: cleavers, lime flower, marigold, nettle.

Wounds: cleavers, clover, myrrh, plantain, St. John's wort, vervain, violet, yarrow, wood betony.

Spleen:
Blockage: angelica, bay, elecampagne, hops, vervain, wormwood.

Teeth:
Abscess: sage, mallow, myrrh.

Throat:
Sore: chamomile, elder, lovage, marigold, thyme, sage.
Laryngitis: chamomile, hyssop, lovage, juniper, sage, thyme.

Thyroid:
Overactive: lemon balm, motherwort, valerian.
Underactive: nettle.

Tongue:
Burning: chamomile, lavender.
Ulcers: mallow, meadowsweet, myrrh, plantain, sage.

Travel sickness: feverfew, milk thistle, mint.

Urinary system:
Bed wetting: St John's wort.
Bleeding: cleavers, meadowsweet, nettle, plantain, St John's wort, wood betony, Yarrow.
Cystitis: angelica, birch, burdock, cleavers, hops, marigold, meadowsweet, thyme, juniper, plantain, St John's wort, vervain, violet, yarrow.

Diuretic:

Warming: angelica, broom, cleavers, dandelion, fennel, guelder rose, hops. juniper, lovage, nettle, wormwood, yarrow.

Cooling: burdock, meadowsweet.

Stones: cleavers, dandelion, nettle, vervain.

Urethritis: cleavers, marigold, meadowsweet, plantain, St John's wort, thyme, vervain.

Responding to viral infections with herbal medicine

This advice is intended as guidance for healthy adults and children. For those with compromised immunity, lung disease, or elders and parents of children under 1-year old consultation with their local favourite herbalist is advised for extra guidance and support.

Make sure you have

- A thermometer in the house.
- Someone on call who can keep a check on you, make you tea etc.
- A large thermos flask for making herbal teas in.
- A hot water bottle, a washing up sized bowl suitable for foot baths.
- Ingredients for soup, either chicken or miso with tofu and seaweed.

Herbal remedies to keep at home

- Cold and flu antiviral tea; elderflower, yarrow, lime flower, and thyme, combined in equal parts.
- Ginger root, cinnamon, honey, and plenty of lemons. Mustard powder.
- Garlic, two or three bulbs.
- Chamomile flowers, at least 100g.
- Inhalation mix combination of chamomile two parts, Thyme two parts and juniper berries one part. A bottle of elderberry juice or elderberry immune tonic, alternatively a homemade leaf and bark tincture (see notes below).

- Echinacea tincture, best from a whole plant fresh extract, 300ml.
- Elecampagne root (*Inula helenium*) and valerian root (*Valeriana officinalis*), 100g of each.

Prevention

Hand washing and surface cleaning are sensible but do not need to be done excessively. Soap and water is as good as anything else for hands, and tea tree and lavender essential oils can be added to basic hand washes or creams to make them more effective as both are powerfully antiviral and antibacterial. Add twenty drops each of lavender and tee tree oil to each 100mls of hand soap. Add twenty drops of each to 500mls of water to make a wash or spray, a teaspoon of liquid soap added to the water will enable the oils to disperse.

Full medical protection grade masks may be effective, others less so.

Good nutrition is essential; vitamin D (2,000–4,000 iu) should be supplemented in the winter, its absorption is enhanced by also taking vitamin K2.

Drink herbal teas daily; they are the easiest way to saturate the body with antimicrobial and immune modulating compounds, all herbs contain some of each.

Propolis gives protection if you are going amongst potentially infectious people, sucking tablets is best but capsules also work, take up to three daily. People with underlying health conditions should consider using propolis continuously.

Elderberry immune tonic, elderberry juice, or linctus work well, and can be drunk with some hot water added and honey and lemon to taste.

Taking medicinal mushrooms helps strengthen immunity in vulnerable people: *Coriolus versicolor* for general support, *Cordyceps sinensis* for lung support, and reishi for those with adrenal exhaustion. Garlic is the universal protector and should be taken daily. Raw is best, and may be sliced in yoghurt or honey, or do as the French do and swallow one clove daily with your main meal. Garlic must be continued throughout the illness to prevent secondary infections.

Fever

Fever is not a disease. It is the healing response of the vital force and should not be suppressed. Avoid using antipyretics, even in children. They should only be used if the temperature exceeds 40°C, and 38.5°C in young babies. Only use paracetamol for COVID-19, Ibuprofen and other NSAIDs may make it worse. Normal temperature taken in the mouth for two minutes is between 36 and 37 degrees, which gets higher over the day. Some adults run hotter and some colder, find out what your resting pulse rate and temperature is in normal health.

Watch for the first signs of viral infection; you will feel fluey, feel chilled especially at night, suffer sudden fatigue after even slight exercise, you may develop a dry cough, and have a headache. Even though you are ill at this point and can infect others, you won't have a fever.

Rest and stay at home.

Do not think that you are indispensable and unable to infect others because you don't have a fever. Drink lots of water, preferably in the form of herbal teas. Fast; remember "feed a cold and starve a fever". Digestion shuts down above 37.5°C.

Acute conditions require high doses and lots of herbs, this is when the thermos flask comes in handy, take herbal teas or tonics every two hours.

Stages of fever

First stage

Feelings of weakness, looking pale, getting tired after minimal exercise, feeling fluey, a mild headache, and feeling slightly chilled; temperature is usually still normal, possibly slightly lower than usual.

Stay warm, don't exercise.

1. DRINK the cold and flu antiviral tea with fresh ginger and elderberry juice added. Make it with two heaped teaspoons per cup (5g), and try to drink a cup every two hours.
2. TAKE 10ml of elderberry tonic three times a day, alternatively 10ml of pure elderberry juice with 5ml of echinacea tincture added three times a day.
3. MAKE DECOCTION—"Three root decoction": 2 teaspoons each of valerian root and Elecampagne root, decocted for 10 minutes with 2cm of sliced fresh ginger root. Add honey and lemon to taste, drink two or three cups daily.
4. STEAM USING THE INHALATION MIX, or just chamomile flowers alone. Use 30g to 2 litres of boiling water. Either steam under a towel or under a blanket for ten minutes, run a warm bath and then pour the liquid from the steam through a sieve into the bath. For children and babies, give the anti viral tea with a little honey, dilute it with half water but get them to drink it continuously.
5. HERBAL BATH make up the inhalation mix or chamomile as above, and put into a warm or tepid bath. Baths are perfect for children.

Second stage

The patient will feel sleepy, the skin is hot and dry to the touch, the pulse is fast and pushes up. Keep the room well aired. Drink the herbal tea freely. If uncomfortable or the temperature rises too high (above 40°C) sponge down using tepid (not cold) water, add a little cider vinegar to it and a couple of drops of lavender essential oil.

Drink the antiviral tea, adding ginger and cinnamon, or make up a thermos of ginger and cinnamon tea—2cm of cinnamon quill, 2cm finely sliced ginger root, a dessertspoonful of honey, put in a large thermos, drink throughout the day.

Make up a mustard footbath, with two tablespoons of mustard or one of mustard powder added to a couple of litres of hot water in a suitable bowl, washing up bowls are perfect. This will help when feeling chilled, and will aid the fever to move onto the final stage.

Meadowsweet, elderflower, yarrow and vervain teas are natural anti-fever herbs, and can be drunk freely at this stage or added to the flu/antiviral tea. They won't interfere with the natural fever process, but will reduce excessive temperatures, as will the herbs in the antiviral tea mix.

Third stage

This final stage is marked by sweating, and it often alternates with the second stage.

- Continue to drink plenty of the herbal teas.
- Alternate the warming mustard footbath or steams when feeling shivery, with the cooling sponging down with tepid water when feeling hot.
- If coughing is severe use the inhalation mix, especially before sleep.
- If the lungs are sore and painful use a mustard poultice—spread mustard (mix powder with oil and vinegar into a paste, spread 1cm thick layer onto cotton, fold it over making an enclosed pad, place on chest, back or sides for no more than 15 minutes at a time, place a hot water bottle over it, it can increase expectoration, so don't do it before sleeping. Re use by moistening with hot water and re apply, it may be used multiple times.
- For painful coughing make a ginger, liquorice and cinnamon tea with honey and sip throughout the day from the thermos.
- If wheezing occurs mix the lavender oil—20 drops to 10ml base oil—and massage it into the chest, ribs, shoulders, and back for ten minutes.
- Use the 'inhalation mix' as a steam for 10 minutes under a towel twice daily, 30g to 2 litres, if you don't have the inhalation mix just use chamomile flowers on their own.

Recovery

Allow at least as much time for the recovery as for the fever stages. Not resting at this point will increase the risk of secondary infection or pneumonia.

Fever depletes proteins, so have high protein snacks little and often: chicken soup or miso, tofu, and seaweed soup along with oat cakes and tahini are simple and tasty. Iron and zinc may be depleted, so take them as supplements, snack on dark chocolate and nuts, and return to exercise slowly.

Herbs such as liquorice will give energy and heal the lungs; sage, dandelion root, lovage, chicory root and burdock root all help recovery as does milk thistle.

Herbal info

Cold and flu antiviral tea: elderflower, lime flower, thyme and yarrow, all are diaphoretic, so help to lower the temperature through sweating. Other useful diaphoretics are mint, rosemary, and melissa, all of which you may have growing in the garden. Boneset (*Eupatorium perf.*) has always been considered effective for reducing viral aches and pains, and to also help reduce the temperature. It may be added to the mix if required.

Vervain: (Verbena officinalis.)
It may be added to the flu tea and is especially helpful for headaches and joint pains and to reduce the fever. It is relaxing and restorative, and especially helpful if there is an ongoing headache or nerve pain. It works particularly well as a footbath—20g infused in 1 litre of hot water for 1 hr and added to a footbath of hot water.

Echinacea: (Echinacea purpurea/angustifolia.)
Best to use a fresh tincture of the whole plant, to take in large doses during the fever 5–10ml three times a day, and in small doses during recovery, 5–10ml once a day. Especially helpful if the symptoms return or there is low grade ongoing fatigue and lethargy, less effective as a long term preventative.

Elecampagne root: (Inula helenium *rt.*)
A very good restorative herb that should be continued for a couple of weeks afterwards. It works well as a preventative, taken as part of a herbal tonic, or taken each morning as a decoction with lemon and elderberry juice. It is especially helpful for those with underlying lung conditions, such as asthma.

Elderberries: (Sambucus nigra *fructa.*)
Elder berries are high in vitamin C, high in immune stimulant bioflavonoids, and have been shown in trials to reduce recovery time. They contain compounds that block viral attachment to ACE-2 linkages on cell walls disabling their attack. These compounds are highest in the leaves and bark, to reduce the risk of elder bark, leaves or berries causing vomiting they must be cooked or decocted. There is no evidence whatsoever that anyone has suffered a "cytokine storm" from taking elder in any of its forms. If you can't get elderberry, make a leaf and bark decoction: 75g elder leaves to 1 litre, boil until reduced by half. Then add 50g elder bark, bring to the boil and simmer for ten minutes. Strain off the liquid and add an equal amount of brandy to preserve. Take 10 ml four times a day of the tincture. If you prefer not to have any alcohol in it, the decocted liquid can be used at a dose of 5ml three or four times a day, and it will last up to a week if kept in the fridge.

Chamomile flowers
They are always available, and if you can get nothing else, they will do everything all of the other herbs put together can do. They relieve pain, are immune stimulant, and are anti viral and anti inflammatory. Give them to children as teas with honey, baths and steams, make strong infusions and drink them throughout the day.
   A chamomile bath is the one reward of being sick.

Medicinal mushrooms

Medicinal mushrooms are excellent for restoring immune function, they should ideally be taken in a dose of 2–5g a day. That is between four and ten capsules a day. It does depend on the size, age, and weight of the patient. For people of a small stature, and children, I find two capsules twice daily adequate. Take *Coriolus versicolor* as a general tonic, *Cordyceps sinensis* if there is lung weakness, and reishi if there is adrenal exhaustion.

Garlic

The most powerful antimicrobial available, especially good for bacterial secondary infections of the lungs or blood, best taken fresh, putting six cloves into a jar of honey is a good way of making a useable and palatable remedy, of which a teaspoon a day is an appropriate dose.

Onions

If garlic is unavailable, use onions. They need to be taken raw, and are easily made into a syrup that even children will love, and it will clear infection from the chest. Layer chopped onions between layers of sugar, or honey as an alternative, leave for 3–4 hours, then strain off the liquid syrup. Take 2 teaspoonfuls every 2 hours.

Foraging

Using herbs that are growing in the garden or the countryside is a particularly effective way of getting the freshest possible form of medicine:

ROSEMARY, use as a tea, bath, or steam. Antiviral, diaphoretic, warming. Specific also for pain, a bath made with 300g fresh rosemary cuttings gently decocted in 3 litres of water in a closed pan for 10 min and added to a hot bath is pain relieving and restorative.

BAY, Commonly found as hedging or as an ornamental, do not confuse with the unscented laurel. Tea made with one fresh leaf to a cup for lung infections, and 200g decocted gently in 2 litres of water for a herbal bath.

MARIGOLD FLOWERS, use as an infusion, or add 200g fresh flowers to 2 litres to make a bath, a particularly good antiviral and diaphoretic herb.

LEMON BALM, *Melissa officinalis* makes a fantastic antiviral fresh tea, use a sprig per cup, helps with headaches and pain.

BIRCH LEAVES, the leaves and twigs make a pain and fever relieving tea, they also make a good herbal bath.

CLEAVERS (*Galium aparine*), gather a large handful of the fresh herb, crush and cover with 2 pints cold spring water, leave overnight and drink in divided doses over the following day. Restores, cleanses, detoxifies, reduces fevers, and aids sleep.

REFERENCES

Introduction

1. Culpeper, N. (1652) *Culpeper's Complete Herbal*. Reprint (1995). Ware, Herts: Wordsworth Library.
2. Grieve, M. (1931) *A Modern Herbal*. Reprint (1971). New York: Dover Publications.

Chapter 1

1. Edelstein, E.J., Edelstein, L. (1945) *Asclepius: a collection and interpretation of testimonies. De Antiodes*, XIV, p.42. (ET 595) Baltimore: Johns Hopkins Press.

Chapter 2

1. Rusten, J., Cunningham, I.C. (2002) *Theophrastus characters Herodas, Mimes.* Loeb Classical library. Cambridge, Massacuesetts, London: Harvard university press.
2. Edelstein, E.J., Edelstein, L. (1945) *Asclepius: a collection and interpretation of testimonies. Aristedes, Oratio*, XLVIII, p.21. (ET 602) Baltimore: Johns Hopkins Press.
3. Ibid. *Oratio*, XXXIX, p.118. (ET 409)

Chapter 3

1. Hesiod *"Theogony"* Trans. Stanley Lombardo. Comp. Robert Lamberton. (1993) *Works and days and Theogony*. (117) 61–90. Indianapolis: Hacket company.

Chapter 7

1. Culpeper (1669) *'An Astrologo-Physical Discourse of the Human Vertues in the Body of Man'* in *Pharmacopoeia Londinensis or the London Dispensary*. London: G. Sawbridge.
2. Ibid.
3. Ibid.
4. Culpeper, N. (1652) *The English Physitian, or an astrologo-physical discourse of the vulgar herbs of this nation*. London. Reprint: (1995) *Culpeper's Complete Herbal*, p.300. Ware, England: Wordsworth.
5. Plato. *Gorgias*. Trans; (1960) p.106. Hamilton, W, Emlyn-Jones, C. London: Penguin.

Chapter 8

1. Hedley, C., Shaw, N. (2021) *Amazing plants: A collection of the teachings of Herbalists*

Christopher Hedley and Non Shaw. (All the following Hedley quotes are from this publication) London: Aeon books.

2. Culpeper, N. (1652) *Galen's Art of Physick*, Ch 59. London: Cole.
3. Hedley, C., Shaw, N. (2021)
4. Culpeper, N. (1652) *Galen's Art of Physick*, Ch 59. London: Cole.
5. Hedley, C., Shaw, N. (2021)
6. Culpeper, N. (1652) *The English Physitian, or An astrologo-physical discourse of the vulgar herbs of this nation*. London. Cole. Reprint: (1995) *Culpeper's complete Herbal*, p.254. Ware, England: Wordsworth.
7. Hedley, C., Shaw, N. (2001)
8. Culpeper, N. (1652) *Galen's Art of Physick*, Ch 59. London: Cole.

Chapter 9

1. Culpeper, N. (1652) *The English Physitian or An Astrologo-Physical discourse of the vulgar herbs of this nation*. London. Cole. Reprint: (1995) *Culpeper's Complete Herbal*, p.300. Ware, England: Wordsworth. (All citations from Culpeper in this chapter are from this publication.)

Chapter 14

1. Tobyn, G. (1997) *Culpeper's medicine*, p.151. Shaftesbury, England: Element books.

Herbal

Borage

1. Gerard, J. (1636) *Gerard's Herball The essence thereof distilled by Marcus Woodward from the edition of TH. Johnson, 1636.* Reprint (1990) p.185. Ed: Woodward, M. London: Studio Editions.
2. Ibid.
3. Fernie, W.T. (1897) *Herbal Simples Approved for Modern uses of cure, A straightforward A–Z guide to natural healing.* Reprint (2014) p.51. London: Createspace independent publishing platform.

4. Gerard, J. (1636). Ibid.
5. Messegue, M. (1981) *Health secrets of plants and herbs*, p.39. London: Pan Books Ltd.

Burdock

1. Messegue, M. (1981) *Health secrets of plants and herbs*, p.73. London: Pan Books Ltd.

Chamomile

1. De Cleene, M., Lejeune, M-C. (1999) *Compendium of symbolic and ritual plants in Europe*, Vol II, p.169. Ghent. Man & Culture publishers.
2. Grieve, M. (1931) *A Modern Herbal*. Reprint (1971) Vol 1, p.186. New York: Dover publications.

Cleavers

1. Pughe, J. (1861) *The Physicians of Myddfai*, Abergavenney. The Welsh Manuscript Society. Extract from: Hoffmann. D. (1978) *Welsh herbal medicine* Aberteifi. Abercastle publications.
2. Coffin, A.I. (1855) *Botanic guide to health, and the natural pathology of disease*. London: Cousins.

Clover

1. De Cleene, M., Lejeune, M-C. (1999) *Compendium of symbolic and ritual plants in Europe*, Vol II, p.176. Ghent. Man & Culture publishers.
2. Fernie, W.T. (1897) *Herbal Simples Approved for modern uses of cure A straightforward A–Z guide to natural healing*. Reprint (2014) p.80. London: Createspace independent publishing platform.
3. Ibid.
4. Bartram, T. (1995) *Encyclopedia of Herbal medicine*. Christchurch, Dorset: Grace publishers.
5. Coffin, A.I. (1855) *Botanic guide to health, and the natural pathology of disease*. London: Cousins.

Comfrey

1. Grieve, M. (1931) *A Modern Herbal*. Reprint (1971) Vol 1, p.218. New York: Dover publications.

Cowslip

1. Pechey, J. (1706) *The compleat herbal of physical plants*. London: Bronwicke. Reprint (2018) p.60. London: Forgotten books & co Ltd.
2. Hatfield, G. (2007) *Hatfield's Herbal*, p.83. London: Penguin.
3. Treben, M. (1980) *Health through God's pharmacy*, p.22. Steyr, Austria: Ennsthaler.
4. Ibid.

Dandelion

1. Hatfield, G. (1994) *Country remedies', Traditional East Anglian plant remedies in the twentieth century*. Appendix: p.119. Woodbridge, Suffolk: The Boydell press.

Dock

1. Hatfield, G. (2007) *Hatfield's Herbal*, p.102. London: Penguin.
2. Grieve, M. (1931) *A Modern Herbal*. Reprint (1971) Vol.1, p.259. New York: Dover publications.
3. Hatfield, G. (1994) *Country remedies', Traditional East Anglian plant remedies in the twentieth century*. p.50. Woodbridge, Sufolk: The Boydell press.
4. Grieve, M. (1931) *A Modern Herbal*. Reprint (1971) Vol.1, p.259. New York: Dover publications.

Elder

1. Evelyn, J. (1664) *Sylva, or A Discourse of Forest trees and the propagation of timber*. London: J. Martin. Also see; Grieve, M. (1931) *A Modern Herbal*. Reprint (1971) Vol.1, p.269. New York: Dover publications.

2. De Cleene, M., Lejeune, M-C. (1999). *Compendium of symbolic and ritual plants in Europe*. Vol.1, p.228. Ghent. Man & Culture publishers.
3. Blockwich, M. Dr. (1677) *The anatomy of the Elder*. London. Reprint (2010) p.29. Apenzel. BerryPharma.
4. Ibid., p.47.
5. Fernie, W.T. (1897) *Herbal Simples Approved for Modern uses of cure A straightforward A–Z guide to natural healing*. Reprint (2014) p.114. London: Createspace independent publishing platform.

Elecampagne

1. Fernie, W.T. (1897) *Herbal Simples Approved for Modern uses of cure A straightforward A–Z guide to natural healing*. Reprint (2014) p.117. London: Createspace independent publishing platform.
2. Ibid., p.118.
3. Ibid., p.118.
4. Parkinson, J. (1640) *Theatrum botanicum*. London. Reprint (2014) p.92. Bruton-Seal, J. Seal, M. *The herbalist's Bible, John Parkinson's lost classic rediscovered*. Ludlow: Merlin Unwin Books Ltd.
5. Fisher, C. (2018) *Materia Medica of Western Herbs*. London: Aeon.
6. Hoffmann, D. (1978) *Welsh herbal medicine*, p.46. Aberteifi: Abercastle publications.
7. Fernie, W.T. (1897) *Herbal Simples Approved for Modern uses of a cure A straightforward A–Z guide to natural healing*. Reprint (2014) p.117. London: Createspace independent publishing platform.

Fennel

1. Hildegard von Bingen. Trans: Throop, P. (1998). *Hildegard von Bingen's Physica*, p.39. Rochester: Healing Arts Press.
2. Fisher, C. (2018) *Materia Medica of Western Herbs*, p.19. London: Aeon.
3. Hildegard von Bingen. Trans: Throop, P. (1998). *Hildegard von Bingen's Physica*, p.40. Rochester: Healing Arts Press.

4. Pechey, J. (1706) *The compleat Herbal of Physical Plants.* Reprint (2018) p.86–87. London: Forgotten Books Ltd.
5. Messegue, M. (1981) *The Health secrets of plants and herbs*, p.119. London: Pan Books Ltd.

Fenugreek

1. Fisher, C. (2018) *Materia Medica of Western Herbs*, p.195. London: Aeon.
2. Messegue, M. (1981) *The Health secrets of plants and herbs*, p.122. London: Pan Books Ltd.

Feverfew

1. Fernie, W.T. (1897) *Herbal Simples Approved for Modern uses of cure A straightforward A–Z guide to natural healing.* Reprint (2014) p.130. London: Createspace independent publishing platform.
2. Pechey, J. (1706) *The compleat herbal of physical plants.* London: Bronwicke. Reprint (2018) p.91. London: Forgotten books & co Ltd.
3. Ibid.
4. Bartram, T. (1995) *Encyclopedia of Herbal medicine*, p.182. Christchurch, Dorset: Grace publishers.

Guelder rose

1. Grieve, M. (1931) *A Modern Herbal.* Reprint (1971) Vol.1, p.381. New York: Dover publications.

Hawthorn

1. Messegue, M. (1981) *Health secrets of plants and herbs*, p.143. London: Pan Books Ltd
2. Tarrant, R.J. (2004) *P. Ovidi Nasonis Metamorphoses.* Oxford Classical Texts. Oxford: Oxford Univ. Press.
3. Graves, R. (1948) *The White Goddess.* London: Faber. Reprint (1999). p.203. London: Faber.

Hops

1. Hildegard von Bingen. Trans: Throop, P. (1998) *Hildegard von Bingen's Physica*, p.36. Rochester: Healing Arts Press.
2. Fisher, C. (2018) *Materia Medica of Western Herbs*, p.127. London: Aeon.

Hyssop

1. Fernie, W.T. (1897) *Herbal Simples Approved for Modern uses of cure A straightforward A–Z guide to natural healing.* Reprint (2014) p.181. London: Createspace independent publishing platform.
2. Fisher, C. (2018) *Materia Medica of Western Herbs*, p.234. London: Aeon.

Juniper

1. Fisher, C. (2018) *Materia Medica of Western Herbs*, p.148. London: Aeon.
2. Pengelley, A. (2004) *Constituents of medicinal plants*, p.23,32. Wallingford, Oxfordshire: CAB international.
3. De Cleene, M., Lejeune, M-C. (1999) *Compendium of symbolic and ritual plants in Europe*, Vol.1, p.366. Ghent. Man & Culture publishers.
4. Fisher, C. (2018) *Materia Medica of Western Herbs*, p.148. London: Aeon.

Lavender

1. Pengelley, A. (2004) *Constituents of medicinal plants*, p.23. Wallingford, Oxfordshire: CAB international.
2. Grieve, M. (1931) *A Modern Herbal.* Reprint (1971) Vol.II, p.472. New York: Dover publications.
3. Hildegard von Bingen. Trans: Throop, P. (1998) *Hildegard von Bingen's Physica*, p.22. Rochester: Healing Arts Press.

Lemon balm

1. Fisher, C. (2018) *Materia Medica of Western Herbs*, p.243. London: Aeon.

Limeflower

1. Hedley, C. (1996) Personal communication.
2. Barker, J. (1994) Personal communication.
3. Messegue, M. (1981) *Health secrets of plants and herbs*, p.170. London: Pan Books Ltd.
4. Ibid.
5. Fisher, C. (2018) *Materia Medica of Western Herbs*, p.422. London: Aeon.
6. Messegue, M. (1981) *The Health secrets of plants and herbs*, p.171. London: Pan Books Ltd.

Lovage

1. Pechey, J. (1706) *The compleat Herbal of Physical Plants*. Reprint (2018) p.144. London: Forgotten Books Ltd.
2. Grieve, M. (1931) *A Modern Herbal*. Reprint (1971) Vol.II, p.500. New York: Dover publications.

Mallow

1. Fernie, W.T. (1897) *Herbal Simples Approved for Modern uses of cure A straightforward A–Z guide to natural healing*. Reprint (2014) p.207. London: Createspace independent publishing platform.
2. Chalwin, C. (1999) Personal communication.

Marigold

1. Grieve, M. (1931) *A Modern Herbal*. Reprint (1971) Vol.I, p.517. New York: Dover publications.
2. Fisher, C. (2018) *Materia Medica of Western Herbs*, p.61. London: Aeon.

Meadowsweet

1. Parkinson, J. (1640) *Theatrum botanicum*. London: Reprint: Bruton-Seal, J. Seal, M. (2014) *The herbalist's Bible, John Parkinson's lost classic rediscovered*, p.140. Ludlow: Merlin Unwin Books Ltd.

Milk Thistle

1. Gerard, J. (1636) *Gerard's Herball The essence thereof distilled by Marcus Woodward from the edition of TH. Johnson, 1636.* Ed, Woodward, M. (1990) London: Studio editions.
2. Grieve, M. (1931) *A Modern Herbal*. Reprint (1971) Vol.I, p.797. New York: Dover publications.
3. Williamson, E. (2003) *Potter's New Cyclopaedia of Botanical Drugs & Preparations*, p.298. Walden, Essex: C.W. Daniel & Co.
4. Fisher, C. (2018) *Materia Medica of Western Herbs*, p.85. London: Aeon.
5. Messegue, M. (1981) *The Health secrets of plants and herbs*, p.274. London: Pan Books Ltd.

Mistletoe

1. Grieve, M. (1931) *A Modern Herbal*. Reprint (1971) Vol.II, p.548. New York: Dover publications.

Motherwort

1. Grieve, M. (1931) *A Modern Herbal*. Reprint (1971) Vol.II, p.556. New York: Dover publications.
2. Parkinson, J. (1640) *Theatrum botanicum*. London: Reprint: Bruton-Seal, J. Seal, M. (2014) *The herbalist's Bible, John Parkinson's lost classic rediscovered*, p.34. Ludlow: Merlin Unwin Books Ltd.
3. Williamson, E. (2003) *Potter's New Cyclopaedia of Botanical Drugs & Preparations*, p.300. Walden, Essex: C.W. Daniel & Co.
4. Fisher, C. (2018) *Materia Medica of Western Herbs*, p.239. London: Aeon.
5. Parkinson, J. (1640) *Theatrum botanicum*. London. Reprint: Bruton-Seal, J. Seal, M. (2014) *The herbalist's Bible, John Parkinson's lost classic rediscovered*, p.34. Ludlow: Merlin Unwin Books Ltd.
6. Ibid.

Mugwort

1. Tobyn, G., Denham, A., Whitelegg, M. (2011) *The western Herbal Tradition*, p.127. London: Churchill Livingstone.
2. Gerard, J. (1636) *Gerard's Herball The essence thereof distilled by Marcus Woodward from the edition of TH. Johnson, 1636.* Ed, Woodward, M. (1990) London: Studio editions.

Also see: Grieve, M. (1931) *A Modern Herbal*. Reprint (1971) Vol.II, p.557. New York: Dover publications.

Myrrh

1. Williamson, E. (2003) *Potter's New Cyclopaedia of Botanical Drugs & Preparations*, p.309–310. Walden, Essex: C.W. Daniel & Co.

Nettle

1. De Cleene, M., Lejeune, M-C. (1999) *Compendium of symbolic and ritual plants in Europe*, Vol.II, p.417. Ghent. Man & Culture publishers.
2. Bartrum, T. (1995) *Encyclopedia of Herbal Medicine*, p.309. Christchurch, Dorset: Grace Publishers.
3. Grieve, M. (1931) *A Modern Herbal*. Reprint (1971) Vol.II, p.575. New York: Dover publications.
4. Dodoens, R. (1619) *A New Herbal: or Historie of Plants*. London. Online. Available: http/library.wellcome.ac.uk/EEBO.
5. Treben. M. (1980) *Health through God's pharmacy*, p.42. Steyr, Austria. Ennsthaler.

Plantain

1. Pliny the Elder. Jones, W.H.S. Trans: (1949–1962) *Pliny Natural History, with an English translation in 10 volumes*. London: W. Heinemann.

Rose

1. Throop, P. (Trans) (1998) *Hildegard von Bingen's Physica*, p.21. Rochester, VT: Healing Arts Press.
2. Gerard, J. (1975) *The Herbal or General History of Plants*. New York: Dover publications.

Rosemary

1. Grieve, M. (1931) *A Modern Herbal*. Reprint (1971) Vol.II, p.682. New York: Dover publications.

2. Fisher, C. (2018) *Materia Medica of Western Herbs*, p.251–252. London: Aeon.

Sage

1. Messegue, M. (1981) *Health secrets of plants and herbs*, p.256–258. London: Pan Books Ltd.
2. De Cleene, M., Lejeune, M-C. (1999) *Compendium of symbolic and ritual plants in Europe*, Vol.1, p.668. Ghent. Man & Culture publishers.
3. Ibid., p.666.
4. Gerard, J. (1975) *The Herbal or General History of Plants*. New York: Dover publications
5. Messegue, M. (1981) *The Health secrets of plants and herbs*, p.257. London: Pan Books Ltd.
6. Fisher, C. (2018) *Materia Medica of Western Herbs*, p.254. London: Aeon.
7. Ibid.
8. Throop, P. (Trans) (1998) *Hildegard von Bingen's Physica*, p.51. Rochester, VT: Healing Arts Press.
9. Messegue, M. (1981) *The Health secrets of plants and herbs*, p.259. London: Pan Books Ltd.

St John's wort

1. De Cleene, M., Lejeune, M-C. (2003) *Compendium of symbolic and ritual plants in Europe*, Vol.II, p.455. Ghent. Man & Culture publishers.
2. Fisher, C. (2018) *Materia Medica of Western Herbs*, p.141. London: Aeon.
3. De Cleene, M., Lejeune, M-C. (2003) *Compendium of symbolic and ritual plants in Europe*, Vol.II, p.457. Ghent. Man & Culture publishers.
4. Fisher, C. (2018) *Materia Medica of Western Herbs*, p.142. London: Aeon.

Thyme

1. Parkinson, J. (1640) *Theatrum botanicum*. London. Reprint: Bruton-Seal, J. Seal, M. (2014) *The herbalist's Bible, John Parkinson's lost classic rediscovered*, p.208. Ludlow: Merlin Unwin Books Ltd.

2. De Cleene, M., Lejeune, M-C. (1999) *Compendium of symbolic and ritual plants in Europe*, Vol.I, p.696. Ghent. Man & Culture publishers.
3. Parkinson, J. (1640) *Theatrum botanicum*. London. Reprint: Bruton-Seal, J. Seal, M. (2014) *The herbalist's Bible, John Parkinson's lost classic rediscovered*, p.208. Ludlow: Merlin Unwin Books Ltd.
4. Ibid.
5. Ibid.
6. Treben, M. (1980) *Health through god's pharmacy*, p.45. Steyr: Ennsthaler.

Valerian

1. Gerard, J. (1975) *The Herbal or General History of Plants*. New York: Dover Publications.
2. Fernie, W.T. (1897) *Herbal Simples Approved for Modern uses of cure A straightforward A–Z guide to natural healing*. Reprint (2014) p.359. London: Createspace independent publishing platform.
3. Fisher, C. (2018) *Materia Medica of Western Herbs*, p.436. London: Aeon.
4. Fox, W. (1920) *The working-man's Model Family Botanic Guide to health*, 22nd edn. Sheffield: W. Fox and Sons.

Vervain

1. Parkinson, J. (1640) *Theatrum botanicum*. London. Reprint: Bruton-Seal, J. Seal, M. (2014) *The herbalist's Bible, John Parkinson's lost classic rediscovered*, p.218. Ludlow: Merlin Unwin Books Ltd.
2. Fisher, C. (2018) *Materia Medica of Western Herbs*, p.442. London: Aeon.
3. De Cleene, M., Lejeune, M-C. (1999) *Compendium of symbolic and ritual plants in Europe*, Vol.II, p.530. Ghent. Man & Culture publishers.
4. Pechey, J. (1706) *The compleat herbal of physical plants*. London, Bronwicke. Reprint (2018) London: Forgotten books & c Ltd.
5. Parkinson, J. (1640) *Theatrum botanicum*. London. Reprint: Bruton-Seal, J. Seal, M. (2014) *The herbalist's Bible, John Parkinson's lost classic rediscovered*, p.218. Ludlow. Merlin Unwin Books Ltd.

6. Messegue, M. (1981) *Health secrets of plants and herbs*, p.286. London: Pan Books Ltd.
7. Bartrum, T. (1995) *Encyclopedia of Herbal Medicine*, p.443. Christchurch, Dorset: Grace Publishers.
8. Parkinson, J. (1640) *Theatrum botanicum*. London. Reprint: Bruton-Seal, J. Seal, M. (2014) *The herbalist's Bible, John Parkinson's lost classic rediscovered*, p.218. Ludlow. Merlin Unwin Books Ltd.

Violets

1. Matthioli, PA. (1554) PetriAndreae Matthioli *Medici Senensis Commentarii, in Libros Sex Pedacii Dioscoridis Anazarbei, De material Medica*. Venice. See: Tobyn, G. Denham, A. Whitelegg, M. (2011) *The Western Herbal Tradition*, p.337–348. London: Elsevier.
2. Throop, P. (Trans) (1998) *Hildegard von Bingen's Physica*, p.54. Rochester, VT: Healing Arts Press.
3. Messegue, M. (1981) *The Health secrets of plants and herbs*, p.289. London: Pan Books Ltd.
4. Gerard, J. (1975) *The Herbal or General History of Plants*. New York: Dover Publications.
5. Ibid.
6. Matthioli, P.A. (1554) Petri Andreae Matthioli *Medici Senensis Commentarii, in Libros Sex Pedacii Dioscoridis Anazarbei, De material Medica*. Venice. See: Tobyn, G. Denham, A. Whitelegg, M. (2011) *The Western Herbal Tradition*, p.337–348. London: Elsevier.
7. Leyel, C.F. (1943) *The truth about herbs*. London: Andrew Dakers Limited.
8. Fisher, C. (2018) *Materia Medica of Western Herbs*, p.449. London: Aeon.

Willow

1. Graves, R. (1948) *The White Goddess*, p. 203. London: Faber. Reprint (1999) London: Faber.
2. Matthioli, P.A. (1554) Petri Andreae Matthioli *Medici Senensis Commentarii, in Libros Sex Pedacii Dioscoridis Anazarbei, De material Medica*. Venice.

Wood avens

1. Grieve, M. (1931) *A Modern Herbal*. Reprint (1971) Vol.1. New York: Dover publications.
2. Pechey, J. (1706) *The compleat herbal of physical plants*. London: Bronwicke. Reprint (2018) London: Forgotten books & co Ltd.
3. Ibid.

Wood betony

1. Pechey, J. (1706) *The compleat herbal of physical plants*. London: Bronwicke. Reprint (2018) London: Forgotten books & co Ltd.
2. Grieve, M. (1931) *A Modern Herbal*. Reprint (1971) Vol.I, p.97. New York: Dover publications.
3. Hunger, F.W.T. (1935) *The herbal of Pseudo-Apuleius from the ninth century manuscript in the abbey of Monte Cassino*. Leyden: E J Brill.

4. Grieve, M. (1931) *A Modern Herbal*. Reprint (1971) Vol.I, p.98. New York: Dover publications.

Wormwood

1. Throop, P. (Trans) (1998) *Hildegard von Bingen's Physica*, p.56–57. Rochester, VT: Healing Arts Press.
2. Fisher, C. (2018) *Materia Medica of Western Herbs*, p.56. London: Aeon.

Yarrow

1. Throop, P. (Trans) (1998) *Hildegard von Bingen's Physica*, p.59. Rochester, VT: Healing Arts Press.
2. Gerard, J. (1975) *The Herbal or General History of Plants*. New York: Dover Publications.
3. Treben, M. (1980) *Health through God's pharmacy*, p.50. Steyr: Ennsthaler.

BIBLIOGRAPHY

Apollodorus, (1997) *The Library of Greek Mythology*. Translated by Robin Hard. Oxford: Oxford University Press.

Bartram, T. (1995) *Encyclopedia of Herbal Medicine*. Christchurch, Dorset. Grace publishers.

Blochwich, M. (1677) *The Anatomy of the Elder*. London: 2010 (edn). Apenzel. BerryPharma.

Breverton, T. (2012) *The Physicians of Myddfai*. Carmarthenshire: Cambria Books.

Brooke, E. (1992) *A Woman's Book of Herbs*. London: The Women's Press.

Bruton-Seal, J., Seal, M. (2014) *The Herbalist's Bible, John Parkinson's lost classic rediscovered*. Ludlow: Merlin Unwin Books.

Cambell, J. (1993) *The Hero with a thousand faces*. London: Fontana Press.

Coffin, A.I. (1855) *Botanic guide to health, and the natural pathology of disease*. London: Cousins.

Culpeper, N. (1651) *A Guide for Midwives, or A guide for women, in their conception, bearing and suckling their children*. London: Peter Cole.

Culpeper, N. (1652) *Galen's Art of Physick*, London: Cole.

Culpeper, N. (1652) *The English Physitian, or An astrologo-physical discourse of the vulgar herbs of this nation*. London: Peter Cole. (1995 edn) *Culpeper's Complete Herbal*. Ware, England: Wordsworth.

Culpeper, N. (1655) *Culpeper's Astrologicall Judgement of Diseases from the Decumbiture of the Sick*. London: Peter Cole.

Culpeper, N. (1669) *'An Astrologo-Physical Discourse of the Human Vertues in the Body of Man'* in *Pharmacopoeia Londinensis or the London Dispensary*. London: G. Sawbridge.

Densmore, F. (1974) *How Indians use Wild Plants for Food, Medicine & Crafts*. New York: Dover.

De Cleene, M., Lejeune, M.C. (1999) *Compendium of symbolic and ritual plants in Europe Vol I, Vol II*, Ghent: Man & Culture publishers.

Dodoens, R. (1619) A New Herbal: or Historie of Plants, London: Online. Available: http// library.wellcome.ac.uk/EEBO.

Edelstein, E.J., Edelstein, L. (1945). *Asclepius: a collection and interpretation of testimonies*. Baltimore: Johns Hopkins Press.

Evelyn, J. (1664) *Sylva, or A Discourse of Forest trees and the propagation of timber*. London: J. Martin.

Fernie, W.T. (1897) *Herbal Simples Approved for Modern uses of cure A straightforward A-Z guide to natural healing Reprint*. (2014) London: Createspace independent publishing platform.

Flaws, B. (1995) *The Secret of Chinese Pulse Diagnosis*. Boulder, Co: Blue Poppy Press.

Fisher, C. (2018) *Materia Medica of Western Herbs*. London: Aeon Books.

Fox, W. (1891) *The Model Botanic Guide to Health*. Sheffield: William Fox and Sons.

Gardiner, P. Osborn, G. (2005) *The Serpent Grail*. London: Watkins.

Gerard, J. (1636) *The Herbal or General Historie of Plants*. London: Reprint: (1975) New York: Dover publications.

Gerard, J. (1636). Gerard's Herball The essence thereof distilled by Marcus Woodward from the edition of T.H. Johnson, 1636. Ed, Woodward, M. 1990 London. Studio editions. P. 185.

Graves, R. (1948) *The White Goddess*. London: Faber and Faber.

Graves, R. (1955) *The Greek Myths*. London: Penguin.

Grieve, M. (1931) *A Modern Herbal*. Vol.I & II. Reprint: 1971. New York. Dover publications.

Griggs, B. (1981) *Green Pharmacy, A History of Herbal Medicine*. London: Hale.

Guarneri, M. (2006) *The Heart Speaks*. New York: Fusion press.

Hakim, G.M., Chishti, N.D. (1988) *The Traditional healer*. Wellingborough: Thorsons.

Hart, G.D. (2000) *Asclepius, the God of Medicine*. London: Royal Society of medicine press Ltd.

Hatfield, G. (1994) *Country remedies*. Woodbridge, Suffolk: The Boydell Press.

Hatfield, G. (1999) *Memory, Wisdom and Healing, The history of domestic plant medicine*. Stroud, Gloucester: Sutton Publishing Ltd.

Hatfield, G. (2007) *Hatfield's Herbal, The secret history of British plants*. London: Allen lane.

Hedley, C. Shaw, N. (2021) *Amazing things, plants: A collection of the teachings of Herbalists Christopher Hedley and Non Shaw*. London: Aeon Books.

Hildegard Von Bingen. (1998) *Physica* Trans; Throop, P. Rochester, V.T: Healing Arts Press.

Hoffmann, D. (1978) *Welsh Herbal Medicine*. Aberteifi: Abercastle Publications.

Kneipp, S. (1896). *My Will. A legacy to the healthy and the sick*. London: Grevel & Co.

Kingsley, P. (1999) *In the dark places of wisdom*. Point Reyes, Calf: The Golden Sufi Center.

Lamberton, R. (1993) *Works and days and Theogony*. Indianapolis: Hacket company.

Leyel, C.F. (1943) *The truth about herbs*. London: Andrew Dakers Limited.

Lee, P.J. (2000) *We Borrow The Earth, An intimate portrait of the Gypsy Shamanic Culture*. London: Thorsons.

Lowry, A. E. (2010) *Sexual Healing: Gender and Sexuality in the Healing Cult of Asklepios* Bloomington IL: Illinois Wesleyan University, Digital Commons@IWU.

Maciocia, G. (1987) *Tongue diagnosis in Chinese Medicine*. Seattle, Wash: Eastland press.

Manniche, L. (1989) *An Ancient Egyptian Herbal*. London: British Museum Press.

Matthioli, P.A. (1554) PetriAndreae Matthioli *Medici Senensis Commentarii, in Libros Sex Pedacii Dioscoridis Anazarbei, De material Medica*. Venice.

Messegue, M. (1981) *Health Secrets of Plants and Herbs*. London: Pan Books Ltd.

Parkinson, J. (1640) *Theatrum botanicum*. London. Reprint: Bruton-Seal, J., Seal, M. (2014) *The herbalist's Bible, John Parkinson's lost classic rediscovered*. Ludlow. Merlin Unwin Books Ltd.

Paterson, J.M. (1996) *Tree Wisdom*. London: Thorsons.

Pechey, J. (1706) *The compleat Herbal of Physical plants*. London. Bronwicke Reprint: 2018. London. Forgotten books & co Ltd.

Pengelley, A. (2004) *The Constituents of Medicinal Plants*. Wallingford, Oxford: CAB International.

Plato. *Gorgias*. Trans; 1960 Hamilton, W, Emlyn-Jones, C. London: Penguin.

Pliny the Elder. Jones, W.H.S. Trans: (1949–1962) *Pliny Natural History, with an English translation in 10 volumes*. London: W. Heinemann.

Pole, S. (2006) *Ayurvedic Medicine, The principles of traditional practice*. London: Elsevier.

Pughe, J. (1861) *The Physicians of Myddfai*, Abergavenney. The Welsh Manuscript Society. Republished (1978) Burnham on Sea: Llanarch press.

Rusten, J. Cunningham, I.C. (2002) *Theophrastus characters Herodas, Mimes*. Loeb Classical library. Cambridge, Massacuesetts, London: Harvard university press.

Tarrant, R.J. (2004) P. *Ovidi Nasonis Metamorphoses.* Oxford Classical Texts. Oxford: Oxford Univ. Press.

Throop, P. (Trans) (1998) *Hildegard von Bingen's Physica.* Rochester, VT: Healing Arts Press.

Tick, E. (2001) *The Practice of Dream Healing.* Wheaton Illinois: Quest Books.

Tobyn, G. (1997) *Culpeper's Medicine.* London: Element books.

Tobyn, G. Denham, A. Whitelegg, M. (2011) *The Western Herbal Tradition.* London: Churchill Livingstone.

Treben, M. (1980) *Health through God's Pharmacy.* Steyr, Austria: Ennsthaler.

Weed, S. (1989) *Healing Wise.* New York: Ash Tree publishing.

Weiss, R.F. (1988) *Herbal Medicine.* Beaconsfield: Beaconsfield publishing limited.

Warren-Davis, D. (2021) *The Hand reveals, A complete guide to Cheiromancy, The Western Tradition of Handreading.* London: Aeon Books.

Williamson, E. (2003) *Potter's Herbal Cyclopaedia.* London: C W Daniel.

Woolley, B. (2004) *The Herbalist.* London: Harper Collins.

INDEX